Rickettsial and Chlamydial Diseases of Domestic Animals

Titles of related interest from Pergamon Press

PERGAMON VETERINARY HANDBOOK SERIES

Series Editor: A. T. B. Edney

BROWN
Aquaculture for Veterinarians: Fish Husbandry and Medicine

ANDERSON & EDNEY
Practical Animal Handling

EMILY & PENMAN
Handbook of Small Animal Dentistry

SHERIDAN & McCAFFERTY
The Business of Veterinary Practice

WILLS & WOLF
Handbook of Feline Medicine

Other books

BURGER
The Waltham Book of Companion Animal Nutrition

GOLDSCHMIDT & SHOFER
Skin Tumors of the Dog and Cat

ROBINSON
Genetics for Cat Breeders, 3rd Edition
Genetics for Dog Breeders, 2nd Edition

STEPHEN
Trypanosomiasis: A Veterinary Perspective

THORNE
The Waltham Book of Dog and Cat Behaviour

Journals

Annual Review of Fish Diseases

Comparative Immunology, Microbiology and Infectious Diseases

Veterinary Dermatology
The official journal of the European Society of Veterinary Dermatology and the American College of Veterinary Dermatology

Rickettsial and Chlamydial Diseases of Domestic Animals

Edited by

ZERAI WOLDEHIWET
Department of Veterinary Pathology, University of Liverpool

and

MIODRAG RISTIC
Professor Emeritus, ProtaTek International Inc., St Paul, Minnesota, U.S.A.

PERGAMON PRESS

OXFORD · NEW YORK · SEOUL · TOKYO

UK	Pergamon Press Ltd, Headington Hill Hall, Oxford OX3 0BW, England
USA	Pergamon Press, Inc., 660 White Plains Road, Tarrytown, New York 10591-5153, USA
KOREA	Pergamon Press Korea, KPO Box 315, Seoul 110-603, Korea
JAPAN	Pergamon Press Japan, Tsunashima Building Annex, 3-20-12 Yushima, Bunkyo-ku, Tokyo 113, Japan

First edition 1993

Library of Congress Cataloging-in-Publication Data

Rickettsial and chlamydial diseases of domestic animals/edited by Zerai Woldehiwet and Miodrag Ristic.—1st ed.
p. cm.
Includes index.
1. Rickettsial diseases in animals. 2. Chlamydia infections in animals. I. Woldehiwet. Zerai. II. Ristic, Miodrag, 1918–
SF809.R52R53 1993
636.089'6922—dc20 92-34988

ISBN 0-08-040831-1

DISCLAIMER

Whilst every effort is made by the Publishers to see that no inaccurate or misleading data, opinion or statement appear in this book, they wish to make it clear that the data and opinions appearing in the articles herein are the sole responsibility of the contributor concerned. Accordingly, the Publishers and their employees, officers and agents accept no responsibility or liability whatsoever for the consequences of any such inaccurate or misleading data, opinion or statement.

Drug and Dosage Selection: The Authors have made every effort to ensure the accuracy of the information herein, particularly with regard to drug selection and dose. However, appropriate information sources should be consulted, especially for new or unfamiliar drugs or procedures. It is the responsibility of every veterinarian to evaluate the appropriateness of a particular opinion in the context of actual clinical situations, and with due consideration to new developments.

Printed in Great Britain by BPCC Wheaton Co Ltd Exeter

Contents

List of Contributors

I. D. Aitken Animal Disease Research Association, Moredun Institute, 408 Gilmerton Road, Edinburgh EH17 7JH, U.K.

P. A. Bobade Faculty of Veterinary Science, University of Zimbabwe, PO Box MP 167 Mount Pleasant, Harare, Zimbabwe

E. Camus Mission Antilles Guyane, Inra Duclos B#1232, 97184 Pointe A Pitre Cedex, Guadeloupe, French West Indies

G. A. Cullen Poultry Department, Central Veterinary Laboratory, New Haw, Weybridge, Surrey KT15 3NB, U.K.

W. J. Foreyt Animal Disease Research Unit, 337 Bustad Hall, WSU Pullman, WA 99164-7030, U.S.A.

T. W. French Department of Pathology, NYSCVM, Cornell University, Ithaca, NY 14853-6401, U.S.A.

J. R. Gorham Animal Disease Research Unit, 337 Bustad Hall, WSU Pullman, WA 99164-7030, U.S.A.

J. W. Harvey College of Veterinary Medicine, University of Florida, Gainesville, FL 32610, U.S.A.

C. J. Holland ProtaTek Reference Laboratory, 574 East Alamo, Suite 90, Chandler, AZ 85225, U.S.A.

B. Kaltenboeck Veterinary Microbiology and Parasitology, School of Veterinary Medicine, Louisiana State University, Baton Rouge, LA 70803-8416, U.S.A.

J. E. Madigan School of Veterinary Medicine, Department of Medicine, University of California at Davis, Davis, CA 95616-8737, U.S.A.

A. S. Nash Department of Veterinary Medicine, University of Glasgow Veterinary School, Bearsden Road, Bearsden, Glasgow G61 1QH, U.K.

M. Ristic ProtaTek International Inc., 1491 Energy Park Drive, St Paul, MN 55108, U.S.A.

G. R. Scott University of Edinburgh, Department of Tropical Animal Health, CTVM, Easter Bush, Nr Roslin, Midlothian EH25 9RG, U.K.

J. Storz Veterinary Microbiology and Parasitology, School of Veterinary Medicine, Louisiana State University, Baton Rouge, LA 70803-8416, U.S.A.

G. Uilenberg Institute D'Elevage et de Medicine Veterinaire, des Pays Tropicaux, Department du CIRAD, 10 rue Pierre-Curie-94700, Maisons-Alfort, France

L. Wanduragala ProtaTek International, Inc., 1491 Energy Park Drive, St Paul, MN 55108, U.S.A.

Z. Woldehiwet Department of Veterinary Pathology, University of Liverpool, Veterinary Field Station, Leahurst, Neston, Wirral L64 7TE, U.K.

Preface

A considerable number of important diseases of domestic animals are caused by organisms in the orders Rickettsiales and Chlamydiales. Although rickettsiae and chlamydiae are obligate intracellular parasites, they are now classified as Gram-negative bacteria. Nevertheless, because of their biology and their unusual host–parasite interaction, there is a need to treat them separately. Most of the rickettsiae which affect animals, with the possible exception of *Coxiella burnetii* and *Neorickettsia helminthoeca,* have ticks as intermediate hosts. In contrast, several rickettsiae which affect human beings are transmitted by lice and fleas. The global distribution of animal rickettsiosis is, therefore, dictated by the ecology of their arthropod hosts. For example, *Anaplasma marginale* is widely distributed by virtue of the fact that it has a wide range of intermediate vectors. In contrast, *Cytoecetes phagocytophila,* the causative agent of tick-borne fever, is limited to temperate areas where the tick, *Ixodes ricinus,* resides while *Cowdria ruminantium,* the causative agent of heartwater, is limited to tropical Africa and the Caribbean which are inhabited by certain species of the *Amblyomma* tick. In contrast, infections caused by chlamydiae and the rickettsial agent, *Coxiella burnetii,* have no such limitations because they do not require an intermediate host. The diseases caused by these organisms are of great economic significance and some cause very serious zoonoses (Q fever, psittacosis).

Nearly all of the tick-borne rickettsial diseases covered in this book are endemic to tropical and semi-tropical regions of the world. While most of the projected increases in livestock production are expected to take place in these regions, the uncontrolled disease situation has hindered and discouraged investment in food animal production by private and public sectors. Although some of the rickettsial diseases, such as anaplasmosis and Rocky Mountain spotted fever, have been well known and intensely studied, the group of leukocytic rickettsiae, and diseases they cause, are relative newcomers to the field. The pathogenic potential of members of the genus *Ehrlichia* has been clearly recognized only during the past 30 years and some species, e.g. *Ehrlichia risticii,* the causative agent of equine monocytic ehrlichiosis (Syn., Potomac horse fever), and *Ehrlichia platys,* the etiologic agent of canine infectious cyclic thrombocytopenia, have been discovered more recently. It is interesting to note that the only commercially available and effective vaccine against Potomac horse fever was developed within three years after the discovery of the causative agent in 1984. This achievement was made possible by an early understanding of the mechanism of protective immunity of this disease. We hope that the information made available will help speed the day when many other diseases covered in this book will be brought under control by immunologic techniques similar to those which have long been successful against a wide range of pathogenic viruses and bacteria.

The importance of *Chlamydia psittaci* as a cause of several disease syndromes of domestic animals and man is well established. Chlamydiae were first recognized as causing atypical pneumonia in human beings and because the disease was regarded to have been contracted from parrots, the name psittacosis was used to describe these human infections. It is now recognized that *Chlamydia psittaci* causes several economically important diseases in domestic animals and birds, including avian chlamydiosis, enzootic abortions in ruminants, respiratory infections, encephalitides, polyarthritis, conjunctivitis and a diversity of other diseases in a wide range of animal hosts.

The recent recognition of human ehrlichiosis and the advent of molecular biology has created a new interest in animal rickettsiae. Although diseases caused by rickettsial and chlamydial agents are covered in text books of veterinary microbiology and a number of review articles concerning specific rickettsial and chlamydial diseases are occasionally published in scientific journals, we are not aware of any publication in the English language which deals specifically with rickettsial and chlamydial diseases of domestic animals and birds. Consequently, the aim of this book is to fill this gap by providing up-to-date information on the etiology, epidemiology, pathogenesis, diagnosis, control and the public health significance of the most important rickettsial and chlamydial diseases of domestic animals and birds.

This state-of-the-art material is provided by an international authorship represented by scientific eminence, intense professional experience and comprehensive knowledge of the respective subject matter. This book should serve as a valuable source of information for research workers, graduate and undergraduate students in veterinary and agricultural sciences, practicing veterinarians, and

allied professionals involved in animal production and disease control. It is obvious that the emergence of Lyme's disease and human ehrlichiosis has greatly contributed to an increase in the scientific interest in tick-borne zoonoses in the U.S.A., Western Europe and elsewhere. Ehrlichiosis is now recognized as one of the most recent zoonoses. In view of the zoonotic nature of many other rickettsial and chlamydial diseases covered, this book should also serve as an authoritative reference text for medical and public health workers.

The editors offer their sincere thanks and appreciation to the contributors for their efforts and cooperation in the realization of this volume. Among the many people who deserve our thanks, we would like to mention the following: From ProtaTek International, Inc., Dr Maxwell Khondowe for his review of one manuscript, and Ms Kelly Landwehr, whose secretarial standards of perfection approach the ideal, and from the Department of Veterinary Pathology University of Liverpool, Dr F. T. W. Jordan for reviewing one manuscript and Mrs Linda Greatwich for secretarial support.

Finally, the editors wish to thank Mrs. Marion Jowett and her associates at Pergamon Press for their courtesy, continuous assistance and cooperation.

ZERAI WOLDEHIWET
AND MIODRAG RISTIC

1

The Rickettsiae

Z. WOLDEHIWET AND M. RISTIC

Taxonomic Position and Nomenclature

In the latest edition of *Bergey's Manual of Determinative Bacteriology*, the rickettsiae are classified as Gram-negative bacteria.[1] This taxonomic position is based on several important criteria which make these organisms more related to the Gram-negative bacteria. Historically the rickettsiae were regarded as intermediates between bacteria and viruses. Their dependence on cells and the ability of some of them to pass through filters that would normally retain bacteria led earlier workers to regard them as viruses.[2] These observations led to the suggestion that the rickettsiae should be regarded as "intermediate" organisms between the bacteria and the viruses. It was argued then that like the bacteria they have a single chromosome. Several reports then followed which showed differences between viruses, rickettsiae and bacteria in terms of their biochemistry and intracellular parasitism. Zinsser and Schoenbach,[3] for example, observed that rickettsiae continued to multiply even when the respiration of their host cells was reduced. Bovarnick and Snyder[4] demonstrated for the first time that purified *Rickettsia prowazekii* and *R. mooseri* can oxidize amino acids. The same group of workers[5] further showed that these purified organisms were capable of transaminating and oxidizing glutamate. Bovarnick[6] confirmed that these organisms derived adenosine triphosphate (ATP) from the oxidation of glutamate, indicating an independent generation of energy. These observations have been subsequently confirmed in other species.[7,8,9,10]

The morphological similarities between the rickettsiae and bacteria were recognized early and ultrathin sections viewed by electron microscopy revealed that rickettsiae are structurally similar to Gram-negative bacteria.[11,12] The fine structure of the rickettsiae includes a typical outer layer, consisting of the cell wall and cytoplasmic membrane and cytosolic ribosomal and DNA structures.[13,14,15]

Division by binary fission has been demonstrated in stained smears and electron-microscopic preparations from several species of rickettsiae.[16,17,18] Further studies on the chemical composition of their cell walls established that the rickettsiae are similar to Gram-negative bacteria. For example, the presence of a lipopolysaccharide layer, typical of Gram-negative bacteria, was suspected because of the endotoxicity of dead rickettsiae.[19] The presence of these lipopolysaccharides as well as other components typical of Gram-negative bacteria such as muramic acid, glucosamine and diaminopimelic acid has been demonstrated in several rickettsial species.[20,21,22,23,24] The composition of the LPS of *Coxiella burnetii*, for example, includes 2-keto-3-deoxyoconate (KDO), which is a common constituent of bacterial LPS and β-hydroxymiristic acid, a specific component of Gram-negative bacterial LPS.[22,25] Thus the multiple structures, including the cytoplasmic membrane, a lipid bilayer and second bilayered membrane, the outer membrane, which characterize Gram-negative bacteria as well as the presence of muramic acid and the absence of teichoic acid, typical of Gram-positive bacteria, suggest that the rickettsiae are Gram-negative bacteria.

Studies on rickettsial DNA have further confirmed the closeness of the rickettsiae to Gram-negative bacteria. The molecular weights and guanine plus cytosine (G + C) contents of the rickettsial DNA are closer to those of Gram-negative bacteria. For example, the DNA of the spotted fever group of rickettsiae has a molecular weight of $1.0–1.5 \times 10^9$ kDa and that of *C. burnetii* is 1.04×10^9 kDa.[26] These are similar to the molecular weights of Gram-negative bacteria such as *Escherichia coli* whose genome size is 2.4×10^9kDa.[26] The G + C content of the DNA of the typhus group of rickettsiae, *Rickettsia prowazekii*, *R. typhi* and *R. canada*, is 29–30%, and the spotted fever group, *R. rickettsii*, *R. conorii* and *R. ackari*, is 32–33%,[26,27,28,29] a figure closer to Gram-negative bacteria than the Gram-positive bacteria. The G + C content of *C. burnetii* and *Rochalimaea quintana* are 42.7% and 39.3% respectively.[26] DNA/DNA hybridization studies between the rickettsiae and other Gram-negative bacteria will help elucidate further the relatedness of Gram-negative bacteria and the rickettsiae.

Differences Between Animal Rickettsiae and Those Affecting Man

The term rickettsiae is often used in reference to the well-studied human pathogens which cause typhus, spotted fever and scrub typhus.[30] This group of organisms is relatively well-characterized. However, most of the rickettsiae which affect animals and birds do not fit into this group. These include *Coxiella burnetii,* which causes Q fever in man and abortions in animals, and several tick-transmitted organisms which, with the exception of *Ehrlichia sennetsu* and *Ehrlichia canis,* are not known to affect humans. Although several members of the genus *Rickettsia* have animal reservoirs, the only member of the genus which is known to cause overt clinical disease in domestic animals is *Rickettsia rickettsii.*[31]

One of the most important characteristics which has been used in the early classification of rickettsiae has been their antigenic structure. The most commonly used serological test to identify the typhus and spotted fever rickettsiae is the Weil–Felix reaction which is based on the reaction of sera from primary, but not secondary, rickettsial infection with the somatic antigens of three strains of *Proteus,* OX 19, OX 2, and OX K. Bacteria which are not members of the genus *Rickettsia* do not stimulate the Weil–Felix reaction and there is no evidence of the presence of other antigens shared by the rickettsiae which cause typhus and spotted-type fevers in man detectable by other tests. Unlike the typhus, spotted and scrub typhus rickettsiae, which grow in the cytoplasm and sometimes in the nuclei, all of the animal rickettsiae grow in the phagolysosomes or phagocytic vacuoles. For example, the Ehrlichieae grow in membrane-bounded vacuoles in the cytoplasm of leucocytes,[32,33] and the *Anaplasma* and *Aegyptianella* spp. grow in vacuoles within the red blood cells.[34,35] *Coxiella burnetii* grows only within phagolysosomes.[36] The only other animal rickettsiae which may grow outside a clearly defined vacuole are those in the genus *Haemobartonella* and the genus *Eperythrozoon.* These organisms may grow in shallow or deep indentations on the surfaces or within the cytoplasm of red blood cells with or without the apparent presence of a bounding membrane or vacuole.[37,38]

The rickettsiae are now classified in the order Rickettsiales comprising three families Rickettsiaceae, Bartonellaceae and Anaplasmataceae. These three families are composed of 17 genera containing more than 45 species, most of which are animal pathogens. All three families contain animal pathogens. The most important rickettsiae which affect domestic animals and birds are shown in Table 1.1.

This table does not include other organisms which had only been occasionally cited in the past and whose taxonomic relationship to the well-known species is not known. These include *R. suis* which was observed in pigs by Donatien and Gayot in 1942[39] and *Ehrlichia bovis* which was first isolated by Donatien and Lestoquard[40] from circulating mononuclear cells of cattle in Morocco after *Hyaloma* ticks brought from Iran were allowed to feed on the cattle. *Ehrlichia*

TABLE 1.1. *Rickettsial species affecting animals and birds*

Family	Tribe	Genus	Species
Anaplasmataceae		*Anaplasma* (A.)	*marginale*
			centrale
			ovis
			caudatum
		Aegyptianella (A.)	*pullorum*
		Haemobartonella (H.)	*felis*
			canis
			muris
		Eperythrozoon (Ep.)	*ovis*
			suis
			wenyoni
Rickettsiaceae	Rickettsieae		
		Rickettsia (R.)	*conorii*
			rickettsii
		Coxiella (C.)	*burnetii*
	Ehrlichieae		
		Ehrlichia (E.)	*canis*
			equi
			risticii
			platys
		Cytoecetes (C.)	*phagocytophila*
			ondiri
		Cowdria (C.)	*ruminantium*

ovis was described as occurring in the peripheral blood monocytes of Moroccan sheep.[41] Raghavarhari and Reddy[42] associated an organism present in ovine blood in India which they gave the name *Cytoecetes ovis* var. *decani,* with a disease known as tick-borne fever. The organism was not characterized further and, therefore, it is not known whether it is related to *Cytoecetes (Ehrlichia) phagocytophila* and since no typical *Cytoecetes ovis* has been described, its name has been regarded as illegitimate by the latest edition of Bergey's Manual of Determinative Bacteriology.[43] Another organism, *Rickettsia belgaumi*, present in the monocytes of sheep and goats in India was reported to infect guinea pigs and white mice.[44] *Cytoecetes microti*[45] was observed on one occasion in the granulocytes and lymphocytes of a vole in Massachusetts, and *Rickettsia delphi* was isolated from the leucocytes of a splenectomized Iranian gerbil.

The Biology of Rickettsiae

Rickettsiae are fastidious obligate intracellular bacteria. Although they are obligate intracellular parasites, they are metabolically independent.[4]

Morphology and Staining Characteristics

Rickettsiae are pleomorphic coccobacilli that may range from 300 to 700 nm by 1500 to 2000 nm in size. Because they grow in cytoplasmic vacuoles, *Coxiella burnetii* and members of the tribe *Ehrlichieae* appear as compact inclusions with various numbers of individual organisms. In the *Ehrlichieae* in particular, the berry-like appearance of these inclusions has led to the use of the terms morulae, initial bodies, and elementary bodies.[46,47]

The rickettsiae are Gram-negative but do not stain well with aniline dyes. The preferred staining methods are those of Gimenez,[48] Machiavello[49] and Giemsa. The first two methods are widely used for staining the members of the genus *Rickettsia* and *Coxiella burnetii* but the animal pathogens which infect red blood cells (*Anaplasma* spp., *Haemobartonella* spp. and *Eperythrozoon* spp.) and white blood cells (*Ehrlichia* spp., *Cytoecetes* spp., *Cowdria ruminantium* etc.) are better stained with Giemsa. Other staining methods that can be used to demonstrate rickettsiae in tissues include general nucleic acid stains such as acridine orange, or immunological stains such as immunofluorescence and immunoperoxidase, which can reveal the morphology of the organisms within infected cells. All members of the family Rickettsiaceae stain deep orange with acridine orange in low pH buffers.[50] Immunological methods of staining are particularly useful in differentiating pathogenic rickettsiae from commensals in arthropod tissues.

Ultrastructure

The ultrastructure of the rickettsiae is that of Gram-negative bacteria. Ultrathin sections of several members of the family Rickettsiaceae reveal that they possess typical multilayered envelopes representing the cell wall and cytoplasmic membranes.[15,51] In some species the cell wall is surrounded by a slime layer, which appears as a halo surrounding the rickettsiae within cells.[13] There is significant variation from species to species as to the thickness of the cell wall, being strongly bound to host cells and thick in some and relatively thin in others.[13] For example, in *R. prowazekii, R. rickettsii* and other members of the typhus and spotted fever causing rickettsiae the cell wall is thicker than the cytoplasmic membrane whereas the reverse is the case in *R. tsutsugamushi,* thus explaining the difficulty of obtaining *R. tsutsugamushi* without losing viability. The morphology of *Coxiella burnetii* is characterized by the presence of vegetative and sporogenic forms.[52] Very limited electron-microscopic studies have been carried out on the intracellular rickettsiae which affect animals. These rickettsiae are highly cell-associated and the limited published ultrastructural studies have relied on ultrathin sections of infected cells. There is a great deal of variation in their size and electron density. Limited studies on ultrathin sections of *Cowdria ruminantium,* separated from infected tissues by Percoll gradient centrifugation, and *C. phagocytophila,* separated from infected leucocytes by Percoll and Renografin density centrifugation, and *E. sennetsu* and *E. risticii*, separated from infected $P388D_1$ cells by Renografin density centrifugation, confirm that they maintain their cell wall and cytoplasmic membranes[10,53,54] but further characterizations are lacking.

Growth in the Arthropod Vector

In general, when rickettsiae are ingested by arthropod vectors after a blood meal on an infected mammalian host, they enter the epithelial cells of the mid-gut where they multiply. While in some species the rickettsiae multiply only in the midgut and are excreted through the faeces,[55] it cannot be excluded that in others there may be rickettsial multiplication in other tissues too.[56] With some exceptions the multiplication of the rickettsiae in the midgut does not have any significant effect on the arthropod itself. An important exception in this respect is the fatal effect of *R. prowazekii* on the vector louse, *Pediculus humanus corporus*. Heavy infection of gut cells of the louse results in the rupture of epithelial cells and death of infected lice within 10 to 14 days.[57] In most rickettsial infections the vector arthropods remain infected for life and some can transfer infection trans-stadially while others will pass on the infection trans-ovarially. The transmission of the rickettsiae to the mammalian host will depend on the feeding habits of the arthropod. For example, in scrub typhus only the larval stage (chiggers) of the vector mites will transmit *R. tsutsugamushi* to man because this stage feeds on a host only once while infection is acquired trans-ovarially. Finally, while yet to be definitely confirmed, it is now increasingly evident that *Anaplasma marginale* is biologically transmitted by the male *Dermacentor andersoni* ticks.[58]

Growth in the Animal Host

Almost all rickettsiae gain access to their mammalian host through a bite by an infected arthropod vector. There are a few exceptions to this. *C. burnetii* does not require an arthropod vector and the portal of entry is usually the oropharynx. Another exception is that of *Neorickettsia helminthoeca*, which requires a trematode and salmon fish as intermediate hosts and gains access to its canine host by ingestion. After gaining entry to the mammalian host, the rickettsiae multiply in specified target cells which may vary from one species to another. In general the rickettsiae affecting animals multiply in cells of the reticulo-endothelial system. They are believed to be taken up by a process of phagocytosis, which is mediated by rickettsial factors.

Growth in Cell Culture

While the classical rickettsiae are readily cultivated in the yolk sacs of embryonated eggs and cell culture systems, cultivating animal rickettsiae has proven to be difficult. These organisms have an unusual target cell specificity. Of the members of the tribe *Ehrlichieae, E. canis* was successfully cultivated in monocytic cultures derived from dogs in 1971.[59] Similarly *Neorickettsia helminthoeca* and *E. sennetsu* have been cultivated in canine monocytic cultures.[60,61] Recently *Cowdria ruminantium* has been cultivated in bovine endothelial cells.[62] *E. risticii* has also been cultivated in human histiocyte U937 cells and mouse macrophage $P388D_1$ cells.[63] The other members which infect mainly granular leucocytes, *E. equi, Cytoecetes phagocytophila* and *C. ondiri* have not been cultivated in cell culture systems, but short-term cultures in infected leucocytes have been used for antigenic studies.[64,65] Similarly, there has been no success in cultivating the rickettsiae which infect erythrocytes, although temporary blood cultures have been used to study the biology of these organisms.[66]

Multiplication and "Development"

The mode of multiplication of the rickettsiae has been extensively studied in those which grow in yolk sacs and cell culture systems. All the members of the genus *Rickettsia* multiply in the cytoplasm and sometimes in the nucleus, while *Coxiella burnetii* multiplies within phagosomes. There are no apparent stages of "development" in the classical rickettsiae, but transformations from vegetative to sporogenic forms have been described in *C. burnetii*. There is very limited information on the modes of multiplication in the animal rickettsiae, but electron-microscopic evidence indicates that they divide by binary fission.[33] Initial observations that there were different morphological variants of the *Ehrlichieae* gave rise to the use of such names as elementary bodies, morulae and initial bodies, which are traditionally used to describe the developmental stages of chlamydia[46,47] and attempts were made to establish stages of development similar to those of the members of the order *Chlamy-*

diales. Despite the morphological similarities with chlamydiae and the possible existence of a developmental cycle, the ehrlichiae differ from them significantly.

Recent phylogenetic and metabolic studies have clearly shown that they are closely related to the members of the family Rickettsiaceae. At least three members of the tribe *Ehrlichiaeae, E. risticii, E. canis,* and *E. sennetsu,* are capable of generating energy from glutamine, unlike the chlamydiae which are energy parasites,[10] and a recent comparison of the 16S rRNA of *E. risticii* with that of *R. prowazekii, R. rickettsii, C. burnetii* and *Wolbachia persica* showed that *E. risticii* is closely related to *R. prowazekii*.[67]

Metabolism and Biochemical Activities

Because of the obligate intrecellular nature oí rickettsiae, it had been difficult to study the metabolism of these organisms. Bovarnick and Snyder (1949)[4] produced the first evidence of an independent rickettsial metabolic activity by showing that purified *R. prowazekii* and *R. mooseri* can oxidize amino acids. Earlier, Zinsser and Schoenbach[3] had observed that rickettsiae continued to multiply even when the respiration of their host cells was reduced. It was later confirmed that these organisms derived adenosine triphosphate (ATP) from the oxidation of glutamate, indicating an independent generation of energy.[6] Since then metabolic activities have been demonstrated in several species. In general, the members of the family in which metabolic activities have been investigated possess catabolic enzymes which are necessary for deriving energy but the type of enzymes present may differ. For example, while *R. typhi* free from host cells contained demonstrable enzymes involved in the catabolism of glutamate and tricarboxylic acid intermediaries, it lacked detectable glycolytic enzymes.[8] This contrasts with the presence of several enzymes including glycolytic enzymes in *C. burnetii*.[7,9] There is very little information on the metabolism of the other intracellular rickettsiae which affect animals, but recently Weiss *et al.*[10] showed that *Ehrlichia risticii* and *E. sennetsu* separated from host cells were capable of using glutamine oxidation to generate ATP *in vitro*.

Molecular Biology

Over the last decade major developments in genetic engineering have opened the way to understanding the molecular basis of the biology of bacteria. The progress in this area has also been reflected in studies related to rickettsiae. The molecular composition of animal rickettsiae in relation to their nucleic acids and the way their proteins are synthesized is being unravelled. The level of knowledge of the molecular biology of the rickettsial organisms affecting animals is varied. While in some the genes responsible for crucial antigenic proteins are known and the DNA is being mapped, no progress has been reported in others. The level of work on individual animal rickettsiae is well covered in the relevant chapters. It is quite clear that molecular techniques are now increasingly being used in the diagnosis of rickettsial infections and in studying their epidemiology. For example, DNA probes are likely to detect low number of rickettsiae in carrier animals and in vector ticks.[68,69,70,71]

Molecular techniques are also being used to differentiate strains. The cleavage patterns of rickettsial DNA after digestion with restriction endonucleases have been widely used to differentiate strains of various rickettsiae including *R. prowazekii*,[72] *C. burnetii*[73] and *A. marginale*.[74] Similarly, cloned DNA probes have also been used to differentiate strains of *R. prowazekii*,[72] *A. marginale*[75] and *Eperythrozoon suis*.[76]

When the sequence of the whole or part of the genome is known, it is possible to use the polymerase chain reaction (PCR) technique to amplify rickettsial DNA. For example, Tzianabos *et al.*[77] used PCR to detect *R. rickettsii* and *R. conorii* DNA in clinical specimens. The inability to obtain pure organisms has hindered progress in understanding the molecular biology of the other animal rickettsiae, notably the members of the tribe *Ehrlichieae*. Recently, Dutta *et al.*[78] have cloned and expressed the genome which encodes for some important antigens of *E. risticii*.

Antigenic Composition

The antigenicity of members of the genus *Rickettsia* was recognized very early, and rickettsial antigen preparations are routinely used to establish diagnosis by serological means. However, detailed studies on the antigenic composition have been limited to specific pathogens which affect humans, notably *Coxiella burnetii* and some members of the genus *Rickettsia*. In the early 1940s and 1950s, agglutinating and complement fixing antigens were demonstrated in a number of rickettsial infections including *C. burnetii* and *A. marginale* in animals. Most subsequent antigenic studies of that period endeavored to establish species- and type-specific antigens for diagnostic purposes. Several workers used physical and chemical means to separate antigens into soluble and insoluble fractions and to test these fractions with antibodies raised against homologous or heterologous strains. The ability to separate rickettsiae from host cells by density gradient centrifugation and the subsequent breakdown of their proteins by sodium dodecyl-sulfate (SDS) followed by electrophoresis in polyacrylamide gels (SDS-PAGE) introduced a new method in analyzing the chemical composition of rickettsiae. SDS-PAGE followed by immunoblotting techniques has further improved our understanding of the antigenic composition of these intracellular bacteria.

Types of Antigens

The early indication that rickettsial antigens may be classified into soluble and insoluble fractions, and/or species- and type-specific ones, was further elaborated to indicate that the antigenic components are of protein and lipopolysaccharide (LPS) nature. Several workers showed that members of the genus *Rickettsia* contained many polypeptides of different molecular weights, but, because of their location in their cell wall, it was thought that some proteins are likely to be more antigenically important than others. For this purpose, extrinsic labelling of surface proteins by radioactive iodine and precipitation with immune sera was used to identify the dominant surface proteins of *R. prowazekii,*[79] *A. marginale*[66] and *R. tsutsugamushi.*[80]

Radio-labelling has also been used to identify the chemical composition of the antigens. For example, incorporation of radiolabelled galactose into bands of proteins of *R. prowazekii* and *R. conorii* was used to establish that they are glycoproteins.[79] After the demonstration that the cell wall of the rickettsiae contained lipopolysaccharides (LPS) similar to that found in Gram-negative bacteria, the role of LPS in pathogenesis as well as in immunogenesis was investigated most notably in *C. burnetii* and *R. prowazekii*. The antigenicity of LPS is tested by the presence of antigenic bands in SDS-PAGE after treatment with proteinase K. In this way, it has been shown that the surface proteins and the LPS are immunodominant, and that several polypeptides are shared within species or even among groups of species (e.g. spotted type group), while others may be limited to strains or types. The use of monoclonal antibodies and the cloning of genes encoding for the various antigens and their expression in appropriate vectors will unravel the role of the different antigens.

Role of Monoclonal Antibodies

Monoclonal antibodies are increasingly being used to identify epitopes which are specific for species and strains and to determine surface antigens responsible for protective immunity.[81] For example, Anacker *et al.*[82] used monoclonal antibodies to demonstrate the antigenic heterogeneity in strains of *R. rickettsii*, and Feng *et al.*[83] used monoclonal antibodies to demonstrate whether or not antigens of *R. conorii* were T-cell dependent. Williams *et al.*[84] produced monoclonal antibodies against a 28 kDa protein which was shared by phase I and phase II variants of *C. burnetii*, but a phase I specific monoclonal antibody was directed against a putative surface LPS. Furthermore, it was observed that the major component which differentiated phase I and phase II was the LPS, and that the surface LPS of phase I variants is a virulence and antigenic determinant.[85]

Role of Molecular Biological Techniques

Recombinant DNA technology is now increasingly being used to clone specific genes which encode for specific antigens and to produce (express) the required antigens in a suitable vector system (*Escherichia coli*). This is bound to revolutionize antigenic studies. Genes which encode for the immunologically dominant surface proteins of several rickettsiae which affect animals and humans have been cloned and some of their antigens expressed in suitable vectors. For example, Krause *et al.*[86] cloned genes of *R. prowazekii* and expressed rickettsial antigens in *E. coli*; McDonald *et al.*[87] expressed cloned antigens of *R. rickettsii* for use as a vaccine for Rocky Mountain spotted fever and Stover *et al.*[88] cloned the major antigen gene of *R. tsutsugamushi*. Experimental recombinant vaccines have been produced against *R. rickettsii*[89] and against *R. conorii*.[90] Dutta *et al.*[78] have also expressed antigens of *E. risticii* in *E. coli*.

Pathogenicity

Modes of Entry

With the exception of *Coxiella burnetii*, which gains entry through the oro-nasal route, the rickettsiae are injected into the blood stream or the vascular epithelium of their mammalian host.

In the classical typhus and spotted type fevers affecting man, the portal of entry is usually the skin following the injection of the saliva of infected arthropods or the deposition of rickettsiae-bearing faeces. Following a period of rickettsemia, the organisms are disseminated to other tissues, via the circulatory and lymphatic system, allowing the rickettsiae to infect the endothelial cells of the blood vessels. Severe damage to the endothelial cells results in thrombosis and cellular infiltration, giving rise to the typical rash which accompanies the disease. The pathogenic mechanisms of the rickettsiae which affect animals differ in several significant ways. With the exception of *C. burnetii*, they invade either the red blood cells or circulating white blood cells. The pathogenesis of these organisms will, therefore, vary according to the target tissues predominantly affected. In those which affect the red blood cells, the pathological reactions involve the immune-mediated destruction and sequestration of infected red blood cells, leading to anemia and autoimmune reactions. In those which affect the white blood cells there are variable degrees of reductions in the number of circulating white blood cells, due to immune-mediated destruction and sequestration of infected cells.

One of the features of rickettsial infections is their capacity to cause a carrier state, in which the organisms are maintained in the host, without apparent ill health. Often the organisms reside within the macrophages or other antigen-presenting cells and this may be their main strategy of evading immune recognition and elimination.

Virulence Factors

The febrile responses that accompany rickettsial infections may be due to the LPS endotoxins released from dead rickettsiae or cellular factors. Some rickettsial species are characterized by a degree of heterogeneity in terms of virulence and antigens. In some rickettsiae, plasmids have been identified[91] but their role in encoding for virulence is not known. After demonstrating that certain types of plasmids were only present in strains of *C. burnetii* which caused chronic endocarditis in man and abortions in goats, Samuel and coworkers[91] suggested that plasmids may be virulence determinants. There is no sufficient explanation as to why there is such a wide range of differences in the severity of disease caused by various strains of the same species. Classical concepts of the rough to smooth variation in Gram-negative bacteria have been invoked to explain the change from Phase I to Phase II in infections by *Coxiella burnetii*. It appears that these phase variations in *C. burnetii* are determined by the host as Phase II occurs only after adaptation to embryonated eggs but reverts back to Phase I when inoculated into its original animal host. The main difference between phase I and phase II variants of *C. burnetii* appears to be in the composition and antigenicity of their LPS.[85] In contrast, the main difference between high and low virulence strains of *R. rickettsii* resides in specific polypeptides and not the LPS.[82] Hanson[92] found that gamma interferon had different effects on three strains of *R. tsutsugamushi* which differed in their virulence to mice. Among the other animal rickettsiae too, there is reported to be a wide range of variation in the virulence of different strains. For example, Tuomi[93] reported that strain variations in *C. phagocytophila* have no parallel in nature. Some strains are more virulent to sheep but less so to cattle and vice versa[93,94] but their virulence determinants are not known. It is possible to attenuate some rickettsiae by passage but it is not clear what virulence determinants are deleted by passage.

Target Tissues

The rickettsiae which affect animals are characterized by a high degree of cytotropism. All of the members of the tribe *Ehrlichieae* invade the circulating leucocytes and/or thrombocytes, and some may also invade the endothelial cells of the capillaries. Members of the genera *Aegyptianella, Anaplasma, Eperythrozoon* and *Haemobartonella* infect erythrocytes. According to the predominant type of leucocytes affected, the ehrlichiae may be divided into two major groups. Those which invade mainly the mononuclear cells and those which infect mainly professional granulocytes. The former includes *E. canis* which usually infects mononuclear cells and occasionally granulocytes. The latter includes *C. phagocytophila, C. ondiri* and *E. equi*. *C. ruminantium* parasitizes mainly capillary endothelial cells but when present in the blood it is mainly found in the granulocytes.

Mechanisms of Immunity

The rickettsiae and other obligate intracellular organisms have unusual features which allow them to survive in environments hostile to other organisms. Some of them may even reside in cells of the immune system. For example, the preferred target cells of some members of the tribe *Ehrlichieae, Ehrlichia equi, Cytoecetes phagocytophila, C. ondiri,* and *Cowdria ruminantium*, are the polymorphonuclear cells and monocytes which are the primary phagocytes in peripheral blood. Other members such as *Ehrlichia canis* invade lymphocytes. Other rickettsiae may also exist in cells inaccessible to the immune system.[95]

Role of Humoral Immune Responses

Several workers had reported that mixing immune sera with rickettsial organisms *in vitro* reduced their infectivity to cell cultures, embryonated eggs or experimental animals. For example, Abinanti and Marmion[96] showed that *C. burnetii* mixed with antibodies was not infectious to experimental animals. Various studies showed that antibodies enhance the uptake of rickettsiae by macrophages and granulocytes. Gambril and Wisseman[97] demonstrated that preincubation of *Rickettsia mooseri* with human convalescent serum enhanced phagocytosis and destruction of the rickettsiae by human macrophages. Similarly, Kishimoto and Walker[98] found that immune serum rendered *C. burnetii* more susceptible to phagocytosis by guinea pig peritoneal macrophages, and Lewis *et al.*[99] found that the addition of immune serum greatly reduced the multiplication of *Ehrlichia canis* in macrophage cultures. Other workers reported similar enhancement of polymorphonuclear and macrophage phagocytosis of *C. burnetii* by the addition of immune serum.[100,101] Passive transfer of immune sera is reported to enhance the clearance of rickettsiae in animals experimentally infected with *R. mooseri*[102] and *R. tsutsugamushi.*[103]

Role of Macrophages

The role of macrophages in the immune system was first elaborated by the elegant experiments carried out by Mackaness.[104] Gambril and Wisseman[97] demonstrated that antibodies were useful in conjunction with macrophages in antirickettsial immunity. Macrophages activated by lymphokines or interferon are more effective against rickettsiae *in vitro* than resting nonactivated macrophages. Infection of mice with *R. tsutsugamushi* or *R. conorii* results in generation of macrophage populations capable of killing the rickettsiae *in vitro.*[105] The macrophages are activated by humoral factors (lymphokines and interferons) produced by lymphocytes and other cells. For example, Kodama *et al.*[106] established a T cell line which secreted gamma interferons specific to *R. tsutsugamushi*. However, it is still unclear how several of the rickettsiae manage to multiply in the macrophages themselves. Their capacity to grow within the macrophages themselves may explain several of the phenomena that accompany rickettsial infections. For example, because the macrophage is infected, its capacity to process and present other antigens may be impaired resulting in immunosuppression. The macrophage may become the target of cytotoxic T cells, again resulting in immunosuppression.

Macrophages which have been activated by interferons or other lymphokines are likely to be more effective against rickettsial infections. For example, normal resting macrophages appear to have no bactericidal effect on *C. burnetii*, but opsonization with immune serum and, more importantly, activation by interferon render them more effective against the organism.[107] Park and Rikihisa[108] recently showed that the addition of recombinant IFN alpha to murine macrophages rendered them refractory to *in vitro* infection with

Ehrlichia risticii, and Hanson[109] reported that recombinant gamma interferon inhibited the infection of cultured BALB/c mouse fibroblasts by *R. tsutsugamushi*. Interferons appear to induce antirickettsial activity either by inhibiting entry of rickettsiae into susceptible cells or by clearing intracellular rickettsiae.[109]

Role of T-cells

The role of T lymphocytes in the development of antirickettsial immunity has been investigated in natural and experimental infections. The participation of T helper cells in antirickettsial immune responses has been the subject of several investigations. If the antigens are T cell dependent, the cellular immune response starts with the recognition of these antigens by T-helper lymphocytes when presented to them directly or often in association with Class II MHC coded molecules of antigen-presenting cells (macrophages). This is followed by the transformation of the helper T cells and secretion of lymphokines (e.g. IL-2, 3, 4 and 5) which in turn will activate other regulatory and effector cells (macrophages, B cells and cytotoxic T cells).

That rickettsiae activate T helper lymphocytes to divide (blastogenesis) and to produce lymphokines which may act on macrophages or other cells has been demonstrated in several rickettsial infections affecting man and animals.

Because rickettsial antigens may be expressed on cell surfaces, the cytotoxic T cells which recognize foreign antigen with the Class I major histocompatibility complex (MHC Class I) antigen may be important in clearing rickettsial infections.[95] Several *in vitro* tests have been used to measure cellular immune responses. These include the lymphocyte transformation test, the macrophage or leucocyte migration inhibition test and the chromium release assay. On the basis of these tests, several workers have concluded that cellular immune responses are important in clearing rickettsial infections. Cellular responses have been demonstrated in animal infections due to *Anaplasma marginale,*[110,111] *Ehrlichia canis,*[112] *Cytoecetes phagocytophila*[113] and *Coxiella burnetii.*[95]

In general, there is substantial data suggesting that all the effector arms of the immune system are involved in eliminating or containing rickettsial infections.

Survival within Hostile Environment

Apart from the specific immune elimination, bacteria are generally cleared by the action of polymorphonuclear cells and macrophages by the generation of toxic products of oxygen and killing of bacteria by nonoxidative means with the help of low pH. Several of the rickettsiae which infect animals and man are capable of multiplying within macrophages. The mechanisms of survival of organisms within the hostile environment of the macrophage has been the subject of several studies. Various mechanisms of survival within macrophages have been postulated for several intracellular bacteria. Weiss[30] speculated that members of the genus *Rickettsia* might escape the action of the lysosomes by their active penetration into the cytoplasm and by avoiding the vacuoles.

What is intriguing is how the ehrlichiae and *C. burnetii* survive and multiply within phagocytic vacuoles. Many bacteria would not survive the low pH generated by the fusion of lysosomes within phagosomes. Intricate mechanisms for the inhibition of action of lysosomes have been elaborated for the chlamydiae and other intracellular organisms. Hirsch[114] suggested that organisms which multiply inside phagocytic vacuoles have the ability to escape their destruction by partial or complete inhibition of the process of fusion with macrophage lysosomes. Escape mechanisms of this nature have been described in Chlamydia,[115] *Mycobacterium tuberculosis* and *Toxoplasma gondii*.[116] There is also some evidence that some of the animal ehrlichiae, which reside within phagocytic vacuoles, may inhibit fusion of lysosomes.[117,118] It has been demonstrated that the phagosomes in which *C. burnetii* resides contain acid phosphatase and 5′-nucleotidase[119,120] which are lethal to other bacteria. Parasites which multiply within phagosomes may possess some means of removing or neutralizing these toxic products. For example, it has been shown that *Leishmania donovani* produces acid phosphatase to neutralize oxygen produced by neutrophils.[121] Among the animal rickettsiae which grow in neutrophils and macrophages there is very limited information on how they avoid lysis. However, there is evidence which suggests that *C. burnetii* prefers low pH for its multiplication.[122] The endospore-like SCVs of *C. burnetii* appear to be designed for this purpose.[52]

Immunosuppression and Misdirected Immune Responses

Because several rickettsiae invade cells involved in the immune responses of the host, it was suspected that they may play an immunosuppressive role and that the immune responses directed at rickettsiae might cause collateral damage to the immune system itself. Both clinical and experimental data have been presented to show that infections with some of the rickettsiae are often followed by severe infections by other agents. For example, lambs infected with *C.*

phagocytophila, the causative agent of tick-borne fever, often develop tick pyemia due to secondary staphylococcal infection.[123] The susceptibility to staphylococci is due to the reduced capacity of infected neutrophils to phagocytose and kill staphylococci.[124,125] Infection of dogs with *Ehrlichia canis* is often complicated by one or more disease-causing agents, most notably the hemoparasite *Babesia canis.*[47] Infection with members of the tribe *Ehrlichieae* is often characterized by lymphoid depletion and reduction of circulating lymphocytes.[47,126,127] The lymphocytopenia accompanying tick-borne fever affects all lymphocyte subpopulations.[128]

Several mechanisms of rickettsia-induced immunosuppression have been described. These include the down regulation of cellular and humorol responses to other antigens by suppressor cells[95] and the production of prostaglandins by macrophages and polymorphonuclear cells (PMN). For example, Koster *et al.*[129] attributed the unresponsiveness caused in chronic infections with *C. burnetii* to suppressor T cells which secrete lymphokines, which in turn stimulate monocytes to produce prostaglandins. Recently, Walker and Hoover[130] demonstrated that murine PMN incubated with *R. prowazekii* secreted higher quantities of the immunosuppressive prostaglandin PGE_2 than PMN incubated without rickettsiae.

Several workers have shown that infection with rickettsiae results in a transient suppression of the proliferative responses of lymphocytes to other unrelated antigens or mitogens.[126,127,131,132] The hypergammaglobulinemia and plasmacytosis that accompany infections with *E. canis* are believed to be immune-mediated.[133] In most cases of canine tropical pancytopenia it is difficult to demonstrate *E. canis,* but the syndrome is usually fatal, even after drug therapy, suggesting that the disease is immunopathological in nature.[134]

Global Distribution and Transmission

With the exception of *C. burnetii* and *Neorickettsia helminthoeca,* the rickettsiae have an arthropod host and a mammalian host. Although *C. burnetii* has been detected in ticks and other arthropods, they do not appear to transmit it by injection. *Neorickettsia helminthoeca* requires a trematode, and salmon fish as intermediate hosts. Dogs acquire infection by ingesting raw salmon infested with the encysted metacercariae of the trematode *Nanophyetus salmincola.*[135,136] *C. burnetii* is distributed worldwide, but the geographical distribution of tick-borne rickettsiae is limited by the ecology of the arthropod vectors. While the rickettsiae such as *A. marginale* with a wide range of arthropod vectors are widely distributed, those transmitted by temperate ticks are limited to

TABLE 1.2. *Global distribution of animal rickettsiae*

Species	Vector	Geographic distribution
Aegyptianella pullorum	*Persicargas walkerae*	Africa
Anaplasma		
A. centrale	Ticks and biting flies	Africa, Asia, Australia and North Central and South America
A. marginale		
A. ovis		
Coxiella		
C. burnetii	None	Worldwide
Cowdria		
C. ruminantium	*Amblyomma* spp.	Africa, Caribbean
Cytoecetes		
C. ondiri	Not known	East Africa
C. phagocytophila	*Ixodes ricinus*	Europe
Ehrlichia	Ticks	
E. bovis	*Hyaloma* spp., *Amblyomma* spp., *Rhipicephalus* spp.	Africa, Asia, and South America
E. canis	*Rhipicephalus sanguineus.*	Africa, Asia, North America
E. equi	Ticks/flies?	North America
E. ovis	*Rhipicephalus* spp.	Africa, Asia
E. platys	Ticks/flies?	North America
E. risticii	Not known	North America
Eperythrozoon	Ticks/flies?	
Ep. bovis		
Ep. ovis	*Culex* spp., *Aedes* spp., ticks?	Worldwide
Ep. suis		
Ep. wenyonii		
Haemobartonella	Ticks/flies?	
H. canis	*Rhipicephalus sanguineus*	Worldwide
H. felis	Not known	Worldwide
Neorickettsia		
N. helminthoeca	Trematode (*Nanophyetus salmincola*)	North America
Rickettsia	Lice/feas/ticks/mites	
R. akari	*Liponyssoides sanguineus*	North America, Russia, Central and Southeast Asia
R. australis	*Ixodes holocyclus*	Australia
R. canada		Canada
R. conorii	*Amblyomma* spp., *Rhipicephalus* spp.	Africa, Middle East, Southern Europe
R. prowazekii	*Pediculus* spp.	Worldwide
R. rickettsii	*Amblyomma* spp., *Dermacentor* spp., *Ixodes* spp., *Rhipicephalus* spp.	North and South America
R. tsutsugamushi	Mites (*Xenopsylla cheopis*)	Asia, Australia
R. typhi		Worldwide

temperate climates. The rickettsiae in the latter category include *C. phagocytophila,* the causative agent of tick-borne fever which is transmitted by the temperate tick *Ixodes ricinus.* Similarly *C. ruminantium,* which is transmitted by tropical ticks such as the *Amblyomma* spp., is limited to tropical areas of the world. The modes of transmission and the epidemiology of the important animal rickettsiae are described in the relevant chapters. Table 1.2 shows the main vectors and the geographical distribution of the most important rickettsiae which have animals as their main hosts or reservoirs of human infections.

References

1. WEISS, E. and MOULDER, J.W. 1984. The Rickettsias and Chlamydias. In: *Bergey's Manual of Systematic Bacteriology,* pp. 687–739. KRIEG, N.R. and HOLT, J.G. (Eds), Williams and Wilkins, Baltimore/London.
2. DAVIS, G.E. and COX, H.R. 1938. A filter-passing infectious agent isolated from ticks. IV. Human infection. *Publ. Hlth. Rep., USA, Wash.* **53:** 2259.
3. ZINSSER, H. and SCHOENBACH, E.B. 1937. Studies on the physiological conditions prevailing in tissue cultures. *J. exp. Med.* **66:** 207.
4. BOVARNICK, M.R. and SNYDER, J.C. 1949. Respiration of typhus rickettsiae *J. exp. Med.* **89:** 561–565.
5. BOVARNICK, M.R. and MILLER, J.C. 1950. Oxidation and transamination of glutamate by typhus rickettsiae. *J. biol. Chem.* **184:** 661–676.
6. BOVARNICK, M.R. 1956. Phosphorylation accompanying the oxidation of glutamate by the Madrid E strain of typhus rickettsiae. *J. biol. Chem.* **220:** 353–000.
7. PARETSKY, D., CONSIGLI, R.A. and DOWNS, C.M. 1962. Studies on the physiology of rickettsiae. III. Glucose phosphorylation and hexokinase activity in *Coxiella burnetii. J. Bact.* **88:** 1205–1210.
8. COOLBAUGH, J.C., PROGAR, J.J. and WEISS, E. 1976. Enzymatic activities of cell extracts of *Rickettsia typhi. Infect. Immun.* **14:** 298–305.
9. WEISS, E. 1982. The biology of rickettsiae. *A. Rev. Microbiol.* **36:** 345–370.
10. WEISS, E., WILLIAMS, J.C., DASCH, G.A. and KANG, Y.H. 1989. Energy metabolism of monocytic *Ehrlichia. Proc. natn. Acad. Sci. U.S.A.* **86:** 1674–1678.
11. ANDERSON, D.R., HOPPS, H.E., BARILE, M.F. and BERNHEIM, B.C. 1965. Comparison of the ultrastructure of several rickettsiae, ornithosis virus and mycoplasma in tissue culture. *J. Bact.* **90:** 1387–1404.
12. ANACKER, R.L., PICKENS, E.G. and LACKMAN, D.B. 1967. Details of the ultrastructure of *Rickettsia prowazekii* grown in chick yolk sac. *J. Bact.* **94:** 260–262.
13. SILVERMAN, D.J. and WISSEMAN, C.L., JR 1978. Comparative ultrastructural study on the cell envelope of *Rickettsia prowazekii, R. rickettsii* and *R. tsutsugamushi. Infect. Immun.* **21:** 1020–1023.
14. SILVERMAN, D.J. and WISSEMAN, C.L., JR 1979. *In vitro* studies on rickettsiae–host cell interactions. Ultrastructural changes induced by *Rickettsia rickettsii* infection of chicken embryo fibroblasts. *Infect. Immun.* **26:** 714–727.
15. SILVERMAN, D.J. and WISSEMAN, C.L., JR and WADDELL, A. 1980. *In vitro* studies on rickettsiae–host cell interactions. Ultrastructural study of *Rickettsia prowazekii. Infect. Immun.* **29:** 778–790.

16. SCHAECHTER, M., TOUSIMIS, A.J., COHN, Z.A., ROSEN, H., CAMPBELL, J. and HAHN, F.E. 1957. Morphological, chemical and serological studies of the cell walls of *Rickettsia mooseri*. *J. Bact.* **74:** 822–829.
17. KORDOVA, N. 1959. Filterable particles of *Coxiella burnetii*. *Acta Virol.* **3:** 25–36.
18. KOKORIN, I.N. 1969. Biological peculiarities of the development of rickettsiae. *Acta Virol.* **12:** 31–35.
19. WISSEMAN, C.L., JR 1968. Some biological properties of rickettsiae pathogenic for man. *Zentbl. Bact. Parasitenk Infect., Hyg. Abr. Orig.* **206:** 299–313.
20. PERKINS, H.R. and ALLISON, A.C. 1963. Cell-wall constituents of rickettsiae and psittacosis–lymphogranuloma organisms. *J. gen. Microbiol.* **30:** 469–480.
21. MYERS, W.F., ORMSBEE, R.A., OSTERMAN, J.V. and WISSEMAN, C.L. JR 1967. The presence of diaminopimelic acid in the rickettsiae. *Proc. Soc. exp. Biol. Med.* **125:** 459–462.
22. BACA, O.G. and PARETSKY, D. 1974. Partial chemical characterization of a toxic lipopolysaccharide from *Coxiella burnetii*. *Infect. Immun.* **9:** 959–961.
23. SCHRAMEK, S., BREZINA, R. and TARASEVICH, I.V. 1976. Isolation of lipopolysaccharide antigen from *Rickettsia* species. *Acta. Virol.* **20:** 270.
24. SCHRAMEK, S., BREZINA, R. and KAZAR, J. 1977. Some biologic properties of an endotoxic lipopolysaccharide from the typhus group rickettsiae. *Acta Virol.* **21:** 439–441.
25. SCHRAMEK, S. and BREZINA, R. 1976. Characterization of endotoxic lipopolysaccharide from *Coxiella burnetii*. *Acta. Virol.* **20:** 152–158.
26. MYERS, W.F., BACA, O. and WISSEMAN, C.L., JR 1980. Genome size of the rickettsiae *Coxiella burnetii*. *J. Bact.* **144:** 460–461.
27. TYERYAR, F.J., JR WEISS, E., MILLER, D.B., BOZEMAN, F.M. and ORMSBEE, R.A. 1973. DNA base composition of rickettsiae. *Science* **180:** 415–417.
28. SCHRAMEK, S. 1972. Deoxyribonucleic acid base composition of members of the typhus group of rickettsiae. *Acta Virol.* **16:** 447.
29. MYERS, W.F., and WISSEMAN, C.L., JR 1981. The taxonomic relationship of *Rickettsia canada* to the typhus and spotted fever groups of genus *Rickettsia*. In: *Rickettsiae and Rickettsial Diseases,* pp. 313–325. BURGDORFER, W. and ANACKER, R.L. (Eds), Academic Press, New York.
30. WEISS, E. 1973. Growth and physiology of rickettsiae. *Bact. Rev.* **37:** 259–283.
31. GREENE, C.E., BURGDORFER, W., CAVAGNOLO, R., PHILIP, R. and PEACOCK, M.G. 1985. Rocky Mountain spotted fever in dogs and its natural differentiation from canine ehrlichiosis. *J. Am. Vet. Med. Ass.* **186:** 465–472.
32. HILDEBRANDT, P.K., CONROY, J.D., MCKEE, A.E., NYINDO, M.B.A. and HUXSOLL, D.L. 1973. Ultrastructure of *Ehrlichia canis*. *Infect. Immun.* **7:** 265–271.
33. WOLDEHIWET, Z. and SCOTT, G.R. 1982. Stages in the development of *Cytoecetes phagocytophila,* the causative agent of tick-borne fever. *J. comp. Path.* **92:** 469–474.
34. RISTIC, M. and WATRACH, A. 1961. Studies in anaplasmosis. II. Electron microscopy of *Anaplasma marginale* in deer. *Am. J. vet. Res.* **22:** 109–116.
35. GOTHE, R., 1967. Ein Beitrag zur systematischen Stellung von *Aegyptianella pullorum* (Carpano 1928). Z. *Parasitenkinde* **29:** 119–129.
36. BURTON, P.R., STUECKEMANN, J., WELSH, R.M. and PARETSKY, D. 1978. Some ultrastructural effects of persistent infection by the rickettsia *Coxiella burnetii*. *Infect. Immun.* **21:** 556–566.
37. TANAKA, H., HALL, W.T., SCHEFFIELD, J.B. and MOORE, O.H. 1965. Fine structure of *Haemobartonella muris* as compared with *Eperythrozoon coccoides* and *Mycoplasma pulmonis*. *J. Bact.* **90:** 1735–1749.

38. SIMPSON, C.F., GASKIN, J.M. and HARVEY, J.W. 1978. Ultrastructure of erythrocytes parasitized by *Haemobartonella felis*. *J. Parasit.* **64:** 504–511.
39. DONATIEN, A. and GAYOT, G. 1942. Conjunctivite rickettsienne du porc. *Bull. Soc. Path. Exot.* **35:** 325.
40. DONATIEN, A. and LESTOQUARD, F. 1936. *Rickettsia bovis* nouvelle espiece pathogene pour le boeuf. *Bull. Soc. Path. Exot.* **29:** 1057–1061.
41. LESTOQUARD, F. and DONATIEN, A. 1936. Sur une nouvelle Rickettsia du mouton. *Bull. Soc. Path. Exot.* **29:** 105–108.
42. RAGHAVARHARI, K. and REDDY, A.K.M. 1959. *Cytoecetes ovis* var. *decani* (n.sp.) as the cause of tick-borne fever in sheep in India. *Ind. J. vet. Sci.* **29:** 69–86.
43. RISTIC, M. and HUXSOLL, D.L. 1984. Tribe II Ehrlichieae Philip 1957. In: *Bergey's Manual of Determinative Bacteriology*, pp. 704–710. KRIEG, N.R. and HOLT, J.G. (Eds), Williams and Wilkins, Baltimore/London.
44. MANJREKAR, S.L. 1954. Rickettsia of domesticated animals. *Ind. J. vet. Sci. Anim. Husb.* **24:** 217–222.
45. TYZZER, E.E. 1938. *Cytoecetes microti* N.G. (n.sp.). A parasite developing in granulocytes and infective for small rodents. *Parasitology,* **30:** 242–257.
46. FOGGIE, A. 1951. Studies on the infectious agent of tick-borne fever in sheep. *J. Path. Bact.* **63:** 1–15.
47. EWING, S.A. 1969. Canine ehrlichiosis. *Adv. vet. Sci.* **13:** 331–353.
48. GIMENEZ, D.F. 1964. Staining rickettsiae in yolk sac culture. *Stain Tech.* **30:** 135–140.
49. MACHIAVELLO, A. 1937. Estudios sobre tifus exanthematico. III. Un nuevo metado para tenir Rickettsia. *Rev. Chilena. Hig.* **1:** 101–106.
50. KRONVALL, G. and MYHRE, E. 1977. Differential staining of bacteria in clinical specimens using acridine orange buffered at low pH. *Acta path. Scand.* (Sect. B.) **85:** 249–254.
51. WISSEMAN, C.L., JR and WADDELL, A.D. 1975. *In vitro* studies on rickettsiae–host cell interactions. Intracellular growth cycle of virulent and attenuated *Rickettsia prowazekii* in chicken embryo cells in slide chamber cultures. *Infect. Immun.* **14:** 1052–1064.
52. MCCAUL, T.F. and WILLIAMS, J.C. 1981. Developmental cycle of *Coxiella burnetii*: structure and morphogenesis of vegetative and sporogenic differentiation. *J. Bact.* **147:** 1063–1076.
53. NEITZ, W.O., VILJOEN, G.J., BEZUIDENHOUT, J.D., OBEREM, P.T., PUTTERILL, J.F., VERSCHOOR, J.A., VISSER, L. and VERMEULEN, N.M.J. 1986. Isolation of *Cowdria ruminantium* by means of percoll density gradient centrifugation and detection by an enzyme-linked immunosorbent assay. *Ondersterpoort J. vet. Res.* **53:** 63–67.
54. WOLDEHIWET, Z., CARTER, S.D. and DARE, C. 1991. Purification of *Cytoecetes phagocytophila* the causative agent of tick-borne fever from infected ovine blood. *J. comp. Path.* **105:** 431–438.
55. SILVERMAN, D.J., BOESE, J.L. and WISSEMAN, C.L. JR. 1974. Ultrastructure of comparative *Rickettsia prowazekii* from louse midgut cells to faeces: Search for "dormant forms". *Infect. Immun.* **10:** 257–263.
56. ROBERTS, L.W., GAN, E., RAPMUND, G., CHAN, C.T., RAMASAMY, S.M. and WALKER, J.S. 1975. Distribution of *Rickettsia tsutsugamushi* in organs of *Leptotrombidium fletchiri* (Prostigmata: Trombiculidae). *J. Med. Ent.* **12:** 345–348.
57. BOESE, J.L., WISSEMAN, C.L., JR, WALSH, W.T. and FISET, P. 1973. Antibody and antibiotic action on *Rickettsia prowazekii* in body lice across host-vector

interface, with observations on strain virulence and retrieval mechanism. *Am. J. Epidem.* **98:** 262–282.

58. KOCAN, K.M., GOFF, W., STILLER, D., EDWARDS, W., CLAYPOOL, P.L., EWING, S.A., HAIR, J.A. and BARRON, S.J. 1990. Development and transmission of *Anaplasma marginale* by male *Dermacentor andersoni* transferred successively to susceptible calves. Oklahoma State Univ., Pullman, WA and Univ. Idaho, Moscow, ID. *71st Meeting of the Conference* of *Research Workers in Animal Diseases;* Chicago, Ill., Nov. 5–6 1990.
59. NYINDO, M.B.A., RISTIC, M., HUXSOLL, D.L. and SMITH, A.R. 1971. Tropical canine pancytopenia: *in vitro* cultivation of the causative agent, *Ehrlichia canis. Am. J. vet. Res.* **32:** 1651–1658.
60. BROWN, J.L., HUXSOLL, D.L., RISTIC, M. and HILDEBRANDT, P.K. 1972. *In vitro* cultivation of *Neorickettsia helminthoeca,* the causative agent of salmon poisoning disease. *Am. J. vet. Res.* **33:** 1695–1700.
61. HOLLAND, C.J., RISTIC, M., HUXSOLL, D.L., COLE, A.I. and RAPMUND, G. 1985. Adaptation of *Ehrlichia sennetsu* to canine blood monocytes; preliminary structural and serological studies with cell culture-derived *Ehrlichia sennetsu. Infect. Immun.* **48:** 366–371.
62. BEZUIDENHOUT, I.D. 1987. The present state of *Cowdria ruminantium* cultivation in cell lines. *Onderstepoort J. vet. Res.* **52:** 205–210.
63. DUTTA, S.K., SHANKARAPPA, B., THAKER, S.R. and MATTINGLY-NAPIER, B. L. 1990. DNA restriction endonuclease cleavage pattern and protein antigen profile of *Ehrlichia risticii. Vet. Microbiol.* **25:** 29–38.
64. WOLDEHIWET, Z. and SCOTT, G.R. 1982. Immunological studies on tick-borne fever. *J. comp. Path.* **92:** 457–467.
65. JONGEJAN, F., WASSINK, L.A., THIELEMANS, M.J.C., PERIE, N.M. and UILENBERG, G. 1989. Serotypes of *Cowdria ruminantium* and relationship with *Ehrlichia phagocytophila* determined by immunofluorescence. *Vet. Microbiol.* **21:** 31–40.
66. BARBET, A. F., ANDERSON, L.W., PALMER, G.H. and MCGUIRE, T.C. 1983. Comparison of proteins synthesized by two different isolates of *Anaplasma marginale. Infect. Immun.* **40:** 1068–1074.
67. WEISBURG, W.G., DOBSON, M.E., SAMUEL, J.E., DASCH, G.A., MALLAVIA, L.P., BACA, O.G., MANDELCO, L., SECHREST, J.E., WEISS, E. and WOESE, C.R. 1989. Phylogenetic diversity of the rickettsiae. *J. Bact.* **171:** 4202–4206.
68. GOFF, W., BARBET, A.F., STILLER, D., PALMER, G.H., KNOWLES, D.P., KOCAN, K.M., GORHAM, J.R. and MCGUIRE, T.C. 1988. Detection of *Anaplasma marginale* infected tick vectors by using a cloned DNA probe. *Proc. Natn. Acad. Sci. U.S.A.* **85:** 919–923.
69. GOFF, W., STILLER, D., ROEDER, R.A., JOHNSON, L.W., FALK, D., GORHAM, J.R. and MCGUIRE, T.C. 1990. Comparison of detection by DNA probe, complement fixation and indirect immunofluorescence tests for diagnosing *Anaplasma marginale* in suspected carrier cattle. *Vet. Microbiol.* **24:** 381–390.
70. ERIKS, I.S., PALMER, G.H., MCGUIRE, T.C., ALFRED, D.R., and BARBET, A.F. 1989. Detection and quantitation of *Anaplasma marginale* in carrier cattle by using nucleic acid probe. *J. clin. Microbiol.* **27:** 279–284.
71. ABOYTES-TORRES, R. and BUENING, G.M. 1990. Development of recombinant *A. marginale* DNA probes. *Vet Microbiol.* **24:** 391–408.
72. REGNERY, R.L., FU, Z.Y. and SPRUILL, C.L. 1986. Flying squirrel-associated *Rickettsia prowazekii* (epidemic typhus Rickettsiae) characterized by specific DNA fragment produced by restriction endonuclease digestion. *J. clin. Microbiol.* **23:** 189–191.

73. O'Rourke, A.T., Peacock, M., Samuel, J.E., Frazier, M.E., Natvig, D.O., Mallavia, L.P. and Baca, O. 1985. Genomic analysis of phase I and II *Coxiella burnetii* with restriction endonucleases. *J. gen. Microbiol.* **131:** 1543–1546.

74. Krueger, C.M. and Buening, G.M. 1988. Isolation and restriction endonuclease cleavage of *Anaplasma marginale* DNA *in situ* in agarose. *J. clin. Microbiol.* **26:** 906–910.

75. Ambrosio, R.E., Visser, E.S., Koekhoven, Y. and Kocan, K.M. 1987. Hybridization of DNA probes to *A. marginale* isolates from different sources and detection in *Dermacentor andersoni* ticks. *Onderstepoort J. vet. Res.* **55:** 227–229.

76. Oberst, R.D., Hall, S.M., Jasso, R.A., Arndt, T. and Wen, L. 1990. Recombinant DNA probe detecting *Eperythrozoon suis* in swine blood. *Am. J. vet. Res.* **51:** 1760–1764.

77. Tzianabos, T., Anderson, B.E. and McDade, J.E. 1989. Detection of *Rickettsia rickettsii* DNA in clinical specimens by using polymerase chain reaction technology. *J. clin. Microbiol.* **27:** 2866–2868.

78. Dutta, S.K., Shankarappa, B. and Mattingly-Napier, B.L. 1991. Molecular cloning and analysis of recombinant major antigens of *Ehrlichia risticii. Infect. Immun.* **59:** 1162–1169.

79. Ostermann, J.V. and Eisemann, C.S. 1978. Surface proteins of typhus and spotted fever group rickettsiae. *Infect. Immun.* **21:** 866.

80. Tamura, A., Ohashi, N., Urakami, H., Takhashi, K. and Oyangi, M. 1985. Analysis of polypeptide composition and antigenic components of *Rickettsia tsutsugamushi* by polyacrylamide gel electrophoresis and immunoblotting. *Infect. Immun.* **48:** 671–675.

81. Anacker, R.L., List, R.H., Mann, R.E., Hayes, S.F. and Thomas, L.A. 1985. Characterization of monoclonal antibodies protecting mice against *Rickettsia rickettsii. J. infect. Dis.* **151:** 1052–1060.

82. Anacker, R.L., List, R.H., Mann, R.E. and Wiedbrauk, D.L. 1986. Antigenic heterogeneity in high- and low-virulence strains of *Rickettsia rickettsii* revealed by monoclonal antibodies. *Infect. Immun.* **51:** 653–660.

83. Feng, H.M., Walker, D.H. and Wang, J.G. 1987. Analysis of T-cell-dependent and -independent antigens of *Rickettsia conorii* with monoclonal antibodies. *Infect. Immun.* **55:** 7–15.

84. Williams, J.C., Johnston, M.R., Peacock, M.G., Thomas, L.A., Stewart, S. and Portis, J.L. 1984. Monoclonal antibodies distinguish phase variants of *Coxiella burnetii. Infect. Immun.* **43:** 421–428.

85. Hackstadt, T., Peacock, M.G., Hitchcock, P.J. and Cole, R.L. 1985. Lipopolysaccharide variation in *Coxiella burnetii. Infect. Immun.* **48:** 359–365.

86. Krause, D.C., Winkler, H.H. and Wood, D.O. 1985. Plasmid cloning of *Rickettsia prowazekii* antigens in *Escherichia coli* K-12. *Infect. Immun.* **47:** 157–165.

87. McDonald, G.A., Anacker, R.L. and Garjian, K. 1987. Cloned gene of *Rickettsia rickettsii* surface antigen: candidate vaccine for Rocky Mountain spotted fever, *Science* **235:** 83–85.

88. Stover, C.K., Marana, D.P., Dasch, G.A. and Oakes, E.V. 1990. Molecular cloning and sequence analysis of the Sta58 major antigen gene of *Rickettsia tsutsugamushi*: Sequence homology and antigenic comparison of Sta58 to the 60-kilodalton family of stress proteins. *Infect. Immun.* **58:** 1360–1368.

89. McDonald, G.A., Anacker, R.L., Mann, R.E. and Milch, L.J. 1988. Protection of guinea pigs from experimental Rocky Mountain spotted fever with a cloned antigen of *Rickettsia rickettsii. J. infect. Dis.* **158:** 228–231.

90. Vishwanath, S., McDonald, G.A. and Watkins, N.G. 1990. A recombinant *Rickettsia conorii* vaccine protects guinea pigs from experimental boutonneuse fever and Rocky Mountain spotted fever. *Infect. Immun.* **59:** 646–653.
91. Samuel, J.E., Frazier, M.E. and Mallavia, L.P. 1985. Correlation of plasmid type and disease caused by *C. burnetii. Infect. Immun.* **49:** 775–779.
92. Hanson, B. 1991. Comparative susceptibility to mouse interferons of *Rickettsia tsutsugamushi* strains with different virulence in mice and of *Rickettsia rickettsii. Infect. Immun.* **59:** 4134–4141.
93. Tuomi, J. 1967. Experimental studies on bovine tick-borne fever. 2. Differences in virulence of strains of cattle and sheep. *Acta path. microbiol. scand.* **70:** 577–589.
94. Hudson, J.R. 1950. The recognition of tick-borne fever as a disease in cattle. *Br. vet. J.* **106:** 3–17.
95. Jerrels, T.R. 1988. Mechanisms of immunity to *Rickettsia* species and *Coxiella burnetii.* In: *Biology of Rickettsial Diseases,* Vol. II, pp. 79–100. Walker, D.H. (Ed), CRC Press, Boca Raton, Florida.
96. Abinanti, F.R. and Marmion, B.P. 1957. Protective or neutralizing antibody to Q fever. *Am. J. Hyg.* **66:** 173–195.
97. Gambril, M.R. and Wisseman, C. 1973. Mechanisms of immunity in typhus infections: III. Influence of human immune serum and complement on the fate *Rickettsia mooseri* within human macrophages. *Infect. Immun.* **8:** 631–640.
98. Kishimoto, R.A. and Walker, J.S. 1976. Interaction between *Coxiella burnetii* and guinea pig peritoneal macrophages. *Infect. Immun.* **14:** 421–426.
99. Lewis, G.E., Hill, S.L. and Ristic, M. 1978. Effects of canine immune serum on the growth of *Ehrlichia canis* within non-immune canine macrophages. *Am. J. vet. Res.* **39:** 71–76.
100. Brezina, R. and Kazar, J. 1965. Study of the antigenic structure of *Coxiella burnetii.* IV. Phagocytosis and opsonization in relation to phases of *C. burnetii. Acta Virol.* **9:** 268–274.
101. Kazar, J., Skultyetova, E. and Brezina, S. 1975. Phagocytosis of *Coxiella burnetii* by macrophages. *Acta Virol.* **19:** 426–431.
102. Murphy, J.R., Wisseman, C.L. Jr and Fiset, P. 1980. Mechanisms of immunity to typhus infection: Analysis of immunity to *Rickettsia mooseri* infection in guinea pigs. *Infect. Immun.* **27:** 730–738.
103. Shirai, A., Catanzaro, P.J., Philips, S.M. and Osterman, J.V. 1976. Host defenses in experimental scrub typhus: Role of cellular immunity in heterologous protection. *Infect. Immun.* **14:** 39–46.
104. Mackaness, G.B. 1969. The influence of immunologically committed lymphoid cells on macrophage activity *in vivo. J. exp. Med.* **129:** 973–986.
105. Kokorin, I.N., Kabanova, E.A. and Shirokova, E.M. 1980. Role of macrophages in infections with *Rickettsia conorii. Acta Virol.* **24:** 137–143.
106. Kodama, K., Kawamura, S., Yasukawa, M. and Kobayashi, Y. 1987. Establishment and characterization of a T-cell line specific for *Rickettsia tsutsugamushi. Infect. Immun.* **55:** 2490–2495.
107. Hinrichs, D.J. and Jerrels. T.R. 1976. *In vitro* evaluation of immunity to *Coxiella burnetii. J. Immun.* **117:** 996–1003.
108. Park, J. and Rikihisi, Y. 1991. Inhibition of *Ehrlichia risticii* infection in murine peritonal macrophages by gamma interferon, a calcium ionophore and concanavalin A. *Infect. Immun.* **59:** 3418–3423.
109. Hanson, B. 1991. Susceptibility of *Rickettsia tsutsugamushi* Gilliam to gamma interferon in cultured mouse cells. *Infect. Immun.* **59:** 4125–4133.

110. BUENING, G.M. 1973. Cell-mediated immune responses in calves with anaplasmosis. *Am. J. vet. Res.* **34:** 757–763.
111. CARSON, C.A., KAKOMA, I. and RISTIC, M. 1980. Use of peripheral blood leucocytes in the study of cell-mediated immunity in bovine anaplasmosis a review. *Comp. Immun. Microbiol. infect. Dis.* **3:** 277–281.
112. KAKOMA, I., CARSON, C.A., RISTIC, M., HUXSOLL, D.L., STEPHENSON, E.M. and NYINDO, B.A. 1977. Autologous lymphocyte-mediated cytotoxicity against monocytes in canine ehrlichiosis. *Am. J. vet. Res.* **38:** 1557–1559.
113. WOLDEHIWET, Z. and SCOTT, G.R. 1982. Tick-borne fever: Leucocyte migration inhibition. *Vet. Microbiol.* **7:** 437–445.
114. HIRSCH, J.G. 1972. The phagocytic defense system. In: *Microbiol pathogenecity in Man and Animals,* pp. 59–74. SMITH, H. and PEARLE, J.H. (Eds). 22nd Symp. Soc. Gen. Microbiol.
115. FRIIS, R.R. 1972. Interaction of L-cells and *Chlamydia psittaci:* Entry of parasite and host response to its development. *J. Bact.* **110:** 706–721.
116. JONES, T.C. 1974. Macrophages and intra-cellular parasitism. *J. Reticul. Endothel. Soc.* **15:** 439–450.
117. TUOMI, J. and VON BONSDORFF, C.H. 1966. Electron microscopy of tick-borne fever agent in bovine and ovine phagocytising leucocytes. *J. Bact.* **92:** 1478–1492.
118. WELLS, M.Y. and RIKIHISA, Y. 1988. Lack of lysosomal fusion with phagosomes containing *Ehrlichia risticii* in $P388D_1$ cells: Abrogation of inhibition with tetracyclines. *Infect. Immun.* **56:** 3209–3215.
119. BURTON, P.R., KORDOVA, N. and PARETSKY, D. 1971. Electron microscopic studies of the rickettsia *Coxiella burnetii*: Entry, lysosomal response, and fate of rickettsial DNA in L-cells. *Can. J. Microbiol.* **17:** 143–158.
120. BURTON, P.R., STUECKEMANN, J. and PARETSKY, D. 1975. Electron microscopy studies of the limiting layers of the rickettsia *Coxiella burnetii. J. Bact.* **122:** 316–324.
121. REMALEY, A.T., KUHNS, D.B., BASFORD, R.E., GLEW, R.H. and KAPLAN, S.S. 1984. Leishmanial phosphatase blocks neutrophil O_2-production. *J. biol. Chem.* **259:** 1173–1175.
122. HACKSTADT, T. and WILLIAMS, J.C. 1981. Biochemical stratagem for obligate parasitism of eucaryotic cells by *Coxiella burnetii. Proc. Natn. Acad. Sci. U.S.A.* **78:** 3240–3244.
123. TAYLOR, A.W., HOLMAN, H.H. and GORDON, W.S. 1941. Attempts to reproduce the pyaemia associated with tick-bite. *Vet. Rec.* **53:** 339–344.
124. FOGGIE, A. 1956. The effects of tick-borne fever infection on the susceptibility of lambs to staphylococci. *J. comp. Path.* **66:** 278–285.
125. WOLDEHIWET, Z. 1987. Effects of tick-borne fever on some functions of polymorphonuclear cells of sheep. *J. comp. Path.* **97:** 481–485.
126. WOLDEHIWET, Z. 1987. Depression of lymphocyte responses to mitogens in sheep infected with tick-borne fever. *J. comp. Path.* **97:** 637–643.
127. RIKIHISA, Y., JOHNSON, G.J. and BURGER, C.J. 1987. Reduced immune responsiveness and lymphoid depletion in mice infected with *Ehrlichia risticii. Infect. Immun.* **55:** 2215–2222.
128. WOLDEHIWET, Z. 1991. Lymphocyte subpopulations in peripheral blood of sheep experimentally infected with tick-borne fever. *Res. vet. Sci.* **51:** 40–43.
129. KOSTER, F.T., WILLIAMS, J.C. and GOODWIN, J.S. 1985. Cellular immunity in Q fever: Modulation of responsiveness by a suppressor T cell-monocyte circuit. *J. Immun.* **135:** 1067–1072.
130. WALKER, T.S. and HOOVER, C.S. 1991. Rickettsial effects on leukotrine and

prostaglandin secretion by mouse polymorphonuclear leucocytes. *Infect. Immun.* **59:** 351–356.

131. ZACHARY, J.F. and SMITH, A.R. 1984. Experimental porcine eperythrozoonosis: Lymphocyte suppression and misdirected immune responses. *Am. J. vet. Res.* **46:** 821–829.
132. JERRELS, T.R. 1985. Immunosuppression associated with the development of chronic infection with *Rickettsia tsutsugamushi*: adherent suppressor cell activity and macrophage activation. *Infect. Immun.* **50:** 175–182.
133. KAKOMA, I., CARSON, C.A., RISTIC, M., HUXSOLL, D.L., STEPHENSON, E.M. and NYINDO, B.A. 1977. Autologous lymphocyte-mediated cytotoxicity against monocytes in canine ehrlichiosis. *Am. J. vet. Res.* **38:** 1557–1559.
134. BUHLES, W.C., HUXSOLL, D.L. and RISTIC, M. 1974. Tropical canine pancytopenia: Clinical, haematologic, and serologic response of dogs to *Ehrlichia canis* infection, tetracycline therapy, and challenge inoculation. *J. infect. Dis.* **130:** 357–367.
135. CORDY, D.R. and GORHAM, J.R. 1950. The pathology and etiology of salmon poisoning in the dog and fox. *Am. J. Path.* **26:** 617–637.
136. NYBERG, P.A., KNAPP, S.E. and MILEMAN, R.E. 1967. Salmon poisoning disease. IV. Transmission of the disease to dogs by *Nanophyetus salmincola* eggs. *J. Parasit.* **53:** 694–699.

2

The Chlamydiales

J. STORZ AND B. KALTENBOECK

Unique Chlamydial Properties

Chlamydial agents are now recognized as prokaryotic organisms that depend absolutely on the intracellular environment of animal cells for multiplication.[1] These microorganisms have a wide distribution in the kingdoms of warm- and cold-blooded animals. Chlamydiae are of medical interest because of the diverse diseases they cause in man and in animals.[2,3] Some of these diseases are of public health interest and others are of economic importance in farm animals. Chlamydiae are of microbiological interest because of their mode of interaction with eukaryotic host cells, and their specialized life cycle with its unique features of parasitism. The relationship that chlamydiae establish with host cells is an intimate association that has evolved between two very different forms of life. The invasion of host cells by chlamydiae represents the incursion of one genetic system by another system.[4] Chlamydiae have evolved mechanisms to exploit cellular functions, which include mechanisms for penetrating into different host cell compartments, dependence on host energy and precursors, inhibition of lysosome fusion, and states of persistence.[5] Once inside the host cell, they do little damage initially and they may even go unnoticed as chlamydial multiplication advances within the host cell. They change their intracellular form of existence and finally exert cytocidal or cytopathic effects on the infected host cells to facilitate release. Under other conditions chlamydiae may persist with surviving host cells for extended periods.

Classification and Taxonomy

Chlamydiae are classified as the single genus of the eubacterial order Chlamydiales and family Chlamydiaceae.[6,7] The unique developmental cycle, the lack of muramic acid in the cell wall and absolute dependence on host-cell-derived nutrients distinguish chlamydiae from other intracellular bacteria.[8]

Criteria for the Species

Four chlamydial species are currently recognized: *Chlamydia (C.) psittaci*, *C. pecorum*,[168] *C. pneumoniae* and *C. trachomatis*. *Chlamydia trachomatis* mainly infects human beings, possesses glycogen with rigid oval and vacuolar inclusions, and its growth is inhibited by sulfadiazine. *Chlamydia psittaci* and *C. pecorum* infect animals, which can transmit this infection to human subjects, induce pleomorphic, usually dense inclusions without glycogen and their growth is insensitive to sulfadiazine. *Chlamydia pneumoniae* resembles *C. psittaci* but is exclusively a human pathogen.[8] It can be differentiated by the pear-shaped elementary bodies (EB), the distinct DNA, and the serological reactivity in the micro-immunofluorescence test.[9]

Phylogenetic Relationships

The singularity of *Chlamydia*, based on phenotypical, morphological and ecological traits, was confirmed through phylogenetic analysis of the 16S rRNA sequence.[10,11] Chlamydiae were established as a distinct phylum among the 11 phyla of the eubacterial kingdom. The 16S rRNAs from *C. psittaci* strain 6BC and *C. trachomatis* differ by 4%, whereas they differ by about 28% from the 16S rRNA of the closest eubacterial division, represented by *Planctomyces staleyi*. Like chlamydiae, these budding bacteria lack peptidoglycan in their cell walls.

Recently, the phylogenetic relationships among extant chlamydiae were investigated on the basis of the *ompA* locus[12,13] which encodes the major outer membrane protein (MOMP). Slowly evolving genes like *ompA* typically differ by 10–30% between closely related species. This level of nucleotide divergence is better suited for elucidating the phylogenetic relationships within bacterial genera than the small differences between the conserved rRNA sequences.

Four groups of chlamydial *ompA* types were identified in the phylogenetic tree proposed (Table 2.1, Fig. 2.1). This tree was rooted at the branch between the clusters of *C. trachomatis ompA* types (trachoma group) and of *C. pneumoniae* together with *C. psittaci ompA* types.[13] This second cluster was comprised of three major groups of *ompA* types, namely the psittacosis group (types MN, 6BC, A22/M, B577, LW508, FEPN, and GPIC), the pneumonia group *C. pneumoniae* AR388 with the type KOALA) and the polyarthritis group (ruminant and porcine chlamydial types LW613, 66P130, L71, and 1710S with propensity for polyarthritis). This phylogram was essentially congruent with a tree based on a smaller sample of complete *ompA* loci.[12]

TABLE 2.1. *Chlamydial* ompA *Prototypes used for Constructing the Phylogenetic Tree*

ompA type	Host	Host clinical condition
C. psittaci		
MN	Birds, Cattle, Ferret/ Human	Respiratory infection, mastitis
6BC	Birds, Human	Respiratory and systemic infection
A22/M	unknown	unknown
B577	Ruminants, Parakeet, Human	Abortion, seminal vesiculitis, systemic infection
LW508	Cattle	Enteritis
FEPN	Cat, Muskrat, Human	Conjunctivitis, pneumonia, systemic infection
GPIC	Guinea Pig	Conjunctivitis
C. pecorum		
66P130	Cattle	Inapparent intestinal infection
LW613	Cattle	Polyarthritis, encephalitis, pneumonia, conjunctivitis
L71	Swine	Polyarthritis
1710S	Swine	Pneumonia, abortion
C. pneumoniae		
AR388	Human	Respiratory infection
KOALA	Koala	Keratoconjunctivitis
C. trachomatis		
MOPN	Mouse	Pneumonia
S45	Swine	Inapparent intestinal infection
A	Human	Trachoma
B	Human	Trachoma
C	Human	Trachoma
E	Human	Urogential infection
F	Human	Urogenital infection
H	Human	Urogential infection
L1	Human	Lymphogranuloma venereum (LGV)
L2	Human	LGV

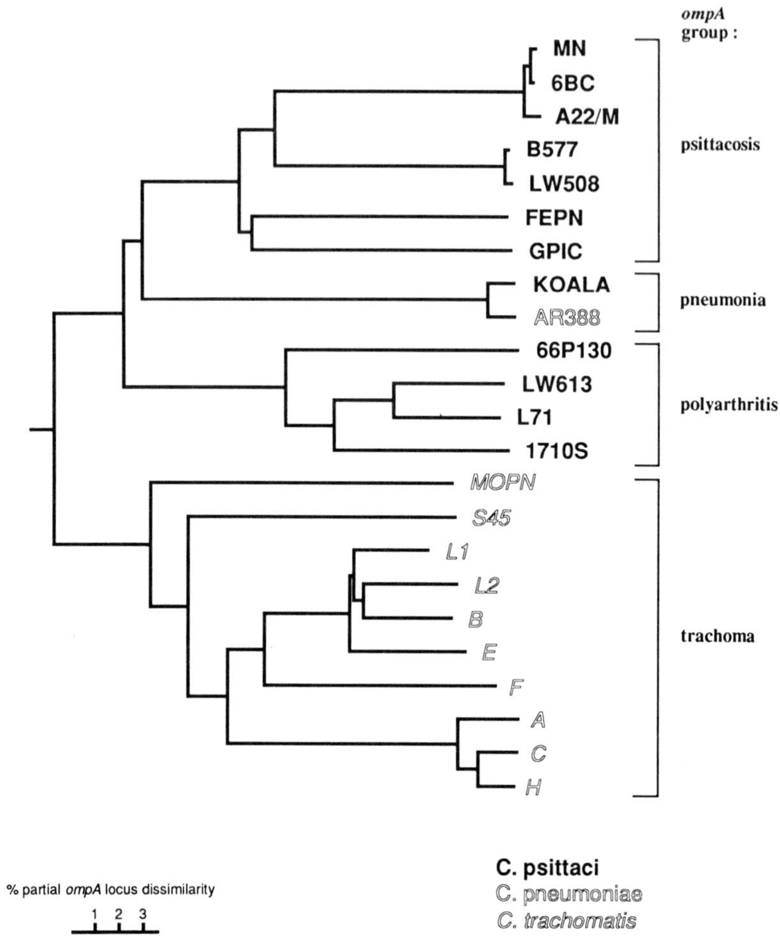

FIG. 2.1. Phylogenetic tree derived from nucleotide sequences on the *ompA* gene of selected prototypes of Chlamydiae.[13]

A phylogenetic tree constructed for a genetic locus does not necessarily represent the evolutionary pathway of the taxa involved. The congruence of the chlamydial *ompA* phylogeny with the chromosomal phylogeny was tested by reconstructing phylograms from two independent sets of chromosomal DNA distance data.[14,15] These chromosomal phylogenies were identical to the *ompA* tree that separated the four major groups of *ompA* types. Human serovars of *C. trachomatis* represented nearly identical chromosomal genotypes, but they had strongly divergent *ompA* loci. The *ompA* phylogeny of human serovars of *C. trachomatis* is not cognate with the evolution of the chromosome. Immunological selection might promote antigenic variation of the MOMP and thus accelerate the evolution of the ompA locus in human strains of *C. trachomatis*.[16]

The phylogenetic analyses suggest that the long-assumed dichotomy between avian and mammalian strains of *C. psittaci* does not exist. The *ompA* types MN, 6BC, and most likely A22/M, were isolated from avian hosts, but the identical *ompA* type BMZ21 was isolated from bovine mastitis. Conversely, *ompA* type B577 represents serovar 1, the prototype of many isolates from sheep and cattle[18] but several avian isolates of this *ompA* type were detected.[13,15]

While the established chlamydial species have less than 10% genomic DNA similarity, extensive DNA divergence exists between human serovars and the mouse biotype of *C. trachomatis*. The data provide an incentive for establishing additional chlamydial species according to the taxonomic criterion that strains of a bacterial genus with more than 30% genomic DNA divergence should be classified as different species.

The analyses of the DNA sequences of 16S rRNA, and *ompA* DNA sequences, genomic DNA distances, as well as the existence of glycogen-positive and -negative chlamydia-like organisms in invertebrates,[19,20] support Moulder's concept of the evolution of chlamydiae.[19–21] He hypothesizes that a host-independent chlamydial ancestor evolved from a peptidoglycan-free eubacterium, which also was ancestral to the *Planctomyces* phylum. The chlamydial ancestors became invertebrate-dependent protochlamydiae, which split into glycogen-positive and -negative lineages. The extant, vertebrate-dependent chlamydiae, evolved from these ancestral lineages.

Genome and Genetic Features

Structure, Size, and Diversity

The genome of chlamydiae is a closed-circular, double-stranded DNA chromosome. The contour length of the *C. trachomatis* and *C. psittaci* chromosome was found to be approximately 345 μm.[22,23,24] These measurements represent an estimated molecular weight of 6.6×10^8 Da corresponding to 1.1×10^6 nucleotide pairs. A molecular weight of 6.6×10^8 Da for *C. trachomatis* and of 9.5×10^8 Da for *C. psittaci* was found by sucrose gradient centrifugation. The reassociation kinetics of denatured DNA yielded somewhat lower molecular weights of 3.3×10^8 for *C. trachomatis* and 4.7×10^8 for *C. psittaci*. Sizing by pulsed-field gel electrophoresis revealed a genome of 1.45×10^6 nucleotide pairs for the chlamydial genome.[25,26]

The molar percentages of guanine plus cytosine (GC) were

assessed from buoyant densities and denaturation temperatures of chlamydial DNA. The consensus is that *C. psittaci* and *C. pneumoniae* generally have a GC content of about 41%, whereas *C. trachomatis* strains have a mean of 44%.[14] The DNA relatedness of the trachoma and LGV biovars of *C. trachomatis* is virtually 100%, but the mouse biovar DNA is less than 30% similar to these biovars. The degree of DNA similarity between *C. trachomatis, C. pneumoniae*, and *C. psittaci* is 10% or less. Similarities between strains of *C. psittaci* range from 93% to about 30%.[27]

Plasmids

A plasmid of 7.4 kb in EB of *C. trachomatis* was detected through DNA hybridization with a cloned plasmid DNA.[28] Closely related plasmids occurred as 10 copies per chromosome equivalent in EB of all human serovars, but not in the murine biotype of *C. trachomatis*. The cloned ECO RI DNA fragments of plasmids isolated from 8 strains of *C. psittaci* were analyzed. Restriction mapping analysis distinguished 4 different 7.5 kb plasmids that were associated with avian, feline, equine, and guinea-pig isolates of *C. psittaci*.[29] The restriction maps of these plasmid types of *C. psittaci* differed from the common plasmid in *C. trachomatis*. The DNA of plasmids of *C. psittaci* significantly cross-hybridized among each other, but minimal homology existed with plasmids of *C. trachomatis*. Plasmids were not found in the Cal-10 and two ovine abortion isolates of *C. psittaci*, and in one isolate of *C. pneumoniae*. A 7.4 kb plasmid was present in chlamydial strains isolated from urogenital infections of Koalas but not in isolates from conjunctival infections.[30,31]

The DNA of the *C. trachomatis* serovar B plasmid had 9 open reading frames (ORF), which coded for polypeptides greater than 10 kDa.[31] A putative origin of replication was identified, and 1 ORF had a 28% sequence homology with the *E. coli* dnaB protein, which is involved in DNA replication. Several plasmid-encoded peptides were found, but their functions have not been defined.[28,28,33] The absence of plasmids in *C. pneumoniae*, several strains of *C. psittaci*, and in a *C. trachomatis* serovar E isolate, implies that the chlamydial plasmid does not provide functions essential for the survival of chlamydiae.[31–34]

Chlamydiophage

A viral infection was identified in reticulate bodies of a *C. psittaci* isolate from ducks.[35] Inclusions of strain N352 contained reticulate bodies with crystalline arrays composed of regular arrangements of a polyhedral virus, which was termed chlamydiophage Chpl. This polyhedron was 22 nm in diameter, and had a single-stranded DNA genome of 4,877 nucleotides.[36] Five major, and 7 other open reading frames (ORFs), were identified based on secondary start sites and overlapping genes. N-terminal amino acid sequencing of the 3′ structural proteins (VP1, VP2, VP3) identified their location on the genetic map. VP1 has a region homologous to the major structural protein gpF of Phi-X174, and ORF4 has two regions homologous to Phi-X174 protein gpA, which is the nicking and closing protein of this phage. These data imply that Chpl evolved from an ancestral microvirus into a member of the *Microviridae*. A new sub-family, the *Chlamydiavirinae*, has been proposed for Chpl, because it is only distantly related to other microviruses, and its host, *C. psittaci*, is a highly specialized bacterium.

The mode of infection of chlamydiae with Chpl is not entirely understood. It may occur by extracellular infection of EB, but intra-inclusion infection of reticulate bodies towards the end of the development cycle may be an alternative mode of spread.[35,36] *In vitro* transmission of Chpl succeeded only to avian strains but not to mammalian strains of *C. psittaci* and not to *C. trachomatis* L2 and *C. pneumoniae* IOL-207. Antibodies to Chpl were found in ducks naturally infected with *C. psittaci*.

Genomes of Chpl were identified by DNA hybridization solely as extrachromosomal DNA. Immunofluorescence staining and *in situ* hybridization demonstrated the simultaneous presence of Chpl DNA and phage antigens but not of DNA without antigens. Apparently, Chpl causes a productive rather than a cryptic intra-inclusion infection. The chlamydiophages can be lost upon passage of the chlamydiae in cell cultures.[36]

Macromolecules and Antigens

Lipopolysaccharides

All chlamydiae share a lipopolysaccharide (LPS) moiety.[37] This major antigen is chemically and serologically related to the LPS of enterobacterial rough mutants of the Re chemotype. Several antigenic determinants cross-react with LPS of *Acinetobacter calcoaceticus*, enterobacterial Re mutants, and the lipid A component. The chlamydial LPS harbors a genus-specific epitope that is not cross-reacting. This property is attributed to the presence of a trisaccharide of 3-deoxy-D-manno-octulosonic acid(KDO) of the sequence KDOp-(2→8)-KDOp-(2→4)-KDO. The 2:8 linkage of two KDO residues is unique for *Chlamydia*. This structure was chemically synthesized within a tetrasaccharide and covalently linked to bovine serum albumin.[38] Monoclonal antibodies against this glycoconjugate antigen had genus-specific reactivity with the chlamydial LPS, thus proving the similarity of the artificial antigen and the natural counterpart.

A chlamydial gene was cloned, which directed the expression of the genus-specific chlamydial LPS epitope in *Escherichia (E.) coli* transformants.[39] Analysis of this clone led to the conclusion that it most likely encodes a single glycosyltransferase that attaches KDO specifically to the hydroxyl group at C-8 of a terminal KDO residue in LPS.

Structural Outer Membrane Proteins

Chlamydiae appear to be deficient in peptidoglycan, which in other gram-negative bacteria confers structural rigidity and osmotic resistance. A supramolecular network of disulfide bonds between outer membrane proteins in chlamydial EB functions as the equivalent of the peptidoglycan layer. The outer membrane of EB consists largely of disulfide-cross-linked MOMP and two cysteine-rich proteins (CRP). The MOMP is not cross-linked in the fragile reticulate bodies (RB) and CRP are synthesized and incorporated into the chlamydial outer membrane only late in the developmental cycle.[40–43]

The approximately 40 kDa MOMP is the most abundant chlamydial protein and accounts for about 60% of the proteinaceous moiety of the EB outer membrane.[40] The reduced MOMP was identified as a pore-forming molecule with an exclusion limit for passive diffusion of solutes with molecular weights of 850 to 2,250 Da.[42] The opening and closing of the pores is controlled through a reduction and oxidation mechanism of disulfide bonds.

The MOMP contains the main epitopic determinants of the serovars in all chlamydial species.[16,44,45] Serovar-specific immuno-accessible MOMP epitopes of *C. trachomatis* serovar B elicited antibodies that protected mice from toxic death after i.v. injection of EB and neutralized infectivity for monkey eyes. In contrast, nonimmuno-accessible subspecies- or species-specific MOMP epitopes, an immuno-accessible genus-specific MOMP epitope, and the chlamydial LPS, did not elicit toxic shock-protective or infectivity-neutralizing antibodies.[46]

The gene encoding the MOMP, *ompA*, of many chlamydial strains has been sequenced.[13,47–50] The *ompA* locus is highly conserved, and the nucleotide divergence between the most distant chlamydial variants is approximately 38%. Four variable domains interrupt highly conserved regions of the *ompA* genes. Variable domains I, II, and IV encode immuno-accessible peptides which represent contiguous species-, subspecies-, and serovar-specific epitopes.[16,44] Seven cysteine residues are present in the conserved regions of the MOMP peptides. An amphipathic peptide between variable domains I and II was found to function as highly effective T helper cell epitope in mice of different genetic background.[51] This peptide is conserved in all chlamydiae with the exception of a valine to isoleucine change in some strains of *C. psittaci*.

The 2 CRP of the chlamydial outer membrane have molecular weights of 12 to 15 kDa, respectively. The loci *envA* encoding small CRP and *envB* encoding large CRP are tandemly arranged on the chlamydial chromosome. The small CRP of *C. psittaci* strain 6BC contains 15 cysteine residues and is 54% identical to *C. trachomatis*.[43] The large CRP contains 37 cysteine residues and is 71% identical to *C. trachomatis*. The positions of the cysteine residues in both CRP are highly conserved. The small CRP are thought to be associated with the EB membrane through a covalently attached lipid portion of the molecule. The molar ratio of EB outer membrane proteins was calculated for the 6BC strain to be about 1 large CRP to 2 small CRP to 5 MOMP.

Adhesion Molecules

Findings by numerous investigators have suggested that carbohydrate and proteinaceous macromolecules of the infectious EB and the host cell participate in chlamydial attachment as initiating event in multiplication. However, experiments for defining chlamydial adhesions through inhibition of bindings by various sugars and glycoproteins have been inconclusive. Several chlamydial adhesins for cellular receptors have been described, but an unambiguous adhesion–receptor pair is still awaiting identification. Monoclonal antibodies to variable domain II and IV epitopes blocked attachment of EB to cells. A temperature sensitive loss of EB adherence was correlated to a temperature-induced conformational change in a conserved, hydrophobic nonapeptide within variable domain IV. Heat-treatment of EB exposed this otherwise inaccessible region to a species-specific monoclonal antibody, with loss of adherence and infectivity.[52] Another thermolabile, surface-exposed protein of 38 kDa was identified and termed chlamydial cytadhesin (CCA) that selectively bound to monolayers of HeLa cells.[53] Viable but not heat- or trypsin-treated EB, inhibited the binding of the CCA to HeLa cells, indicating competition for a common moiety on the host cell membrane.

An *E. coli* plasmid library of the *C. trachomatis* genome was screened for genes involved in attachment to host cells by the whole-cell-binding and cell-membrane-binding characteristics of individual recombinant *E. coli* clones.[54] This assay revealed plasmid-directed expression of novel 18, 28 and 82 kDa proteins, which putatively mediated adherence of recombinant *E. coli* clones to McCoy and human endometrial epithelial cells. The cell-binding specificity of an *E. coli* clone expressing these 3 proteins, paralleled that of EB of *C. trachomatis*.

A possible cellular receptor facilitating chlamydial adhesion was recently identified.[55] Radioactively labelled chlamydiae were layered on thin-layer chromatograms of separated lipids isolated from target cells, and bound bacteria were detected by autoradiography. A specific, high affinity lipid receptor of HeLa 229 cells for *C. trachomatis* and *C. pneumoniae* was phosphatidylethanolamine. The chlamydiae also bound strongly to purified asialo-ganglioside-GM and asialo-GM, but not to other neutral or acid lipids. The relative binding of chlamydiae was modified by divalent cations.

Stress-Response Proteins

A soluble Triton X-100 extract of chlamydial EB elicited a delayed hypersensitivity reaction in the conjunctiva of immune guinea pigs and monkeys. A 57 kDa protein of the Triton X-100 extract but not chlamydial LPS, caused the ocular hypersensitivity response, which was induced with extracts from EB of *C. trachomatis* and *C. psittaci* after sensitization with the guinea pig inclusion conjunctivitis (GPIC) strain of *C. psittaci*. A predominantly mononuclear, macrophage and lymphocyte infiltrate in guinea pig conjunctiva characterized this reaction.[56] This genus-reactive 57 kDa protein, also termed hsp60 was cloned and identified as a member of the family of heat-shock or stress-response proteins, which are among the most highly conserved proteins.[57] It is encoded in the *hypB* or *groEL* locus of the chlamydial hyp or groE operon.[58,59]

Stress-response proteins have vital functions in protein folding, transport and assembly. The hsp60 of all chlamydiae has 4 precisely conserved cysteine residues, which are not present in other *groEL* homologs. While *groEL* is located intracellularly, hsp60 was bound by disulfide linkages to the EB outer membrane and remained loosely associated with it when reduced. These facts have led to the speculation that hsp60 is involved in the rearrangement of the chlamydial outer membrane during the transition from EB to RB.[59] The chlamydial hsp60 is highly conserved among all chlamydiae. Three patterns of anti-hsp60 immunoreactivity of monoclonal antibodies were found: species-specific and genus-specific for chlamydiae, and cross-reactive with other bacteria.[60] The majority of the monoclonal antibodies mapped either to the amino or the carboxyl terminus of hsp60.

A chlamydial homolog of the hsp/0 family of heat-shock proteins was identified by immunoblot analysis of a *C. trachomatis* genomic library.[61] This 75 kDa protein was recognized by a monoclonal antibody, which neutralized chlamydial infectivity and reacted with an immuno-accessible outer membrane protein of EB.

Life or Developmental Cycle of Chlamydiae

The developmental cycle of chlamydiae, which is synonymous with the infectious cycle, proceeds through a series of functional and morphological changes during intracellular multiplication.[62–65] Chlamydiae are structurally and functionally reorganized during multiplication and progress through several morphologies, depending on the stage of multiplication and the function in the developmental cycle. The following forms exist: EB, dispersing forms; RB, dividing reticulate bodies; and condensing forms.[63,64] The developmental cycle may be divided into: Adsorption of infectious EB to receptors in cellular membranes; uptake of EB and their translocation into cytoplasmic sites of host cells; primary reorganization of the infecting EB into a large dispersing form with further differentiation into a RB ready to divide; growth and binary division of RB; secondary reorganization of the RB into infectious EB through a transition stage called condensing forms; and finally release of infectious EB from host cells.

Properties of Elementary Bodies

The extracellular and infectious chlamydial forms, EB, have a diameter of 200 to 280 nm. The internal organization of EB as viewed in thin sections of chlamydial inclusions and of purified particles, is identical[66–68] and has the appearance of a closely packed tuft of fibrils representing genome DNA and histone proteins.[69] The remaining semilunar area contains closely packed, round ribosome-like structures approximately 200 Å in diameter. Elementary bodies have a 90 to 100 Å thick, smooth trilaminar membrane that is rigid and provides high resistance in the extracellular environment. A second, narrower and less distinct, trilaminar plasma membrane is frequently detected beneath the outer cell membrane.[70] Peptidoglycan is not found between the two layers in contrast to other gram-negative bacteria.[65] The EB membrane contains disulfide cross-linked protein complexes, which determine the rigidity of the EB envelope. The eccentrically located electron-dense nucleoid is in contact with the plasma membrane.[40,41,66–68]

Projections are observed on the outside surface of EB of *C. psittaci* in scanning electron microscopy preparations, and "button" structures on the inside surface after freeze-fracture.[66,71] The projections are arranged hexagonally. These projections are distributed over about half the chlamydial surface and are located opposite the concave side of the electron-dense, crescent-shaped chlamydial nucleoid. The localized patches of surface projections opposite the nucleoid confers a polarity to the chlamydial EB.[72] Theoretically, these structures may function as transmembrane pores in the transfer of molecules from cellular to chlamydial sites during the developmental cycle. The significance of the projections is not fully understood, but they may be related to projection-associated binding sites important for attachment to host cells.

Adsorption of EB to, and Uptake by, Host Cells

Chlamydial EB are negatively charged at neutral pH. The MOMP has an isoelectric point of 5.3 to 5.5. Host cells also have a net negative charge at neutral pH. It is hypothesized that the chlamydial ligands are neutralized by electrostatic interaction with host cell receptors, which facilitates binding of EB to host cells, a process that requires cations, particularly Ca^{2+}.[73–75] Mild heating reduces the adsorption rate of EB to host cells. Incubation of host cells with trypsin greatly reduces their ability to adsorb EB. The host cells regenerate their EB-binding function within a few hours of cultivation in trypsin-free medium.[65,76] Trypsin-sensitive components of the host cell surface are thus involved in binding EB. Putative chlamydial adhesins on infectious EB have been described in several reports.[52,53,77,78] Some strains had 2 proteins of 18 and 32 kDa that bound to cell membrane preparations, while others had one at 17 to 19 kDa. The MOMP is also involved in binding EB to cell membranes through variable domains II and IV because monoclonal antibodies to these sites inhibit attachment of EB and neutralize infectivity.[52]

Binding of EB to microvilli was first observed in infections of intestinal epithelial cells and subsequently in cultured L cells.[79] The attached EB of the Cal 10 strain became associated with the bases of the microvilli. The binding of EB to microvilli may help to bridge electronegative barriers.[80] Entry was associated with depressions in the plasma membrane which are known sites of clathrin-coated pits. If gold-labelled $\alpha 2$ macroglobulin was mixed with EB, both were seen in the same coated pits or either one of them in separate coated pits.

Chlamydial uptake by receptor-mediated endocytosis involving the clathrin-coated vesicle pathway is an attractive mechanism, but more evidence must still be furnished to exclude other possible mechanisms.[81–83] Entry of EB into host cells leads to the ultimate presence of a membrane-bound chlamydial form in the cytoplasm of the host cell.

Multiplication of Chlamydiae

During reorganization of the EB into the dispersing form, several characteristic changes occur: the disulfide bonds that cross-link the protein moieties of outer membrane proteins of EB are reduced, making the membrane more fluid.[83] The dense nucleoid of the EB disperses into less electron-dense, filamentous material and becomes mixed with scattered, granular, ribosome-like particles. This process reflects unfolding of the densely packaged chlamydial genome. Division signals the completed change from dispersing form into the RB.[63]

The reorganization from infectious EB to the noninfectious RB proceeds throughout the dispersing form that is seen as a single chlamydial particle within an endosome of cells during the early stage of infection.[63] This chlamydial form is round or ovoid and has a diameter of 400 to 500 nm. It contains a granular matrix that is less electron-dense than the nucleoid of the EB but denser than the RB and is surrounded by an outer trilaminar membrane and an inner, less pronounced plasma membrane. A fine fibrillar network is distributed throughout this form and contains ribosome-like structures.

The RB arise from the dispersing forms as dividing large, and intermediate-sized pleomorphic, noninfectious chlamydial forms that may reach a size of 500 to 1000 nm. They are surrounded by an outer membrane, which contains MOMP monomers that are not disulfide cross-linked and an inner, ill-defined plasma membrane. Fine reticulated fibrils are interspersed with numerous ribosomes as their internal structure.[63,64,84]

The RB are characteristically plastic and predominate throughout most of the development cycle. After numerous divisions by binary fission, the RB become smaller and more circular, and reorganization into condensing forms occurs. This event is marked by condensation of fibrillar material in the center of the smaller RB. The 300 to 500 nm diameter condensing forms have a centrally located, electron-dense nucleoid. The central nucleoid mass is surrounded by an electron-lucent fibrillar zone connected through fibrils with an outer, electron-dense, granulofibrillar matrix of ribosome-like material and fibrils. These forms also have a trilaminar cell membrane and an inner, less prominent plasma membrane. The condensing forms then develop into the mature, infectious EB by polarization of the electron-dense nucleoid to an eccentric location and by further decrease in size. Disulfide cross-linked proteins are formed during this phase. Secondary reorganization and formation of EB occurs in an asynchronous fashion while many dividing RB are still present in chlamydial inclusions producing additional progeny for maturation.[63,64,85]

Proteins Associated with Developmental Cycle

While the morphological aspects of the chlamydial developmental cycle were investigated in detail, the understanding of the molecular mechanism directing these events is only marginal. The gene *sigA* for the putative chlamydial homolog of the sigma-70 and sigma-43 proteins of the RNA polymerase of *E. coli* and *B. subtilis*, respectively, was isolated from the murine strain and from serovar L2 of *C. trachomatis*.[86,87] It was almost identical between these strains, and the deduced protein had 571 amino acid residues and a 67 kDa molecular weight. Four regions of the deduced sigma peptide had as much as 92% sequence identity with sigma-70 of *E. coli*, while other regions were highly divergent.

The 16s and 23s rRNA operons, which are transcribed throughout chlamydial development, have two tandem promoters located approximately 100 bases apart within the 5′ regions of the operons.[86] The two chlamydial rDNA transcripts were not differentially regulated, and they were coordinately expressed 9 h postinfection. The putative tandem promoter sequences near the transcription initiation sites differed substantially from each other and from the *E. coli* promoter sequences.

Identification of proteins and genes expressed early in the chlamydial developmental cycle is a particularly challenging task. A host-free protein synthesis system with chlamydiae isolated by lysis of host cells at various time intervals after infection was used to detect temporally regulated chlamydial proteins as early as 15 min after infection.[88] The same proteins were synthesized by host-free and by intracellular chlamydiae during the initial period of infection. Chlamydial RNA was radiolabelled at different times postinfection. The labelled RNA was employed to probe the same genomic library of *Chlamydia*. Clones were identified that contained sequences which were transcribed in a cycle-dependent manner.

DNA-binding proteins represent another type of protein related to specific stages of chlamydial development.[69,89–91] Proteins separated from EB and RB by polyacrylamide gel electrophoresis and transferred to nitrocellulose, were probed with nick-translated chlamydial DNA. Three putative DNA binding proteins of 58, 25.7 and 17 kDa were detected in EB but not RB. The smaller proteins had physical properties similar to prokaryotic nucleoprotein, and the protein–DNA interaction was principally charge related. The 17 and 25.7 kDa proteins were hypothesized to be involved in compaction of the chlamydial DNA within the EB because they were also found in chromosome preparations isolated from EB. The 58 kDa protein was exclusively associated with the EB outer membrane complex.[89–91] Putative DNA-binding proteins of 18 and 26 kDa were cloned and found to be expressed late in the developmental cycle. They had homology with eukaryotic histone Hl. Both the 18 and 26 kDa products contained a high number of lysine residues. These properties are consistent with DNA-binding proteins.

Characteristics of a Chlamydial Growth Curve

Adsorption of EB to the plasmalemma occurs by specific but yet undefined binding between chlamydial ligands and receptors on the host cell. Through this specific interaction, the host cell is committed to take up the EB, a process that can explain the observation of facilitated uptake whereby chlamydiae preferentially enter host cells.[92–95] The process of entry most likely occurs by receptor-mediated endocytosis via coated pits. Elementary bodies within the endocytic vacuole are then transported to the area of the Golgi apparatus in harmony with primary reorganization. The development of the inclusion at the site of the Golgi is consistent with the coated-pit concept of entry, because the endocytic pathway usually cycles through the Golgi apparatus rather than through lysosomes.

Chlamydiae are relatively efficient in inducing their uptake by different types of host cells. Chlamydiae are taken up by non-professional phagocytes at a rate approximately 10 to 100 times faster than the uptake of latex beads or of *E. coli* cells. The term parasite-specified phagocytosis was coined to stress the chlamydial influence on this enhanced rate of uptake.[93,95] Classical phagocytosis, ultrastructurally, is characterized by particle uptake through pseudopodial enclosure. This process of phagocytosis is inhibited by microfilament inhibitors such as cytochalasin B. Uptake of chlamydiae is unaffected by cytochalasin B, but methylamine and monodansylcadaverine, inhibitors of receptor-mediated endocytosis, block EB uptake.[93,94,95]

Chlamydial infectivity declines after adsorption and uptake. A phase follows when infectivity cannot be detected lasting for about 20–36 h, depending on species and biotype, then infectivity rises rapidly along with the number of extracellular EB. The rise in extracellular infectivity of *C. psittaci* correlates with a decline in host viability, as measured by trypan blue exclusion; and cells are extensively lysed after 40 h of infection.[96] Reorganization of the EB into the dispersing form is comparable to the lag phase, lasts for about 6 to 8 h, and is of much longer duration than the lag period of the typical bacterial growth curve. Multiplication and division of the noninfectious RB corresponds to the exponential growth phase. The estimated mean generation time of *C. psittaci* growing exponentially in L cells is about 2 h. The exponential growth phase lasts from 8–20 h, then the organisms enter the retardation and stationary growth phases, beginning with the appearance of condensing forms, about 20 h after infection and continuing until the host cells die. Emergence of infectivity coincides with the formation of EB. The duration of the developmental cycle differs between chlamydia-host-cell systems.[62,64,65]

Properties and Functions of the Inclusion Membranes

Chlamydial EB are taken up by cells through a process of endocytosis. Importantly, they continue to reside in the cytoplasmic inclusion vacuole, which is bounded by a host plasmalemma-derived unit membrane. This cytoplasmic inclusion membrane expands and is modified as chlamydiae multiply. It continues to play important containment and transport functions throughout chlamydial development.[68,97] The inclusion membranes were considered as part of the inclusion because they were less stable in 0.25 M sucrose solution than the plasmalemma. Isolated inclusions were stable in 5% bovine serum albumin in 10 mM tris-hydroxymethylaminomethane buffer.[97] Chlamydial inclusions behaved similarly whether they were isolated from mouse macrophages or L cells in discontinuous dextran or sucrose gradients, and they exhibited similar detergent sensitivities. Inclusion membranes isolated from infected macrophages had at least 9 proteins in SDS-PAGE. Only 2 of these proteins had mobilities equal to plasmalemma proteins.[95]

Reticulate bodies also have surface projections directly connected with the host cytoplasm. It may be possible that RB within an inclusion communicate and interchange directly with the host cell cytoplasm. It was not resolved whether mitochondria form direct contacts with the inclusion membranes. The morphology of the inclusion membrane as revealed by freeze-replica techniques appears to differ from that of the plasmalemma.[71,97] The P and E faces are reversed because the inclusion membrane is derived from the plasmalemma during endocytosis. The convex surface of the inclusion membrane corresponds to the E face, and the P face represents the concave surface. Membrane particles were not encountered on the convex surface but many are present on the concave surface.

Control of Lysosomes during Chlamydial Infection

Lysosomes are an important hurdle for chlamydiae to clear in becoming successful intracellular parasites. Bacteria that adapted successfully to the intracellular habitat evolved a variety of ways to deal with lysosomes. The typical function of lysosomes is fusion with the endosomes that are formed as the plasmalemma engulfs extracellular particles, including bacteria. Within these fused endosome–lysosome vacuoles, or phagolysosomes, the engulfed particles are digested by acid hydrolases.[96,98,99]

Chlamydiae remain within the endosome, but prevent that endosome from fusing with lysosomes. If fusion occurs, chlamydiae will be digested by the lysosomal enzymes. In fact, endosomes containing chlamydiae that were coated with specific antibodies or that were heated at 90°C for 30 min, fuse with lysosomes and are digested.[99] One hypothesis is that chlamydiae modify the endosomal membrane by insertion of a chlamydial component. Chlamydia-specified protein synthesis is not required to prevent endosome–lysosome fusion, which infers that the putative component must be preformed, perhaps as a surface constituent of the infectious EB. Solid data demonstrating such a component are presently lacking. The second and more intriguing hypothesis is that chlamydiae can recognize and exploit specific receptor sites on the plasmalemma that trigger formation of an endosome that normally does not fuse with lysosomes. Evidence supporting this hypothesis derives from the observation that chlamydiae enter host cells using the coated-pit entry, a pathway not programmed for lysosomal fusion.[80,82,92]

Chlamydial Effects on Host Cells and Release

The findings characterizing the effect of chlamydial multiplication on host cell organelles are virtually limited to ultrastructural observations.[100–102] The organelles within infected cells retain their typical ultrastructural morphology until late in the chlamydial developmental cycle when EB are released by cell lysis. All host cell organelles, including lysosomes, the nucleus, smooth and rough endoplasmic reticula, Golgi apparatus, mitochondria and ribosomes, lose their normal fine ultrastructural features and disintegrate with impending cell lysis. This destruction of host cell organelles is coincident with the release of lysosomal enzymes.[96,97]

As the chlamydial inclusion develops in the central portion of the cell, it gradually forces the organelles of the host cell to peripheral positions. The lysosomes become dislocated to peripheral sites near the plasmalemma.[96,100] In contrast, mitochondria frequently are detected in close association with the inclusion membrane. Mitochondria remain well preserved during chlamydial development until the terminal stage of cell lysis when they swell, and round up as their cristae become distorted and fragmented. Eventually, they disintegrate along with the other host cell organelles, including smooth and rough endoplasmic reticula, ribosomes, cytoskeletal network, nucleus and plasmalemma. The inclusion membrane remains intact, while most of the host cell organelles disintegrate, until the last event of actual release of chlamydiae occurs in cell lysis.[96]

All organelles remain ultrastructurally intact in the non-lytic, exocytotic mechanisms of release observed with some strains of *C. trachomatis* biovar trachoma.[102] The exceptions involve the inclusion membrane, which is extruded with a portion of the plasmalemma during the late stages of the developmental cycle. The inclusion is extruded through focal distention of the plasmalemma without affecting the rest of the host cell surface. These openings are repaired by smooth membranes without the characteristic surface modification of the cell. This release mechanism resembles exocytosis allowing release of infectious chlamydiae without death of the host cell. These observations are pertinent for explaining features of persistent chlamydial infections in cultured cells and in infected human subjects or animals.

Metabolism in Chlamydial Multiplication

Source of Metabolic Energy

The failure to detect mechanisms by which host-free chlamydiae might generate useful energy led Moulder to propose the concept that they are energy parasites.[1,5,62] Recent findings revealed that chlamydiae utilize host cellular energy intermediates. This concept implies that the successful chlamydial parasite sequesters the products of host energy-yielding reactions for its own use. The increase in glucose uptake by chlamydia-infected cells as compared to control cells is significant, and increased utilization coincides with chlamydial multiplication, which is proportional for *C. psittaci* in L cells to the glucose concentration, and APP levels fall while ADP levels rise.[65,103,104] An inhibitor of mitochondrial functions, ethidium bromide, renders FL cells incapable of supporting growth of the

LGV biovar of *C. trachomatis*.[105] Antimycin, an inhibitor of aerobic respiration at the cytochrome level, or other inhibitors of cellular respiration decreased chlamydial yields.[104]

The first demonstration of the use of an energy-rich product of cell metabolism by multiplying chlamydiae was accomplished by Hatch.[106,107] The direct utilization of host cell nucleoside triphosphates by multiplying chlamydiae became evident from analysis of equilibrium labelling of nucleotides in infected cells and from incorporation of labels into 16s chlamydial RNA. The kinetics of CMP:UMP and GMP:AMP labelling of chlamydial 16s RNA indicated that the chlamydial parasite utilized preformed host nucleoside triphosphate pools. Exogenous thymidine was incorporated at a minimal level into chlamydial DNA. The failure of chlamydiae to utilize host thymidine pools efficiently may be due to the concentration of the thymidine triphosphate pools in the nucleus and to the more successful competition of the host for this substrate.[107]

Two enzymes of the pentose-phosphate pathway, glucose-6-phosphate dehydrogenase and 6-phosphogluconate dehydrogenase were detected in mixtures of EB and RB purified from the chicken embryo-propagated Cal 10 strain of *C. psittaci*.[108,109] Furthermore, glutamate is deaminated to α-ketoglutarate and decarboxylated to succinate, partial reactions of the tricarboxylic acid cycle. These reactions do not generate ATP, however RB purified from 6BC-infected L cells transport ATP and ADP but EB do not.

Protein Synthesis and Amino Acid Metabolism

Isoleucine was identified as a limiting factor in chlamydial multiplication.[110] Insufficient levels of this essential amino acid prevented the L cell hosts from dividing. Chlamydial multiplication did not proceed when isoleucine levels were too low to permit L cell growth. An overall reduction in the rate of protein synthesis by both host and parasite resulted from the deficiency of isoleucine. Under these conditions *C. psittaci* persisted in a noninfectious latent state within the host cell. The host cell and the chlamydial parasite competed for the same limiting factor, isoleucine. Addition of isoleucine to starved cells containing chlamydiae in a latent state activated the parasite to complete its cycle. A similar effect was induced by adding cycloheximide, whereby the infection became productive because cycloheximide prevented host protein synthesis and made host isoleucine available for chlamydial protein synthesis and multiplication.[111]

Chlamydial protein synthesis was studied in cycloheximide-treated L cells infected with the meningopneumonitis strain[110] and in emetine-treated FL cells infected with the T'ang strain of *C. trachomatis*.[105] Two micrograms of cycloheximide per ml inhibited over 90% of the protein synthesis of L cells. Incorporation of radioactive amino acid into infected cells treated with cycloheximide 1 h before labelling became clearly evident 14–17 h after infection and reached a maximum at 22–24 h after infection. The rate of ^{14}C-leucine incorporation decreased rapidly as host cells lost viability. The rate of protein synthesis in the developing trachoma strain was low during the first 18 h of the cycle, increased for the next 30 h, and then declined. The complete inhibition by chloramphenicol or chlortetracycline of the cycloheximide-insensitive protein synthesis in infected cells substantiated that it is chlamydia-mediated.

Synthesis of chlamydial cell walls was studied by tracing incorporation of ^{14}C-L-alanine and ^{14}C-L-lysine in the presence of D-cycloserine and penicillin G.[112] D-Cycloserine enhanced incorporation of ^{14}C-L-alanine throughout the developmental cycle but inhibited incorporation of ^{14}C-L-lysine. This drug prevented synthesis of peptidoglycan side chains by inhibiting alanine racimase and by preventing formation of D-alanine. Penicillin G did not affect incorporation of the two amino acids. Penicillin inhibited division of large reticulate forms and formation of EB. The cross-linked peptide subunits of chlamydial walls are presumed to consist of L-alanine–D-glutamine–L-lysine–D-alanine–D-alanine because diaminopimelic acid, that has cross-linking functions in Gram-negative bacteria, was not detectable. Conceivably, penicillin could inhibit the cross-linking of chlamydial cell well peptides, which are attached to a polysaccharide without muramic acid.[112–114]

Nucleic Acid Synthesis

Labelled chlamydia-infected cells were fractionated into nuclear and cytoplasmic fractions, and chlamydial components were sedimented from the cytoplasmic fraction in studies on rate of nucleic acid synthesis.[115,116] The rate of host-RNA synthesis was significantly reduced at the time of maximum chlamydial multiplication. Chlamydial RNA synthesis was detected 10–15 h after infection and reached a maximum 10–15 h later. The RNA species synthesized in the chlamydial compartment of the infected cells had sedimentation values of 4S, 16S and 21S, characteristic of transfer and ribosomal RNA. The 16S and 21S RNA were not detected in uninfected cells. Investigations of the sequential emergence of different RNA species during the developmental cycle of a T'ang strain of *C. trachomatis* detected 23S, 17.2S, 16S, 5S and 4S RNA. The 17.2S RNA was identified in chase experiments as a precursor of the 16S ribosomal RNA. Deeper insight into transcription processes depends on increased understanding of the chlamydial RNA polymerase. The gene of the β' subunit of the holoenzyme was cloned and expressed as a 43 kDa fusion protein.[86,87,118,119]

The rate of cellular DNA synthesis in chlamydial-infected cells was significantly suppressed 20 h after infection, and the degree of inhibition differed among different cell populations. The cytoplasmic inclusion was the site of chlamydial DNA synthesis. Cycloheximide-resistant DNA was detected 10–12 h after infection, the time when division of the meningopneumonitis RB was detected by electron microscopy. The amount of radioactive label incorporated into the DNA of cycloheximide-treated infected cells doubled every 2 h during chlamydial multiplication, indicating a generation time of about 2 h. The exponential rate of DNA synthesis was maintained for 18–20 h of the developmental cycle and then became linear. Inhibitors of DNA synthesis—such as 5′-fluorodeoxy-uridine, aminopterin or hydroxyurea—prevented formation of infectious EB.[120,121]

Lipid and Glycogen Synthesis

Another interesting aspect of host cell dependence of chlamydiae was identified in studies of lipid biosynthesis in chlamydia-infected cells.[122] Host cell lipid synthesis appeared to be inhibited in cells infected with the LGV strain of *C. trachomatis*. This observation suggested that chlamydial agents also exploit the host cell capacity for lipid synthesis. Chlamydiae must derive the three-carbon compounds required for the glycerol moiety of lipids from the host cells, because they were found to lack aldolases for glucose utilization. Phosphatidic acid, glycerol phosphate and dihydroxy acetone were considered sufficient to satisfy the requirements for three-carbon units. By reducing the formation of host cellular diglycerides, which are important in lipid biosynthesis of mammalian cells, chlamydiae could divert phosphatidic acid for the synthesis of cytidine-diphosphate-diglyceride leading to the formation of chlamydial phosphatidylethanolamine.[123] Cycloheximide markedly inhibits the lipid biosynthesis of L cells without affecting chlamydial multiplication. The synthesis of lipids in infected L cells increased 12 h after infection to maximal levels at 25–30 h under conditions when ^{3}H-isoleucine is used to label newly synthesized branched-chain fatty acids and phospholipids.

Iodine-staining carbohydrate accumulates in inclusions of *C. trachomatis* but not in those of *C. psittaci*.[19,124] The carbohydrate is found as glycogen with an average chain length of 14 to 16 glycose moieties.[68] It is mediated by a chlamydia-specific glycogen synthetase which uses ADP-glucose as a substrate. The number of iodine positive inclusions in an infected L-cell culture increases from 18 to 24 h, and the highest amounts of glycogen are found late in the development cycle at about 48–72 h after infection. Ultrastructural analysis implies that the initial glycogen accumulation occurs within RB and is shed into the inclusion space by rupture of RB membranes. Another level of host cell dependence is observed with strains of *C. psittaci*. These strains utilize cellular folic acid or its precursors for chlamydial biosynthetic processes.[125]

Cultivation of Chlamydiae

Experimental Animals

Developing chicken embryos, inoculated into the yok sacs, represented an important host for isolation and propagation of chlamydiae in the past, and they still play a useful role.[126,127] Chicken embryos are incubated at 37°C. Growth rates of some avian *C. psittaci* strains were increased at 39°C.[128] Other investigators prefer to incubate chicken embryos inoculated with strains of *C. trachomatis* at 35°C.[129] Death within 3 days of inoculation is usually nonspecific. Infection is determined by demonstrating red EB in Gimenez-stained impression smears made with yolk-sac membranes of dead or surviving chicken embryos. Some chlamydial strains were adapted to multiply in the cells of the chorioallantoic cavity, which release EB into the allantoic fluid for easy harvest and purification. Three-week old mice, inoculated by various routes, also were used to isolate or propagate chlamydiae.[127]

Susceptibility of Cultured Cells to Chlamydial Infection

Propagation of chlamydiae in cultured cells has been used to isolate these agents from specimens of affected subjects, to quantify infectivity, to obtain purified preparations of EB or RB, to study the metabolism of the parasite and the host cell, and to analyze mechanisms of host–parasite interactions.[65,127,129] The restriction of *C. trachomatis* growth to a few types of cells in naturally occurring human infections is not evident *in vitro* because strains of this species infect a variety of cell types from many animal species. *Chlamydia psittaci*, having a much broader host cell range in nature, infects many mammalian and avian cell cultures. When comparing the susceptibility of cell lines, one should be aware that different optimal cultural conditions prevail for each type of cell in culture and for the different chlamydial species. The nutritional state of the cell is important because chlamydiae depend on the nutrient pools of the host. It was found that medium M199, supplemented with 10% fetal calf serum and 0.5% glucose, promoted development of more chlamydial inclusions than other combinations.[130] Streptomycin and vancomycin can be used at concentrations of up to 500 μm/ml without decreasing the number of inclusions of *C. trachomatis* below that of cultures without antibiotics. Gentamicin can be used at concentrations of 100 μg/ml without reducing chlamydial inclusion counts.[65,127,129] Chlamydiae can also be propagated in large quantities in suspension cultures of various animal cells.[131,132]

Host Cell Range of Chlamydial Infections

While the infectivity of *C. trachomatis* for cultured cells is relatively low, it can be enhanced significantly by treatment of cells with cytoactive agents.[65] The lymphogranuloma biotypes of *C. trachomatis* and most strains of *C. psittaci* infect cultured cells efficiently. The cell types include, among others, fibroblasts, kidney and conjunctival epithelial cells, synovial cells, L cells, McCoy cells, Hela cells, astrocytes, macrophages, liver cells of lizards, a cell line from fat head minnows and mosquito cells.[85,127,129,133,135]

The cell types of *in vivo* infections with *C. trachomatis* are principally epithelial cells. The cells include conjunctival cells, respiratory epithelial cells, columnar and transitional endocervical epithelial cells and urethral epithelial cells. The infections with non-LGV strains remain localized in mucous membranes and are not invasive while the invasive LGV strains also infect macrophages and other cells of the lymphatic system.[2,101]

A wide range of cell types in addition to epithelial cells were found to be productively or nonproductively infected in naturally occurring infections of animals with strains of *C. psittaci*. These cell types were studied in greatest detail in immunotype 2 infections of the intestinal mucosa of the calf and in the inclusion conjunctivitis infection of the conjunctival and genital mucous membranes of guinea pigs.[136–138] Ultrastructural examination of sections from the terminal ileum revealed productive chlamydial infections of the absorptive epithelial cells of tips and intervillous zones, undifferentiated epithelial cells of the crypts, enterochromaffin cells, follicle-associated epithelial or M cells of Peyer's patches, fibroblasts, endothelial cells, macrophages, as well as synovial cells. Strains of *C. psittaci* also infect ciliated epithelial cells and pneumocytes of the respiratory tract of many animal species. Furthermore, *C. psittaci* strains of immunotype 1, involved in placental and fetal infections, cytolytically parasitize endometrial cells, trophoblastic epithelial cells of the placenta and cells of the mammary gland.[127] Epithelial cells of the endocervix are the main target cells in the genital infection of guinea pigs.[138] Liver cells were parasitized extensively in chlamydial infections of frogs.[139]

The following cells were observed to be invaded by chlamydiae *in vivo*, but the developmental cycle always appeared to be interrupted or arrested before dense-centered EB were formed: plasma cells, goblet cells, monocytes, and neutrophilic leukocytes.[136] The chlamydial forms present in these cell types from *in vivo* infections had morphological features of degeneration. Leukocytes were attracted to chlamydia-infected cells and often pavemented infected mucous membranes. Degenerating chlamydial forms were found in macrophages and fibroblasts under certain conditions.

Measuring Chlamydial Infectivity

Chlamydial infectivity has been determined in various assay systems. A plaque assay of cytocidal chlamydial strains with L-cell monolayers has been used for infectivity quantitation and serotyping *C. psittaci* strains.[140–142] Infectivity titrations are commonly done by determining the inclusion forming units in cell cultures. Aliquots of dilutions of chlamydial suspensions are inoculated onto cells on coverslips which are fixed 24–48 h later and Giemsa stained. The most sensitive conditions for infectivity quantitation involve centrifuge-assisted infection, cycloheximide-containing medium, and cell culture systems such as L cell monolayers on round coverslips in flat bottom tubes. The best results in titrating chlamydial suspensions are achieved by fixing cells 40 h after infection, by staining them with the Giemsa or the Gimenez methods, by counting inclusions, and by computing "inclusion forming units". An overlay is not required because cultures are analyzed within the first cycle of multiplication.[110,111,130]

Increase of Host Cell Susceptibility to Chlamydial Infections through Treatment with Cytoactive Agents

Methods used to enhance infectivity of chlamydiae for cultured cells resulted in important observations on the host–parasite relationship. Ionizing radiation was one of several methods used to prepare nondividing cells for chlamydial culture.[143] Irradiated cells no longer divide, but over the course of several days they become large, flattened and multinucleated. An advantage of this system is that the large cytoplasm of irradiated cells allows the development of extensive, easily recognized inclusions.

Additional approaches to enhance chlamydial uptake and infectivity are pretreatment of the cells with the polycation diethylaminoethyl dextran (DEAE-D) or centrifugation of the cells along with the inoculum.[144] A solution containing 20–30 μg/ml of DEAE-D (mol wt 2×10^6) is used to wash the monolayer prior to infection. Treatment with DEAE-D enhanced infectivity of some strains of *C. psittaci* and *C. trachomatis*. Highly infectious strains from avian sources, ovine or bovine abortions, or LGV were not enhanced.[145,146] Chlamydiae have a net negative surface charge (pI 4–5) at neutral pH. Cells also have a net negative charge on their surface. The low spontaneous infectivity of chlamydiae for cultured cells may well be due to their mutually repulsive surface charges. Treatment of cells with the polycation DEAE-D enhanced infectivity of *C. trachomatis* or *C. psittaci* for cells presumably by neutralizing mutually repulsive electrostatic forces.[65] The DEAE-D effect varies quantitatively with both the cell type and the chlamydial strain.

Weiss and Dressler[147] were the first to show that centrifugation could enhance infectivity of obligate intracellular parasites for cultured cells. A 1200-fold increase in infectivity of *C. psittaci* was reported when chlamydiae were centrifuged in the presence of L cell monolayers. Maximum infectivity resulted from centrifugation for 1 h at $2000 \times G$. It was also shown that lower centrifugal forces are satisfactory for enhancing infectivity of chlamydiae.[146] Although centrifuge-enhanced infectivity did increase when centrifugal force was increased, infectivity did not increase after 10 min of centrifugation. Observations are not compatible with EB sedimentation onto cells as the mechanism for centrifuged-enhanced infectivity, and it is theorized that centrifugation may expose cellular receptors.[65,146] Although centrifugation is much more efficient than DEAE-D treatment of cells to enhance infectivity, the effects of centrifugation and DEAE-D are not additive at high centrifugal forces.[146] Centrifuge-enhanced adsorption occurs rapidly, within 10 min or less, and is not dependent on additional time of stationary adsorption.

Cycloheximide consistently enhances chlamydial inclusion formation in treated cells.[110,111] Treatment of L cells with cycloheximide at 2 μg/ml enhanced inclusion formation 1.75-fold for *C. psittaci* strain LW-613 and 2.50-fold for strain B-577.[130,145,146] It is believed that cycloheximide enhances infectivity by increasing the soluble pool of amino acids and by allowing the parasite to compete more effectively for the host cellular pool of nutrients.[110] Consequently, it does not affect adsorption or uptake.

Cytochalasin B has no effect on chlamydial infectivity for either phagocytic or nonphagocytic cells treated with this drug. Cytochalasin B inhibits polymerization of actin and formation of microfilaments. At the levels used (1 μg/ml), cytochalasin B inhibits energy-requiring microfilament activity, including cellular motility and cytoplasmic streaming.[65,93,94] Chlamydial uptake requires energy. Cytochalasin B does not inhibit energy-independent micropinocytosis, a mechanism that functions during uptake of soluble nutrients.

Enhanced infectivity of *C. trachomatis* for HeLa cells treated with cGMP or drugs that enhance intracellular levels of cGMP, namely carbachol and prostaglandin FS2 and E_2, was reported.[148] Treatment of L cells with similar doses of carbachol or cGMP had little, if any, enhancing effect on *C. psittaci* inclusion formation. The lack of inhibitory action alone is important in understanding chlamydia host cell interactions. Although the exact effect of cGMP on phagocytosis is largely unknown, it is generally felt that increased levels of cGMP enhance lysosomal mobilization by stimulating microtubules and phagolysosome formation.

An increase in infectivity of *C. psittaci* for L cells treated with hydrocortisone at levels up to 100 μg/ml was observed.[146,149] Although no effect was found on infectivity of *C. trachomatis* in hydrocortisone-treated mouse macrophages, increased infectivity of *C. trachomatis* in hydrocortisone-treated McCoy cells was observed by others. Enhanced chlamydial infectivity in hydrocortisone-treated cells is difficult to explain. Hydrocortisone is most effective in enhancing chlamydial inclusion formation when given before infection. This drug is known to have a stabilizing effect on plasma and lysosomal membranes and is also known to reduce host cellular RNA and DNA synthesis. Analogous to the theory on cycloheximide-enhanced chlamydial infectivity, it was suggested that reduced host–parasite competition for nutrients allows chlamydiae to prosper.[146]

When cells were treated to depolymerize microtubules, equal infectivity enhancement of *C. psittaci* for L cells was seen when colchicine (1 μg/ml) was used to treat cells 2 h before, at, or 2 h after centrifuge-enhanced adsorption.[146] Results of this experiment are not compatible with the theory that depolymerization of microtubules alters adsorption or uptake. The enhancing effect of colchicine was rapid and appeared to be irreversible. The early events in chlamydial multiplication after uptake proceeded faster in colchicine-treated cells, so the inclusions were larger at 48 h after infection. Evidently, cells with depolymerized microtubules provide favorable conditions for the early phases of chlamydial multiplication.

Persistence of Chlamydial Infections

Persistence as an Epidemiological and Clinical Feature

An important state of the host–parasite interaction in some chlamydial infections is the persistent, clinically inapparent infection, which plays a significant role in spreading the organism within human and animal populations. Persistent infections with *C. psittaci* and *C. pecorum* were recognized in birds, ruminants and swine as intestinal infections and a natural habitat for perpetuation.[3,151–152] Ocular and genital chlamydial infections of guinea pigs often persist with minimal clinical signs.[153] Mouse pneumonitis is a unique example of a naturally occurring persistent infection with the mouse biotype of *C. trachomatis*.[154,155] Respiratory infections with *C. psittaci* and ocular as well as genital infections of people with *C. trachomatis* have features of persistence that facilitate spread of these infections in the population.[150,156] Very little is known about the mechanisms of persistence at the cellular level in the infected human and animal hosts. Gamma interferon possibly plays an important modulating role in naturally occurring persistent infections.[157–159]

Mechanisms Leading to Persistency in Cell Cultures

Several cell culture models of persistence of *C. psittaci* and of *C. trachomatis* were described.[65] Viable cell cultures from which infectious chlamydiae are recovered for long time periods are considered persistently infected. Different conditions and treatments lead to persistence. Cell cultures deprived of essential nutrients for chlamydial multiplication changed into a persistent state which was lost after correction of the nutrient deficiency.[160,161] Isoleucine deprivation clearly demonstrated this phenomenon.[110,111]

One mechanism of immune-mediated persistence in cell culture involves gamma interferon, which stimulates host cells to suppress chlamydial multiplication without eliminating this infection. This interferon induces an enzyme that breaks down tryptophane which is essential for the multiplication of most strains of *C. psittaci*.[157–159]

Specific inhibition of chlamydial multiplication by the addition of 25 μg of aminopterin per ml within 20 h after infection leads to *C. psittaci* persistence in McCoy cells.[162] The addition of folinic acid restores chlamydial multiplication and implicates that C_1 transfer reactions possibly involved in the biosynthesis of methionine by host cells may be the limiting step.

Persistent chlamydial infections also arise under conditions facilitating unrestricted multiplication of chlamydiae and host cells.[65] The mechanisms leading to persistence probably vary, and they are illustrated by the following selected examples. Several types of cell cultures infected with limiting dilutions of *C. psittaci* strains evolved into persistent infections.[163,164] HeLa cells infected with limiting levels of *C. trachomatis* also developed persistence.[165]

Persistent infections were established *in vitro* with the psittacine 6BC strain of *C. psittaci*, and the abortigenic serotype 1 strain B-577. Both persistent states were characterized by cycles of low cytopathic expression and cycles of high cytopathic expression.[163,164] These cycles appeared to be determined, at least in part, by temporary changes in the susceptibility of L cells to chlamydial infection and by the selection of a chlamydial mutant better adapted to the cultural conditions. Immunofluorescence studies, together with centrifugation and cycloheximide treatments, revealed that the persistently infected cultures go through periods of resistance in which infectious EBs may adsorb, but productive infection does not occur.[164] These changes in susceptibility are not absolute, but relative, and can be abolished by cycloheximide treatment: a situation similar to that described for L cells treated with α-interferon and infected with *C. trachomatis*. Efforts to detect an antiviral activity indicative of α-interferon in supernatants collected from persistently infected L cell cultures were unsuccessful.[164] Consequently, the factors responsible for changing the susceptibility of persistently infected cultures remain unknown.

The behavior of the persistently infected L cell population in the model of the avian 6BC strain of *C. psittaci* was explained by assuming that cells are cryptically infected and that the cryptic infection makes the cultures completely resistant to superinfection with exogenous chlamydiae.[163,166,167] Morphological evidence for the presence of a chlamydial cryptic body was not obtained. Theoretically, the presence of a cryptic body should be revealed by specific gene probes or sensitive fluorescent antibody tests. Penicillin-sensitive chlamydial infectivity was required for maintenance of the persistent state of B-577.[164]

Persistent infections of a trachoma biovar of *C. trachomatis* in McCoy cells were established after an initial productive infection which resulted in lysis of most host cells.[165] Medium change and maintenance of these cultures allowed the few surviving cells to establish a fresh monolayer. Chlamydial inclusions were present in only a small fraction of this cell population and uninfected host cells multiplied more rapidly so that inclusion-bearing cells fell below 1%. The proportion of infected cells rose with time and subpassage leading to a phase of host cell lysis and destruction. These host cells were not resistant to superinfection, but a chlamydial substrain emerged that more easily established persistent infections.

References

1. MOULDER, J.W. 1974. Intracellular parasitism: Life in an extreme environment. *J. infect. Dis.* **130:** 300–306.
2. SCHACHTER, J. and DAWSON, C.R. 1978. *Human Chlamydial Infections.* PSG Publishing Co. Littleton, MA.
3. STORZ, J. 1988. Overview of animal diseases. In: *Microbiology of Chlamydia,* BARRON, A.L. (Ed.), pp. 167–192. CRC Press, Inc., Boca Raton, FL.
4. BYRNE, G.I. 1988. Host cell relationships. In: *Microbiology of Chlamydia,* BARRON, A.L. (Ed.), pp. 135–150. CRC Press, Inc., Boca Raton, FL.
5. MOULDER, J.W. 1985. Comparative biology of intracellular parasitism. *Microbiol. Rev.* **39:** 298–337.
6. PAGE, L.A. 1966. Revision of the family *Chlamydiacae* Rake: Unification of the psittacosis–lymphogranuloma–venereum–trachoma group of organisms in the genus *Chlamydia* Jones, Rake and Stearns, 1945. *Int. J. Syst. Bact.* **16:** 223–252.
7. STORZ, J. and PAGE, L.A. 1971. Taxonomy of the chlamydiae. Reasons for classifying organisms of the genus *Chlamydia,* family Chlamydiaceae, in a separate order, Chlamydiales ord. nov. *Int. J. Syst. Bact.* **21:** 332–334.
8. MOULDER, J.W., HATCH, T.P., KUO, C.-C., SCHACHTER, J. and STORZ, J. 1984. Genus *Chlamydia* Jones, Rake, and Stearns, 1945. In: *Bergey's Manual of Systematic Bacteriology,* Vol. 1, pp. 729–739. The Williams and Wilkins Company, Baltimore.
9. GRAYSTON, J.T., KUO, C.-C., CAMPBELL, L.A. and WANG, S.-P. 1989. *Chlamydia pneumoniae* sp. nov. for *Chlamydia* sp. Strain TWAR. *Int. J. Syst. Bact.* **39:** 88–90.
10. WEISBURG, W.G., HATCH, T.P. and WOESE, C.R. 1986. Eubacterial origin of chlamydiae. *J. Bact.* **167:** 570–574.
11. WEISBURG, W.G. 1989. Polyphyletic origin of bacterial parasites. In. *Intracellular Parasitism,* pp. 1–15. MOULDER, J.W. (Ed.), CRC Press, Inc., Boca Raton, FL.
12. CARTER, M.W., AL-MAHDAWI, S.A.H., GILES, I.G., TREHARNE, J.D., WARD, M.E. and CLARKE, I.N. 1991. Nucleotide sequence and toxonomic value of the major outer membrane protein gene of *Chlamydia pneumoniae* IOL-207. *J. gen. Microbiol.* **137:** 465–475.
13. KALTENBOECK, B., KOUSOULAS, K.G. and STORZ, J. 1993. Structure of and allelic diversity and relationships among the major outer membrane protein (*ompA*) genes of the four chlamydial species. *J. Bact.* **175**, in press.
14. COX, R.L., KUO, C.-C., GRAYSTON, J.T. and CAMPBELL, L.A. 1988. Deoxyribonucleic acid relatedness of *Chlamydia* sp. strain TWAR to *Chlamydia trachomatis* and *Chlamydia psittaci. Int. J. Syst. Bact.* **38:** 265–268.
15. FUKUSHI, H. and HIRAI, K. 1989. Genetic diversity of avian and mammalian *Chlamydia psittaci* strains and relation to host origin. *J. Bact.* **171:** 2850–2855.
16. STEPHENS, R.S., WAGER, E.A. and SCHOOLNIK, G.K. 1988. High-resolution mapping of serovar-specific and common antigenic determinants of the major outer membrane protein of *Chlamydia trachomatis. J. exp. Med.* **167:** 817–831.

17. WEISS, E., SCHRAMEK, S., WILSON, N.N. and NEWMAN, L.W. 1970. Deoxyribonucleic acid heterogeneity between human and murine strains of *Chlamydia trachomatis*. *Immun.* **2:** 24–28.
18. PEREZ-MARTINEZ, J.A. and STORZ, J. 1985. Antigenic diversity of *Chlamydia psittaci* of mammalian origin determined by microimmunofluorescence. *Infect. Immun.* **50:** 905–910.
19. RICE, C.E. 1936. The carbohydrate matrix of the epithelial-cell inclusion in trachoma. *Am. J. Opthal.* **19:** 1–8.
20. HARSHBARGER, J.C., CHANG, S.C. and OTTO, S.V. 1977. Chlamydiae (with phages), mycoplasmas, and rickettsiae in Chesapeake Bay bivalves. *Science* **196:** 666–668.
21. MOULDER, J.W. 1988. Characteristics of chlamydiae. In: *Microbiology of Chlamydia,* pp. 3–20. BARRON, A.L. (Ed.). CRC Press, Inc., Boca Raton, FL.
22. KINGSBURY, D.T. 1969. Estimate of the genome size of various microorganisms. *J. Bact.* **98:** 1400–1401.
23. TAMURA, A. 1964. Biochemical studies on the mechanism of infection of meningopneumonitis agent. *A. Rep. Inst. Virus Res.,* Kyoto Univ. **7:** 1–13.
24. SAROV, I. and BECKER, Y. 1969. Trachoma agent DNA. *J. Molec. Biol.* **42:** 581–589.
25. FRUTOS, R., PAGES, M., BELLIS, M., ROIZES, G. and BERGOIN, M. 1989. Pused-field gel electrophoresis determination of the genome size of obligate intracellular bacteria belonging to the genera *Chlamydia, Rickettsiella,* and *Porochlamydia*. *J. Bact.* **171:** 4511–4513.
26. STEPHENS, R.S. 1990. Molecular genetics of chlamydia. In: *Chlamydial Infections,* pp. 63–72. BOWIE, W.R. *et al.* (Eds), Cambridge University Press.
27. CAMPBELL, L.A., KUO, C.-C., and GRAYSTON, J.T. 1987. Characterization of the new *Chlamydia* agent, TWAR, as a unique organism by restriction endonuclease analysis and DNA–DNA hybridization. *J. clin. Microbiol.* **25:** 1911–1916.
28. PALMER, L. and FALKOW, S. 1986. A common plasmid of *Chlamydia trachomatis*. *Plasmid* **16:** 52–62.
29. LUSHER, M., STOREY, C.C. and RICHMOND, S.J. 1989. Plasmid diversity within the genus *Chlamydia*. *J. gen. Microbiol.* **135:** 1145–1151.
30. GIRJES, A.A., HUGALL, A.F., TIMMS, P. and LAVIN, M.F. 1988. Two distinct forms of *Chlamydia psittaci* associated with disease and infertility in *Phascolarctos cinereus* (Koala). *Infect. Immun.* **56:** 1897–1900.
31. TIMMS, P., EAVES, F.W., HUGALL, A.F. and LAVIN, M.F. 1988. Plasmids of *Chlamydia psittaci*: Cloning and comparison of isolates by Southern hybridisation. *FEMS Microbiol. Lett.* **51:** 119–124.
32. STRIPRAKASH, K.S. and MACAVOY, E.S. 1987. Characterization and sequence of a plasmid from the trachoma biovar of *Chlamydia trachomatis*. *Plasmid* **18:** 205–214.
33. JOSEPH, T., NANO, F.E., GARON, C.F. and CALDWELL, H.D. 1986. Molecular characterization of *Chlamydia trachomatis* and *Chlamydia psittaci* Plasmids. *Infect. Immun.* **51:** 699–703.
34. PETERSON, E.M., MARKOFF, B.A., SCHACHTER, J. and DE LA MAZA, L.M. 1990. The 7.5-kb plasmid present in *Chlamydia trachomatis* is not essential for growth of this microorganism. *Plasmid* **23:** 144–148.
35. RICHMOND, S.J., STIRLING, P. and ASHLEY, C.R. 1982. Virus infecting the reticulate bodies of an avian strain of *Chlamydia psittaci*. *FEMS Microbiol. Lett.* **14:** 31–36.
36. STOREY, C.C., LUSHER, M. and RICHMOND, S.J. 1989. Analysis of complete

nucleotide sequence of Chpl, a phage which infects avian *Chlamydia psittaci*. *J. gen. Virol.* **70:** 3381–3390.

37. BRADE, H., BRADE, L. and NANO, F.E. 1987. Chemical and serological investigations on the genus-specific lipopolysaccharide epitope of *Chlamydia*. *Proc. natn. Acad. Sci. U.S.A.* **84:** 2508–2512.
38. FU, F., BAUMANN, M., KOSMA, P., BRADE, L. and BRADE, H. 1992. A synthetic glycoconjugate representing the genus-specific epitope of chlamydial lipopolysaccharide exhibits the same specificity as its natural counterpart. *Infect. Immun.* **60:** 1314–1321.
39. NANO, F.E. and CALDWELL, H.D. 1985. Expression of the chlamydial genus-specific lipopolysaccharide epitope in *Escherichia coli*. *Science* **228:** 742–744.
40. CALDWELL, H.D., KROMHOUT, J. and SCHACHTER, J. 1981. Purification and partial characterization of the major outer membrane protein of *Chlamydia trachomatis*. *Infect. Immun.* **31:** 1161–1176.
41. HATCH, T.P., ALLAN, I. and PEARCE, J.H. 1984. Structural and polypeptide differences between envelopes of infective and reproductive life cycle forms of *Chlamydia spp*. *J. Bact.* **157:** 13–20.
42. BAVOIL, P., OHLIN, A. and SCHACHTER, J. 1984. Role of disulfide bonding in outer membrane structure and permeability in *Chlamydia trachomatis*. *Infect. Immun.* **44:** 479–485.
43. EVERETT, K.D.E. and HATCH, T.P. 1991. Sequence analysis and lipid modification of the cysteine-rich envelope proteins of *Chlamydia psittaci* 6BC. *J. Bact.* **173:** 3821–3830.
44. BAEHR, W., ZHANG, Y.-X., JOSEPH, T., SU, H., NANO, F.E., EVERETT, K.D.E. and CALDWELL, H.D. 1988. Mapping antigenic domains expressed by *Chlamydia trachomatis* major outer membrane protein genes. *Proc. natn. Acad. Sci. U.S.A.* **85:** 4000–4004.
45. FUKUSHI, H. and HIRAI, K. 1988. Immunochemical diversity of the major outer membrane protein of avian and mammalian *Chlamydia psittaci*. *J. clin. Microbiol.* **26:** 675–680.
46. ZHANG, Y.-X., WATKINS, N.G., STEWART, S. and CALDWELL, H.D. 1987. The low-molecular-mass, cysteine-rich outer membrane protein of *Chlamydia trachomatis* possesses both biovar and species-specific epitopes. *Infect. Immun.* **55:** 2570–2573.
47. STEPHENS, R.S., MULLENBACH, G., SANCHEZ-PESCADOR, R. and AGABIAN, N. 1986. Sequence analysis of the major outer membrane protein gene from *Chlamydia trachomatis* serovar L_2. *J. Bact.* **168:** 1277–1282.
48. PICKETT, M.A., EVERSON, J.S. and CLARKE, I.N. 1988. *Chlamydia psittaci* ewe abortion agent: complete nucleotide sequence of the major outer membrane protein gene. *FEMS Microbiol. Lett.* **55:** 229–234.
49. ZHANG, Y.-X., MORRISON, S.G., CALDWELL, H.D. and BAEHR, W. 1989. Cloning and sequence analysis of the major outer membrane protein genes of two *Chlamydia psittaci* strains. *Infect. Immun.* **57:** 1621–1625.
50. YUAN, Y., ZHANG, Y.-X., WATKINS, N.G. and CALDWELL, H.D. 1989. Nucleotide and deduced amino acid sequences for the four variable domains of the major outer membrane proteins of the 15 *Chlamydia trachomatis* serovars. *Infect. Immun.* **57:** 1040–1049.
51. SU, H., MORRISON, R.P., WATKINS, N.G. and CALDWELL, H.D. 1990. Identification and characterization of T helper cell epitopes of the major outer membrane protein of *Chlamydia trachomatis*. *J. exp. Med.* **172:** 203–212.
52. SU, H., WATKINS, N.G., ZHANG, Y.-X. and CALDWELL, H.D. 1990. *Chlamydia*

trachomatis–host cell interactions: Role of the chlamydial major outer membrane protein as an adhesin. *Infect. Immun.* **58:** 1017–1025.

53. JOSEPH, T.D. and BOSE, D.K. 1991. A heat-labile protein of *Chlamydia trachomatis* binds to HeLa cells and inhibits the adherence of chlamydiae. *Proc. natn. Acad. Sci. U.S.A.* **88:** 4054–4058.
54. SCHMIEL, D.H., KNIGHT, S.T., HAULSTON, J.E., CHOONG, J., DAVIS, C.H. and WYRICK, P.B. 1991. Recombinant *Escherichia coli* clones expressing *Chlamydia trachomatis* gene products attach to human endometrial epithelial cells. *Infect. Immun.* 59: 4001–4012.
55. KRIVAN, H.C., NILSSON, B., LINGWOOD, C.A. and RYU, H. 1991. *Chlamydia trachomatis* and *Chlamydia pneumoniae* bind specifically to phosphatidylethanolamine in HeLa cells and to GALNACB1–GALB1–4GLC sequences found in asialo-GM_1 and asialo-GM_2. *Biochem. biophys. Res. Commun.* **175:** 1002–1009.
56. MORRISON, R.P., LYNG, K. and CALDWELL, H.D. 1989. Chlamydial disease pathogenesis. Ocular hyposensitivity elicited by a genus specific 57-KD protein. *J. exp. Med.* **169:** 663–675.
57. MORRISON, R.P., BELLAND, R.J., LYNG, K. and CALDWELL, H.D. 1989. Chlamydial disease pathogenesis. The 57-kD chlamydial hypersensitivity antigen is a stress response protein. *J. exp. Med.* **170:** 1271–1283.
58. KIKUTA, L.C., PUOLAKKAINEN, M., KUO, C.-C. and CAMPBELL, L.A. 1991. Isolation and sequence analysis of the *Chlamydia pneumoniae* GroE operon. *Infect. Immun.* **59:** 4665–4669.
59. CERRONE, M.C., MA, J.J. and STEPHENS, R.S. 1991. Cloning and sequence of the gene for heat shock protein 60 from *Chlamydia trachomatis* and immunological reactivity of the protein. *Infect. Immun.* **59:** 79–90.
60. YUAN, Y., ZHANG, Y.-X., MANNING, D.S. and CALDWELL, H.D. 1990. Multiple tandem promoters of the major outer membrane protein gene (*omp1*) of *Chlamydia psittaci*. *Infect. Immun.* **58:** 2850–2855.
61. DANILITION, S.L., MACLEAN, I.W., PEELING, R., WINSTON, S. and BRUNHAM, R.C. 1990. The 75-kilodalton protein of *Chlamydia trachomatis*: a member of the heat shock protein 70 family: *Infect. Immun.* **58:** 189–196.
62. MOULDER, J.W. 1969. A model for studying the biology of parasitism: *Chlamydia psittaci* and mouse fibroblasts (L cells). *Bioscience* **19:** 875–881.
63. STORZ, J. and SPEARS, P. 1977. *Chlamydiales*: Properties, developmental cycle, and effect on eukaryotic host cells. *Curr. Topics Microbiol.* **76:** 165–212.
64. WARD, MICHAEL E. 1988. The chlamydial developmental cycle. In: *Microbiology of Chlamydia,* pp. 71–95. BARRON, A.L. (Ed.). CRC Press, Boca Raton, FL.
65. MOULDER, JAMES W. 1991. Interaction of chlamydiae and host cell *in vitro*. *Microbiol. Rev.* **55:** 143–190.
66. MATSUMOTO, A. 1973. Fine structures of cell envelopes of *Chlamydia* organisms as revealed by freeze-etching and negative staining techniques. *J. Bact.* **116:** 1355–1363.
67. MATSUMOTO, A. 1976. Electron microscopic studies on the structure of the envelopes of *Chlamydia psittaci*. *J. Electron Microsc.* **25:** 51–52.
68. MATSUMOTO, A. 1988. Structural characteristics of chlamydial bodies. In: *Microbiology of Chlamydia,* pp. 21–45. BARRON, A.L. (Ed.). CRC Press, Boca Raton, FL.
69. WAGAR, E.A. and STEPHENS, R.S. 1988. Developmental form-specific DNA-binding proteins from *Chlamydia* spp. *Infect. Immun.* **56:** 1678–1684.
70. SCHACHTER, J. and CALDWELL, H.D. 1980. Chlamydiae. *A. Rev. Microbiol.* **34:** 285–309.

71. LOUIS, C., NICOLAS, G., EB, F., LEFEBVRE, J. and ORFILA, J. 1980. Modifications of the envelope of *Chlamydia psittaci* during its developmental cycle: Freeze-fracture study of complementary replicas. *J. Bact.* **141:** 868–875.
72. STOKES, G.V. 1978. Surface projections and internal structure of *Chlamydia psittaci*. *J. Bact.* **113:** 1514–1516.
73. KUO, C.-C., WANG, S.-P. and GRAYSTON, J.T. 1973. Effect of polycations, polyanions, and neuraminidase on the infectivity of trachoma-inclusion conjunctivitis and lymphogranuloma venereum organisms in HeLa cells: sialic acid residues as possible receptors for trachoma-inclusion conjunctivitis. *Infect. Immun.* **8:** 74–79.
74. SODERLUND, G. and KIHLSTROM, E. 1982. Physiochemical surface properties of elementary bodies from different serotypes of *Chlamydia trachomatis* and their interaction with mouse fibroblasts. *Infect. Immun.* **36:** 893–899.
75. SCHIEFER, H.G., KRAUSS, H. and SCHUMMER, U. 1982. Anionic sites on *Chlamydia* membranes. *FEMS Microbiol. Lett.* **15:** 41–44.
76. BYRNE, G.I. 1978. Kinetics of phagocytosis of *Chlamydia psittaci* by mouse fibroblasts (L cells): separation of the attachment and ingestion stages. *Infect. Immun.* **19:** 607–612.
77. HACKSTADT, T. 1986. Identification and properties of chlamydial polypeptides that bind eucaryotic surface components. *J. Bact.* **165:** 13–20.
78. WENMAN, W.M. and MEUSER, R.U. 1986. *Chlamydia trachomatis* elementary bodies possess proteins which bind to eucaryotic cell membranes. *J. Bact.* **165:** 602–607.
79. DOUGHRI, A.M., STORZ, J. and ALTERA, K.P. 1972. Mode of entry and release of chlamydiae in infections of intestinal epithelial cells. *J. infect. Dis.* **126:** 652–657.
80. MOORMAN, D.R., SIXBEY, J.W. and WYRICK, P.B. 1986. Interaction of *Chlamydia trachomatis* with human genital epithelium in culture. *J. gen. Microbiol.* **132:** 1055–1067.
81. BYRNE, G.I. and MOULDER, J.W. 1978. Parasite-specified phagocytosis of *Chlamydia psittaci* and *Chlamydia trachomatis* by L and HeLa cells. *Infect. Immun.* **19:** 598–606.
82. WARD, M.E. and MURRAY, A. 1984. Control mechanisms governing the infectivity of *Chlamydia trachomatis* for HeLa cells: mechanisms of endocytosis. *J. gen. Microbiol.* **130:** 1765–1780.
83. PRAIN, C.J. and PEARCE, J.H. 1989. Ultrastructural studies on the intracellular fate of *Chlamydia psittaci* (strain guinea pig inclusion conjunctivitis) and *Chlamydia trachomatis* (strain lymphogranuloma venereum 434): Modulation of intracellular events and relationship with endocytic mechanism. *J. gen. Microbiol.* **135:** 2107–2123.
84. HATCH, T.P., MICELI, M. and SUBLETT, J.E. 986. Synthesis of disulfide-bonded outer membrane proteins during the development cycle of *Chlamydia psittaci* and *Chlamydia trachomatis*. *J. Bact.* **165:** 379–385.
85. STORZ, J., TODD, W.J. and SCHNORR, K.L. 1988. Chlamydial infections: Breach of host cellular barriers. In: *Virulence Mechanisms of Veterinary Bacterial Pathogens*, pp. 161–199. ROTH, J.A. (Ed.). ASM Publishing Co.
86. ENGEL, J.N. and GANEM, D. 1987. Chlamydial rRNA operons: gene organization and identification of putative tandem promoters. *J. Bact.* **169:** 5678–5685.
87. KOEHLER, J.E., BURGESS, R.R., THOMPSON, N.E. and STEPHENS, R.S. 1990. *Chlamydia trachomatis* RNA polymerase major subunit. *J. biol. Chem.* **265:** 13206–13214.
88. PLAUNT, M.R. and HATCH, T.P. 1988. Protein synthesis early in the developmental cycle of *Chlamydia psittaci*. *Infect. Immun.* **56:** 3201–3205.

89. HACKSTADT, T., BAEHR, W. and YING, Y. 1991. *Chlamydia trachomatis* developmentally regulated protein is homologous to eukaryotic histone H1. *Proc. natn. Acad. Sci. U.S.A.* **88:** 3937–3941.
90. TAO, S., KAUL, R. and WENMAN, W.M. 1991. Identification and nucleotide sequence of a developmentally regulated gene encoding a eukaryotic histone H1-like protein from *Chlamydia trachomatis. J. Bact.* **173:** 2818–2822.
91. PERARA, E., GANEM, D. and ENGEL, J.N. 1992. A developmentally regulated chlamydial gene with apparent homology to eukaryotic histone H1. *Proc. natn. Acad. Sci. U.S.A.* **89:** 2125–2129.
92. HODINKA, R.L. and WYRICK, P.B. 1986. Ultrastructural study of mode of entry of *Chlamydia psittaci* into L-929 cells. *Infect. Immun.* **54:** 855–863.
93. GREGORY, W.W., BYRNE, G.I., GARDNER, M. and MOULDER, J.W. 1979. Cytochalasin B does not inhibit ingestion of *Chlamydia psittaci* by mouse fibroblasts (L cells) and mouse peritoneal macrophages. *Infect. Immun.* **25:** 463–466.
94. REYNOLDS, D.J. and PEARCE, J.H. 1990. Characterization of the cytochalasin D-resistant mechanisms of endocytosis utilized by chlamydiae. *Infect. Immun.* **58:** 3208–3216.
95. ZEICHNER, S.L. 1983. Isolation and characterization of macrophage phagosomes containing infectious and heat-inactivated *Chlamydia psittaci.* Two phagosomes with different intracellular behaviors. *Infect. Immun.* **40:** 956–966.
96. TODD, W.J. and STORZ, J. 1975. Ultrastructural cytochemical evidence for activation of lysosomes in the cytocidal effect of *Chlamydia psittaci. Infect. Immun.* **12:** 638–646.
97. MATSUMOTO, A. 1981. Isolation and electron microscopic observations of intracytoplasmic inclusions containing *Chlamydia psittaci. J. Bact.* **145:** 605–612.
98. KORDOVA, N., WILT, J.C. and SADIG, M. 1971. Lysosomes in L cells infected with *Chlamydia* psittaci 6BC strain. *Can. J. Microbiol.* **17:** 955–959.
99. FRIIS, R.R. 1972. Interaction of L cells and *Chlamydia psittaci*: Entry of the parasite and host responses to its development. *J. Bact.* **110:** 706–721.
100. TODD, W.J., DOUGHRI, A.M. and STORZ, J. 1976. Ultrastructural changes in host cellular organelles in the course of the chlamydial developmental cycle. *Zentbl. Bakt. I. Orig.* **236:** 359–373.
101. SWANSON, J., ESCHENBACH, D.A., ALEXANDER, E.R. and HOLMES, K.K. 1975. Light and electron microscopic study of *Chlamydia trachomatis* infection of the uterine cervix. *J. infect. Dis.* **131:** 678–687.
102. TODD, W.J. and CALDWELL, H.D. 1985. The Interaction of *Chlamydia trachomatis* with host cells: Ultrastructural studies of the mechanism of release of biovar II strain from HeLa 229 Cells. *J. infect. Dis.* **151:** 1037–1044.
103. MOULDER, J.W. 1970. Glucose metabolism of L cells before and after infection with *Chlamydia psittaci. J. Bact.* **104:** 1189–1196.
104. GILL, S.D. and STEWART, R.B. 1970. Effect of metabolic inhibitors on the production of *Chlamydia psittaci* by infected L cells. *Can. J. Microbiol.* **16:** 1076–1085.
105. BECKER, Y. and ASHER, Y. 1972. Obligate parasitism of trachoma agent: Lack of trachoma development in ethidium bromide-treated cells. *Antimicrobiol. Agents Chemother.* **1:** 171–173.
106. HATCH, T.P. 1975. Utilization of L cell nucleoside triphosphates by *Chlamydia psittaci* for ribonucleic acid synthesis. *J. Bact.* **122:** 393–400.
107. HATCH, T.P. 1976. Utilization of exogenous thymidine by *Chlamydia psittaci* growing in thymidine kinase-containing and thymidine kinase-deficient L-cells. *J. Bact.* **125:** 706–712.

108. MOULDER, J.W., GRISSO, D.L. and BRUBAKER, R.R. 1965. Enzymes of glucose catabolism in a member of the psittacosis group. *J. Bact.* **89:** 810–812.
109. WEISS, E. 1967. Transaminase activity and other enzymatic reactions involving pyruvate and glutamate in *Chlamydia* (psittacosis–trachoma group). *J. Bact.* **93:** 177–184.
110. HATCH, T.P. 1975. Competition between *Chlamydia psittaci* and L cells for host isoleucine pools: A limiting factor in chlamydial multiplication. *Infect. Immun.* **12:** 211–220.
111. ALEXANDER, J. 1968. Separation of protein synthesis in meningopneumonitis agent from that in L cells by differential susceptibility to cycloheximide. *J. Bact.* **95:** 327–332.
112. TRIBBY, I. 1970. Cell wall synthesis by *Chlamydia psittaci* in L cells. *J. Bact.* **104:** 1176–1188.
113. TAMURA, A. and MANIRE, G.P. 1968. Effect of penicillin on the multiplication of meningopneumonitis organisms (*Chlamydia psittaci*). *J. Bact.* **96:** 875–880.
114. MATSUMOTO, A. and MANIRE, G.P. 1970. Electron microscopic observations on the effects of penicillin on the morphology of *Chlamydia psittaci*. *J. Bact.* **101:** 278–285.
115. SCHECHTER, M. 1966. Synthesis of nucleic acid and protein in L cells infected with the agent of meningopneumonitis. *J. Bact.* **91:** 2069–2080.
116. SCHECHTER, E.M., TRIBBY, I.I.E. and MOULDER, J.W. 1964. Nucleic acid metabolism in L cells infected with a member of the psittacosis group. *Science* **145:** 819–821.
117. GUTTER, B. and BECKER, Y. 1972. Synthesis and maturation of ribosomal RNA during the developmental cycle of trachoma agent, a prokaryotic obligate parasite of eukaryocytes. *J. molec. Biol.* **66:** 239–253.
118. KOEHLER, J.E. and STEPHENS, R.S. 1990. Characterization of *Chlamydia trachomatis* RNA polymerase β' subunit. In: *Chlamydial Infections,* pp. 48–51. BOWIE, W.R. *et al.* (Eds). Cambridge University Press.
119. ENGEL, J.N. and GANEM, D. 1990. A polymerase chain reaction-based approach to cloning sigma factors from eubacteria and its application to isolation of a sigma-70 homolog from *Chlamydia trachomatis*. *J. Bact.* **172:** 2447–2455.
120. TANAMI, Y., POLLARD, M. and STARR, T.J. 1961. Replication pattern of psittacosis virus in a tissue culture system. *Virology* **15:** 22–29.
121. ROSENKRANZ, H.S., GUTTER, B. and BECKER, Y. 1973. Studies on the development cycle of *Chlamydia trachomatis*: Selective inhibition by hydroxyurea. *J. Bact.* **115:** 682–690.
122. FAN, V.S.C. and JENKIN, H.M. 1975. Biosynthesis of phospholipids and neutral lipids of monkey kidney cells (LLC-MK-2) infected with *Chlamydia trachomatis* strain lymphogranuloma venereum. *Proc. Soc. exp. Biol. Med.* **148:** 351–358.
123. REED, S.I., ANDERSON, L.A. and JENKIN, H.M. 1981. Use of cycloheximide to study independent lipid metabolism of *Chlamydia trachomatis* cultivated in mouse L cells grown in serum-free medium. *Infect. Immun.* **31:** 668–673.
124. GORDON, F.B. and QUAN, A.L. 1965. Occurrence of glycogen in inclusions of the psittacosis lymphogranuloma venereum–trachoma agents. *J. infect. Dis.* **115:** 186–196.
125. LIN, H.-S. and MOULDER, J.W. 1966. Patterns of response to sulfadiazine, D-cycloserine and D-alanine in members of the psittacosis group. *J. infect. Dis.* **116:** 372–376.
126. T'ANG, F.F., CHANG, H.L., HUANG, Y.T. and WANG, K.C. 1957. Studies on

the etiology of trachoma with special reference to isolation of the virus in chick embryo. *Medicine* **75:** 429–446.

127. Storz, J. 1971. *Chlamydia and Chlamydia-induced Diseases*. Thomas, Charles C., Publ. Co. Springfield, Il.
128. Page, L.A. 1971. Influence of temperature on the multiplication of chlamydiae in chicken embryos. In: *Trachoma and Related Disorders Caused by Chlamydial Agents,* pp. 40–51. R.L. Nichols, (Ed.).
129. Gordon, F.B., Harper, I.A., Quan, A.L., Treharne, J.D., Dwyer, R.S.C. and Garland, J.A. 1969. Detection of chlamydia (bedsonia) in certain infections of man. I. Laboratory procedures: Comparison of yolk sac and cell culture for detection and isolation. *J. infect. Dis.* **120:** 451–462.
130. Spears, P. and Storz, J. 1979. *Chlamydia psittaci*: Growth characteristics and enumeration of serotypes 1 and 2 in cultured cells. *J. infect. Dis.* **140:** 959–967.
131. Morrison, S.J. and Jenkin, H.M. 1972. Growth of *Chlamydia psittaci* strain meningopneumonitis in mouse L cells cultivated in a defined medium in spinner cultures. In Vitro **8:** 94–100.
132. Perez-Martinez, J.A. and Storz, J. 1986. Propagation of ovine and bovine abortion strains of *Chlamydia psittaci* in suspension cultures of L-cells. *J. vet. Med.* **33:** 346–353.
133. Levitt, D., Danen, R. and Levitt, P. 1986. Selective infection of astrocytes by *Chlamydia trachomatis* in primary mixed neuron-glial cell cultures. *Infect. Immun.* **54:** 913–916.
134. Bard, J.A. and Levitt, D. 1985. Binding, ingestion, and multiplication of *Chlamydia trachomatis* (L_2 Serovar) in human leukocyte cell lines. *Infect. Immun.* **50:** 835–937.
135. Wyrick, P.B. and Brownridge, E.A. 1978. Growth of *Chlamydia psittaci* in macrophages. *Infect. Immun.* **19:** 1054–1060.
136. Doughri, A.M., Altera, K.P. and Storz, J. 1973. Host cell range of chlamydial infection in the neonatal bovine gut. *J. comp. Path.* **83:** 107–114.
137. Soloff, B.L., Rank, R.G. and Barron, A.L. 1982. Ultrastructural studies of chlamydial infection in guinea-pig urogenital tract. *J. comp. Path.* **92:** 547–558.
138. Barron, A.L., White, H.J., Rank, R.G. and Soloff, B.L. 1979. Target tissues associated with genital infection of female guinea pigs by the chlamydial agent of guinea pig inclusion conjunctivitis. *J. infect. Dis.* **139:** 60–68.
139. Newcomer, C.E., Anver, M.R., Simmons, J.L., Wilcke, B.W. and Nace, G.W. 1982. Spontaneous and experimental infections of *Xenopus laevis* with *Chlamydia psittaci*. *Lab. Anim. Sci.* **32:** 680–686.
140. Higashi, N. and Tamura, A. 1960. A plaque assay for meningopneumonitis virus in monolayers of strain L cells. *Virology* **12:** 578–588.
141. Piraino, F. and Abel, C. 1964. Plaque assay for psittacosis virus in monolayers of chick embryo fibroblasts. *J. Bact.* **87:** 1502–1511.
142. Banks, J., Eddie, B., Schachter, J. and Meyer, K.F. 1970. Plaque formation by *Chlamydia* in L cells. *Infect. Immun.* **1:** 259–262.
143. Gordon, F.B., Dressler, H.R., Quan, A.L., McQuilkin, W.T. and Thomas, J.I. 1972. Effect of ionizing irradiation on susceptibility of McCoy cell cultures to *Chlamydia trachomatis*. *Appl. Microbiol.* **23:** 123–129.
144. Harrison, M.J. 1970. Enhancing effect of DEAE-dextran on inclusion counts of an ovine *chlamydia* (Bedsonia) in cell culture. *Aust. J. exp. Biol. med. Sci.* **48:** 207–213.
145. Spears, P. and Storz, J. 1979. Biotyping of *Chlamydia psittaci* based on inclusion morphology and response to DEAE-dextran and cycloheximide. *Infect. Immun.* **24:** 24–232.

146. Dennis, M.W. and Storz, J. 1982. Infectivity enhancement of *Chlamydia psittaci* of bovine and ovine origin for cultured cells. *Am. J. vet. Res.* **43:** 1897–1901.

147. Weiss, E. and Dressler, H. 1960. Centrifugation of rickettsiae and viruses onto cells and its effect on infection. *Proc. Soc. exp. Biol. Med.* **103:** 691–695.

148. Kaul, R. and Wenman, W.M. 1986. Cyclic AMP inhibits developmental regulation of *Chlamydia trachomatis*. *J. Bact.* **168** (2): 722–727.

149. Bushell, A.C. and Hobson, D. 1978. Effect of cortisol on the growth of *Chlamydia trachomatis* in McCoy cells. *Infect. Immun.* **21:** 946–953.

150. Meyer, K.F. 1967. The host spectrum of psittacosis-lymphogranuloma venereum (PL) agents. *Am. J. Opthal.* **63:** 1225/199–1246/220.

151. York, C.J. and Baker, J.A. 1951. A new member of the psittacosis–lymphogranuloma group of viruses that causes infection in calves. *J. exp. Med.* **93:** 587–604.

152. Storz, J. and Thornley, W.R. 1966. Serologische und aetiologische Studien uber die intestinale Psittakose–Lymphogranuloma-Infektion der Schafe. *Zentbl. Vet.* **13:** 14–24.

153. Murray, S. 1964. Guinea pig inclusion conjunctivitis virus. Isolation and identification as a member of the psittacosis–lymphogranuloma–trachoma group. *J. infect. Dis.* **114:** 1–12.

154. Gönnert, R. 1941. Die Bronchopneumonie, eine neue Viruskrankheit der Maus. *Zentbl. Bakt. I. Orig.* **147:** 161–174.

155. Nigg, C. 1942. Unidentified virus which produces pneumonia and systemic infection in mice. *Science* **95:** 49–50.

156. Hanna, L., Dawon, C., Briones, O., Thygeson, P. and Jawetz, E. 1968. Latency in human infections with the TRIC agents. *J. Immun.* **101:** 43–50.

157. Byrne, G.I., Lehmann, L.K. and Landry, G.J. 1986. Induction of tryptophan catabolism is the mechanism for gamma-interferon-mediated inhibition intracellular *Chlamydia psittaci* replication in T24 cells. *Infect. Immunol.* **53:** 347–351.

158. Rothermel, C.D., Rubin, B.Y. and Murray, H.W. 1983. Gamma-interferon is the factor in lymphokine that activates human macrophages to inhibit intracellular *Chlamydia psittaci* replication. *J. Immunol.* **131:** 2542–2544.

159. Rothermel, C.D., Rubin. B.Y., Jaffe, E.A. and Murray, H.W. 1986. Oxygen-independent inhibition of intracellular *Chlamydia psittaci* growth by human monocytes and interferon-activated macrophages. *J. Immunol.* **137:** 689–692.

160. Bader, J.P. and Morgan, H.R. 1961. Latent viral infection of cells in tissue culture: Abortive infection with psittacosis virus. *Proc. Soc. exp. Biol. Med.* **106:** 311–313.

161. Bader, J.P. and Morgan, H.R. 1961. Latent viral infection of cells in tissue culture: Role of water-soluble vitamins in psittacosis virus propagation in L Cells. *J. exp. Med.* **113:** 271–281.

162. Pollard, M. and Sharon, N. 1963. Induction of prolonged latency in psittacosis infected cells by aminopterin. *Proc. Soc. exp. Biol. Med.* **112:** 51–54.

163. Moulder, J.W., Levy, N.J. and Schulman, L.P. 1980. Persistent infection of mouse fibroblasts (L cells) with *Chlamydia psittaci*: Evidence for a cryptic chlamydial form. *Infect. Immun.* **30:** 874–883.

164. Perez-Martinez, J.A. and Storz, J. 1985. Persistent infection of L-cells with an ovine abortion strain of *Chlamydia psittaci*. *Infect. Immun.* **50:** 453–458.

165. Truant, A.I. and Wong, K.H. 1981. Persistent infection of HeLa-229 cells with *Chlamydia trachomatis*. *Curr. Microbiol.* **5:** 105–109.

166. MOULDER, J.W., LEVY, N.J., ZEICHNER, S.L. and LEE, C.K. 1981. Attachment defect in mouse fibroblasts (L cells) persistently infected with *Chlamydia psittaci*. *Infect. Immun.* **34:** 285–291.

167. MOULDER, J.W. 1983. Inhibition of onset of overt multiplication of *Chlamydia psittaci* in persistently infected mouse fibroblasts (L Cells). *Infect. Immun.* **39:** 898–907.

168. FUKUSHI, H. and HIRAI, K. 1992. Proposal of *Chlamydia pecorum* sp. nov. for *Chlamydia* strains derived from ruminants. *Int. J. Syst. Bact.* **42:** 306–308.

3

Anaplasmosis

L. WANDURAGALA AND M. RISTIC

Introduction

Anaplasmosis is an arthropod-borne disease of cattle and other ruminants caused by the intraerythrocytic rickettsiae of the genus *Anaplasma*. According to the eighth edition of Bergey's Manual, the bovine rickettsia, *Anaplasma marginale*, is the representative species of this genus and belongs to the family Anaplasmataceae, order Rickettsiales.[1] During their classic studies on *Babesia (Piroplasma) bigemina,* Smith and Kilbourne observed the occurrence of "intracorpuscular bodies" that were coccus-like and located at the margin of erythrocytes in the blood of infected cattle. They considered these bodies to be a developmental stage of *B. bigemina.*[2] Unaware that they were dealing with a mixed infection of *A. marginale* and *B. bigemina,* other workers too described the occurrence of inclusion bodies in erythrocytes of cattle suffering from piroplasmosis.[3,4,5] Subsequent studies by Theiler conclusively demonstrated that these marginal bodies in the erythrocytes of affected cattle were not developmental stages of *B. bigemina,* but were parasites belonging to another genus of protozoa, *Anaplasma.*[6] The term, *Anaplasma,* implies that the organism is devoid of cytoplasm and the species names '*marginale*' and '*centrale*' refer to the location of the organism within the infected erythrocyte. In the years following this discovery, anaplasmosis has been reported from different geographical regions of the world. In affected cattle the disease causes mortality, abortion and losses in meat and milk production.[7]

The losses attributable to bovine anaplasmosis in the United States (U.S.) has been estimated at U.S.$5 million in California alone to over U.S.$100 million in the whole continental U.S.[8,9] In most regions of the world where anaplasmosis is endemic, it is difficult to determine the losses, mainly due to the lack of records, inability to quantify production losses or the concurrent infection with other hemoparasitic diseases.[10]

Causative Agent

Three species of Anaplasma are in existence, i.e., *A. marginale, A. centrale* and *A. ovis*; the latter being the species infecting sheep and goats. Another member of the family Anaplasmataceae causing anaplasmosis in cattle has been assigned to the genus *Paranaplasma* based on structural and antigenic differences.

Morphology

In infected erythrocytes stained with Romanovsky's stain the marginal *Anaplasma* body appears as a dense, homogenous, bluish-purple, round to oval structure that measures 0.3–1.0 μ in diameter.[6] This marginal body is composed of several subunits (4–8) known as the initial bodies as revealed by staining infected erythrocytes by the acridine orange method.[11] The organism has both DNA and RNA, and the DNA is double stranded.[12]

Electron-microscopic studies using ultrathin sectioning and, subsequently, freeze-fracture, the ultrastructure of the organism has been elucidated.[12,13,14,15] The marginal body, about 1.0 μ in size, appears to be surrounded by a limiting or matrix membrane that separates it from the host erythrocyte cytoplasm. The initial bodies, which are the subunits of the marginal body, are oval or round in shape, measuring 300–400 μm in diameter (Fig. 3.1). Each initial body, an infectious unit, is enclosed in a trilaminar membrane composed of an outer cell wall and an inner plasma membrane. The interior of the initial body contains dark, dense aggregates and strand-like material presumed to be ribosomes and DNA, respectively. Freeze-fracture replication demonstrated the presence of an area of parallel striations with a periodicity of 10.5 nm between the ridges on the limiting membrane of the marginal body. These corrugations may serve to strengthen the limiting membrane.[15]

Cultural Properties

Several attempts have been made over the years, utilizing a variety of culture systems, to propagate *A. marginale in vitro*, but none of the systems provided suitable conditions for active replication of the organism.[16] More recently, a culture technique that enabled maintenance of the organism for 28–60 days was reported.[17,18] Infected erythrocytes resuspended in medium RPMI-1640 containing 25 mM

HEPES, 10% bovine serum and incubated in a candle jar showed a 3- and 10-fold increase of parasitized erythrocytes in 8 and 14 days, respectively. Subculture at 4–5 day intervals, using uninfected bovine erythrocytes, did not result in a significant increase in parasite numbers. Viability of the organism in culture was demonstrated by animal inoculation using a 33 day old culture. Evidence of invasion of new erythrocytes by *A. marginale* in culture was shown by coculturing attenuated *A. marginale* infected ovine erythrocytes with uninfected bovine erythrocytes and subsequently demonstrating the organism in the latter.

There are reports on attempts to propagate *A. marginale* in cells other than those of bovine origin. Rabbit primary bone marrow culture and a stable rabbit bone marrow cell line have been used with limited success.[19,20] Since *A. marginale* infects ticks and multiplies in tick tissue, two groups of workers used a continuous cell line derived from *Dermacentor andersoni* for propagation of the organism.[21,22] One group utilized infected bovine erythrocytes to infect the cell line and reported a substantial increase in the number of parasitized cells in culture.[21] Homogenized midguts from *A. marginale*-infected *Derma-*

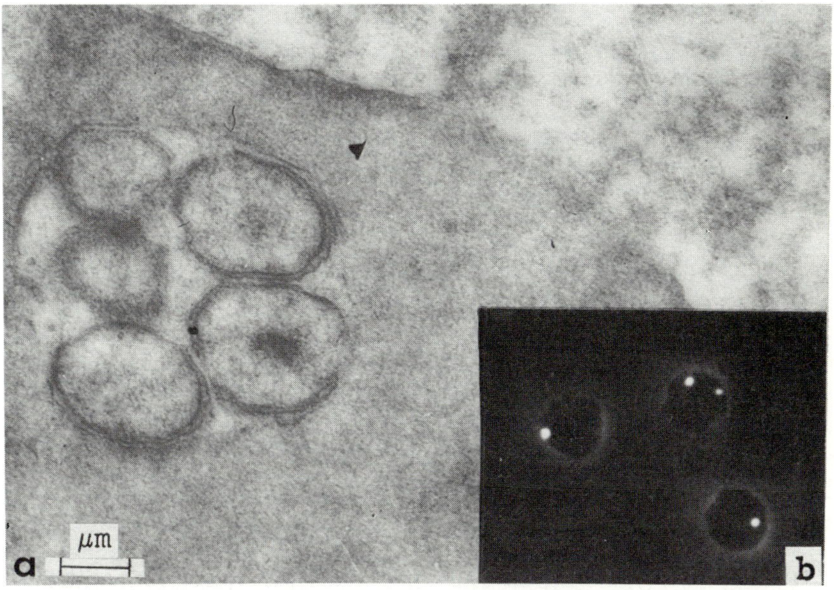

FIG. 3.1. Ultrathin section of an *Anaplasma marginale*-infected bovine erythrocyte. The marginal inclusion body is separated from the cytoplasm of the erythrocyte by a limiting or matrix membrane. The inclusion body contains five subunits known as initial bodies (a) *Anaplasma marginale* bodies stained by the indirect fluorescent antibody method. (b) Electron micrograph (× 42,000) and light microscopy (× 800).

centor variabilis were used by other workers to infect the cell line. They were able to maintain the organism in culture through 22 passages over a period of more than 11 months without the loss of antigenicity or infectivity for the tick cells, although the cultured organism failed to initiate a demonstrable infection in cattle.[22]

Antigenic Characteristics

The antigens of *A. marginale* described thus far can be classified into 2 broad categories, namely, (a) soluble antigens that may be secretory or excretory products and (b) corpuscular antigens which include those associated with the initial body membrane (integral or surface located). Except for antigens of the infected erythrocytes which may be exposed by parasitic damage and are incriminated in autoantibody production, no antigens of parasite origin have been reported on the surface of the erythrocyte.[23,24]

Soluble antigens. A soluble *A. marginale* exoantigen was detected in the serum of cattle in the acute stage of the disease and 1 or 2 days prior to occurrence of peak parasitemia.[25] The same antigen, also found in aqueous lysates of infected erythrocytes, was believed to be a parasite metabolic product which was either a glycoprotein or a lipoprotein. This antigen did not confer protective immunity.[26] Soluble antigens were prepared from infected erythrocytes by hydrochloric acid or protamine sulphate precipitation. The protamine sulphate-precipitated antigen was found to be a component of the damaged erythrocyte and was shown to be responsible for the autoimmunity associated with anaplasmosis.[27]

Corpuscular antigens. Several particulate or corpuscular antigens have been prepared from infected erythrocytes for use in diagnostic tests. The antigens used in complement fixation, capillary tube agglutination and card agglutination tests are relatively crude preparations of *A. marginale* initial bodies.[27]

More recently, purified *A. marginale* initial bodies have been utilized to determine the location of the antibody reactive proteins and to isolate these antigens for characterization and the definition of their role in protection. Nine surface proteins were radiolabelled from *A. marginale* purified initial bodies that were found to be free from most of the bovine erythrocyte components, morphologically intact and infective. Rabbit polyclonal antibody, that was capable of neutralizing the infectivity of *A. marginale* initial bodies, immunoprecipitated 5 of these surface proteins with molecular weights of 105, 86, 61, 36 and 31 kDa, respectively.[28]

Monoclonal antibodies that neutralized the infectivity of *A. marginale* initial bodies also immunoprecipitated a 105 kDa protein.[29]

This protein was shown to consist of two noncovalently linked polypeptides of the same molecular weight and these were designated as AM 105L and AM 105U, respectively. Following cloning of *A. marginale* DNA and expression in *E. coli*, it was seen that the 105 kDa recombinant protein had structural and antigenic homology with the 105L peptide. Proteolytic cleavage of the proteins also showed structural homology of recombinant 105 with 105L and not with 105U; thus showing that they were separate gene products.[30] Subsequently, this complex was referred to as the major surface protein consisting of 2 units with mol wt of 105 and 100 kDa, respectively.

Antigenic Variation

Antigenic variation among different isolates or the extent of the variation, is of particular concern in the formulation of vaccines against the disease. Antigenic differences between *A. centrale* and *A. marginale* became apparent by the variable resistance of cattle vaccinated with *A. centrale* to challenge with *A. marginale*.[31,32] *Anaplasma centrale* infected cattle produced a lesser complement fixing antibody response when tested with *A. marginale* antigen, indicating differences in the antigenic make up.[33]

Stage specific antigens were not seen during the course of *A. marginale* infection.[34] Antigenic similarities between bovine erythrocyte stage and tick stages of the parasite have been demonstrated, but sufficient evidence is not available to warrant the conclusion that antigenic differences exist between these two stages.[35] It has been demonstrated by probing with a panel of 19 monoclonal antibodies that isolates of *A. marginale* from Kenya and Israel and *A. centrale* possessed isolate restricted antigens and genus common antigens.[34] The genus common antigenic epitopes were present on the 36 and 105 kDa surface proteins.[36]

Protective Antigens

Neutralizing antibody against initial body of the *A. marginale* Florida isolate recognized protein antigens, presumably located on the surface of the initial body and having mol wt 105, 86, 61, 36 and 31 kDa, respectively, indicating that all or some of these peptides possessed epitopes that were essential for protection.[28] Cattle immunized with the 105 kDa peptide, which was found to be conserved among several geographical isolates of *A. marginale* and *A. centrale*, were protected against homologous challenge as well as challenge with an antigenically different isolate.[29,34,36] Immunization with a 36 kDa protein, which also is conserved among several isolates of *A. marginale* and *A. centrale*, provided significant protection against challenge exposure.[37]

Epidemiology

In endemic areas a primary infection acquired in calfhood protects the animal for life. In a study conducted in an area with a high prevalence of anaplasmosis, all of the 112 calves observed became infected with *A. marginale* during 4–24 weeks of age and showed only mild signs of the disease.[38] In such areas the vectors are abundant throughout the year and reservoirs of infection, namely, cattle and wild ruminants, are present constantly. This state of enzootic stability prevents disease outbreaks and the balance could be disturbed only by manipulations that can cause fluctuations of vector burden.

Host Range

Anaplasma marginale and *A. centrale* infect cattle; *A. ovis* infects sheep and goats. Other ruminants such as antelope, buffalo, zebra, camel, deer, elk, black wildebeest, duiker and blesbok are also considered to be susceptible to natural infection with *A. marginale.*[16]

Breed and Age Susceptibility

Cattle of all ages and breeds are susceptible to infection. The susceptibility to infection and severity of the disease increase with the age of the animal; the calves being more resistant.

Geographic Distribution

Anaplasmosis is known to occur in Africa, Southern Europe, Australia, South America, Far Eastern and South Eastern Asia and the former Soviet Union. In the United States the disease is endemic in some 40 states.[16]

Transmission

Under natural conditions anaplasmosis is transmitted to susceptible animals both biologically and mechanically from symptomless carrier cattle and other wild ruminants. Several species of ticks, biting flies and mosquitoes are mentioned as vectors of *Anaplasma spp.*[39] The organism can also be transmitted through the use of instruments contaminated with infected blood.[16]

Tick Transmission

Under experimental conditions about 20 species of ticks were shown to be capable of transmitting anaplasmosis. *Dermacentor andersoni, Dermacentor occidentalis* and *Dermacentor variabilis* have been identified as the tick vectors in the United States.[14] *Dermacentor andersoni* and *D. variabilis* acquire infection as nymphs and are able to transmit as adults. No transovarial transmission has been demonstrated.[40] Intrastadial transmission by male ticks feeding on carrier animals, however, has been reported. The fact that not all tick species can transmit all the different geographical isolates of *A. marginale* was demonstrated when an efficient trans-stadial vector of the organism was unable to transmit the Illinois isolate but transmitted the Virginia isolate. Antigenic and morphologic differences among isolates may influence geographical distribution and natural selection of reservoirs where the tick determines the wild animal reservoir.[41]

Development of the parasite in the tick following the ingestion of infected blood has been studied. *Anaplasma marginale* bodies were demonstrated in the gut contents and malpighian tubules of engorged *D. andersoni* nymphs by the fluorescent antibody technique. The organisms seen in groups of 4 or 5 in the malpighian tubules of the nymphs resembled the organism in infected erythrocytes.[42]

Several morphologically distinct stages of the parasite have been demonstrated in the midgut of *D. andersoni* ticks, suggestive of a developmental cycle in the vector. The organisms were usually found in colonies in the midgut cells. Three types of morphologically distinct colonies that appeared in chronological order were reported in nymphs that fed on *A. marginale*-infected animals. Early stages that were observed 5 days after feeding were seen by the electron microscope as small forms, or larger round reticulated forms, that appeared to divide by binary fission, whereas the final stage that appeared after day 20 postfeeding did not show division.[43] Only the organisms in the latter stage of development were infective to cattle, indicating that some developmental stages in the tick may not be infective.[44] Infected adult ticks, after 8 days of feeding, had small numbers of *A. marginale* in the acinar cells of the salivary gland when stained by fluorescent antibody technique. The appearance of the parasite in the acinar cells coincided with a decrease in numbers of organisms detectable in the gut tissue, indicating that transmission occurred via the salivary gland.[45]

Insect Vectors

The role of insects in the transmission of *A. marginale* has been studied and horse flies (Diptera: *Tabanidae*), stable flies (*Stomoxys*), deer flies (*Chrysops*), horn flies (*Siphona*) and mosquitoes of the genus *Psorophora* have been incriminated as potential vectors, based on experimental and epidemiological data.[14] The relative importance of each species of insects in the transmission of *A. marginale* will depend on the geographical locality and the cattle density in a given area.

Transmission of *A. marginale* by insects is presumably mechanical as there is no evidence of a developmental cycle in insect tissues. The fact that insects are able to transmit the agent only for a short time after feeding on an infected animal further supports this assumption. In those species of horseflies studied it was found that the flies remained infective for a period of about 2 h and that 5–10 horsefly bites were needed to transmit the disease after obtaining a partial blood meal from an acutely infected animal.[46]

Reservoirs of Infection

Carrier cattle are the main reservoirs of infection. Wild deer have also been regarded as equally important reservoirs and anaplasma may survive in nature through deer-to-deer transfer via appropriate vectors. Several investigators have demonstrated transmission of infection from deer to cattle.[14]

Pathogenesis

Entry of the organism into the host animal is via the bite of a vector or by experimental inoculation of infected blood. In an experimental infection or in the case of mechanical transmission by insects it is evident that the erythrocyte stage of the organism initiates the infection process. But the stage that the tick transmits, following cyclic development of the organism in the midgut epithelial cells, the muscle cells and the salivary gland acini (although not clear at present) may be morphologically and antigenically different from the erythrocyte stage. The tick stage of the parasite that is presumably transmitted to cattle has been demonstrated as a largely reticulated form that occurs within an inclusion membrane in the cells of the salivary gland.[47] In cattle the site of parasite multiplication is the mature erythrocyte. No extraerythrocytic developmental stage of *A. marginale* in the bovine host has been demonstrated. Erythrocyte-free *A. marginale* initial bodies were found to attach to the erythrocyte membrane when incubated with uninfected bovine erythrocytes.[48] In studies undertaken to define the mechanism of interaction between the initial *Anaplasma* body and the erythrocyte membrane and to identify the parasite proteins responsible for invasion, 3 surface exposed *A. marginale* proteins of mol wt 91, 68 and 29 kDa, respectively, were demonstrated as having an affinity for glycoproteins on the erythrocyte surface. These may act as ligands for the organismal proteins.[49] The initial body enters the erythrocyte by pinocytic vacuolation. First detection of the anaplasma minute bodies, presumably initial bodies, is usually possible 3–4 weeks postinfection. The initial bodies that are closely associated with the erythrocyte membrane divide by binary fission and form into marginal bodies. There was a constant increase in marginal bodies from about the 21st day postinfection. During the ensuing period there was vigorous growth and transfer of initial bodies into uninfected erythrocytes. Changes in membrane potential was observed during ascending parasitemia which may be indicative of loss of erythrocyte membrane function leading to increased fragility.[50] The organisms may invade fresh erythrocytes through intercellular tissue bridges and may not remain free in the plasma prior to invasion. A decrease in the concentration of phospholipids in erythrocyte stroma and increase in serum sialic acid content occurs as a result of initial body interaction with the erythrocyte.[51]

Following recovery and disappearance from erythrocytes of microscopically visible marginal bodies, the animal becomes a symptomless carrier. Blood of carrier animals is infectious for a long period of time, as much as 12 years in one instance. Splenectomy of a carrier animal can lead to relapse of the clinical disease.[16]

Clinical Disease

Prepatent Period

The prepatent period corresponds with the incubation period and this is defined as the interval between exposure to infection and the first appearance of *Anaplasma marginale* bodies in the erythrocytes. Under experimental conditions, the prepatent period varied from 24 to 35 days.[52] The prepatent period is inversely proportional to the size of the inoculum.[14]

Clinical Signs and Symptoms

The clinical signs of anaplasmosis are those that are attributable to severe anemia. They include depression, weakness, high body temperature, labored breathing, inappetence, dehydration, constipation and jaundice. The acute stage of the disease is characterized by elevated temperatures ranging from 103° to 107°F that persist for 3–7 days. With the progress of the disease, the temperature returns to normal and becomes subnormal prior to death. During the febrile stage there is suppression of rumination, dryness of the muzzle, loss of appetite, dullness and depression. The visible mucus membranes appear yellow. There is frequent urination, but the urine is not colored. Constipation is common and feces are dark and often blood-tinged.

Lactating cows show a decrease in milk production and abortion is a common feature in advanced cases of pregnancy. None of the cows experimentally infected in the second trimester of pregnancy aborted, and 5 out of 6 cows infected during the third trimester of pregnancy, exhibited foetal death or abortion.[53] Infected bulls during the acute stage of the disease show a lack of libido and abnormal sperm morphology occasionally accompanied by transitory testicular degeneration.[53]

The severity of the disease increases with age, with the calves under 1 year usually acquiring the mild form of the disease and animals over 3 years of age, the peracute and possibly fatal disease.

Pathology

Postmortem Findings

The macroscopic lesions found at postmortem are those generally associated with acute anemia. The mucus membranes are icteric and there is pallor of tissue. The spleen is often greatly enlarged and its cut surface shows dark pulp and enlarged splenic follicles. The liver may be enlarged with rounded borders and the cut surface appears brownish-yellow to sulphur-yellow. The gall bladder is enlarged and obstructed with dark, thick bile. Petechiae could be observed on the epicardium, pericardium, pleura and diaphragm. The lymph glands are enlarged.[54,55]

Histopathology

Microscopically there is hyperplasia of the bone marrow. The spleen shows a decrease of lymphoblasts and increased vacuolation and degeneration of reticular cells. There is a reduction of the white pulp and accumulation of pigment resembling hemosiderin seen in sections of the spleen. Hepatic changes consist of leukocytic infiltration of Glissons capsule, dilation of portal veins and swelling of endothelial cells.[56]

Hematology

With the appearance of *A. marginale* marginal bodies in the peripheral blood, there is a constant reduction of erythrocyte numbers, hemoglobin content and oxygen capacity. The erythrocyte count may decrease to 2 million or less and the hemoglobin content to below 3.0 gm per 100 ml of blood. Erythrocytes showed increased osmotic and mechanical fragility along with anisocytosis, poikilocytosis and polychromasia.[57] Leukocytosis is usually observed with counts reaching 20,000 per mm^3. Bilirubinemia is observed during the acute stage of infection.

In terminal cases of anaplasmosis there is reduction in the nitrogen and uric acid content of blood and an increase in nonprotein nitrogen. There is a decrease of phospholipid concentration in the erythrocytic stroma and an increase of sialic acid in the serum.[51,58]

During the recovery phase of the disease there is an increase in the number of immature erythrocytes, the predominant ones being normoblasts and reticulocytes.[16]

Immunity

Protective immunity to anaplasmosis was traditionally associated with premunition; the continuous presence of the organism at low levels in clinically recovered animals following primary infection. This concept led to the practice of the procedure termed preimmunization of cattle by the use of virulent *A. marginale* or *A. centrale* in many areas of the world.[14]

Carrier animals are completely protected against homologous challenge but may remain susceptible to heterologous challenge.[59] The mechanism by which the resulting carrier state protects the host, however, has not been clearly understood.

There is evidence that immunity exists in the absence of replicating parasites. Killed, whole organisms or derived fractions have been shown to confer different degrees of protection. Animals treated with either Imidocarb or long acting tetracycline to clear the infection were found to be protected from clinical disease. Only low-level parasitemia and a transient drop in packed cell volume were observed when challenged 8–12 months after treatment.[60,61] Prior to infection challenge no antibodies were detected by the complement fixation test and card agglutination test; but animals became seropositive on 7–21 days postchallenge, suggesting memory stimulation.

A vaccine composed of killed *A. marginale* initial bodies was shown to confer protection. The duration of immunity, however, has not been accurately determined.[62,63] This sterile immunity, however, is short-lasting, requiring multiple vaccination at regular intervals. The vaccinated animals are protected from severe disease and death but not from infection and subsequent development of a carrier state.

Depending upon the manner the protective immunity to anaplasmosis is defined it can be stated that there is a degree of sterile immunity that is short-lasting but life-long protection is afforded only by premunition.

Immune Responses

Evidence has accumulated over the years that the immune response against anaplasmosis is both humoral and cell mediated. Several assay systems have detected anaplasma specific antibodies in animals that are protected following natural or experimental infection.

Antibodies alone (or *per se*) cannot protect animals against anaplasmosis as evidenced by the lack of protection observed when serum from recovered animals was transfused into susceptible cattle.[27] Specific antibodies, however, neutralized the infectivity of the organism *in vitro* as demonstrated in an experiment where purified initial bodies reacted with hyperimmune rabbit serum failed to infect susceptible cattle.[28] Although similar neutralization experiments have not been conducted using bovine immune serum, the results of this study provide an indication of a protective role for specific *A. marginale* antibody. Whether a similar situation can occur *in vivo* where antibody alone can act as the only line of defense is debatable, although complement fixing and agglutinating antibody have also been demonstrated in natural and experimental infections.[27] A recent study has shown that animals immunized with surface membrane components of *A. marginale* exhibited protection that correlated with the antibody levels to the membrane polypeptides.[64] In the host several factors such as the protective environment of the erythrocyte, the manner in which the organism invades fresh cells, immune evasion mechanisms that are inherent to the parasite together with the properties and concentration of protective antibody may influence the neutralization capability of the antibody. Removal of parasites from the circulation takes place by phagocytosis of the entire infected erythrocyte and the organism is rarely observed extracellularly.[27] If the initial bodies are not exposed to the antibody, and parasite antigens are not present on the infected erythrocytes, neutralization, lysis or antibody-mediated phagocytosis may not occur. The occurrence of autohemagglutinins and opsonins directed against the erythrocyte membrane in sera of *A. marginale*-infected animals has been documented. These antibodies may be responsible for the erythrophagocytosis observed in the bone marrow of both infected and noninfected erythrocytes. Such antibodies eluted from erythrocytes of infected animals were shown to be capable of inducing phagocytosis of erythrocytes in an *in vitro* assay. This activity was highest during the peak of anemia.[65]

Cell Mediated Immunity

Except in animals that have received a killed vaccine, delayed type hypersensitivity (DTH) has not been observed in either acutely infected or carrier animals. The DTH observed in the vaccinated animals may be due to the administration of adjuvant in the presence of heterologous erythrocyte antigens, and therefore, not related to protective immunity.[66]

Leukocyte migration inhibition (LMI) was observed in animals infected with virulent *A. marginale* and calves immunized with a killed vaccine.[66]

In another study, the results of leukocyte migration inhibition tests appeared to correlate with protection. Animals showing the LMI response early in the incubation period showed less severe clinical signs. Cattle vaccinated with attenuated *A. marginale* showed a LMI response in 2–3 weeks, as did animals infected with virulent parasites. Animals that received a killed vaccine showed only a low and transient LMI response.[67] The mechanism responsible for the leukocyte migration inhibition or the role the lymphokines, or other factors responsible for this phenomenon, play in protection has not been defined.

Diagnosis

Microscopic Examination of Blood

Routine diagnosis of anaplasmosis is done by microscopic examination of thin blood smears stained with Giemsa. This procedure, though convenient, becomes less reliable when the percentage of parasitized erythrocytes is low and where dye deposits may be mistaken for *A. marginale*. Use of acridine orange (AO) stain can improve detection but this dye stains nucleic acids of immature erythrocytes. In formalin fixed erythrocytes stained with acridine orange and examined under ultra violet light, *A. marginale* appears bright orange.[68] Direct and indirect fluorescent antibody tests have also been used to detect *A. marginale* in erythrocytes. This procedure enables the visualization of marginal bodies and the smaller initial bodies.[69]

Serology

Several antigens, both soluble and particulate, have been used for the detection of antibody in subclinical cases of anaplasmosis and in vaccinated animals. The most widely used serological test is the indirect fluorescent antibody (IFA) test. Despite several proposed modifications of the basic technique, this test has the serious drawback of nonspecific reactivity which makes the interpretation of the results difficult, especially in sera with low levels of antibodies.[70] Three other tests, namely complement fixation (CF), capillary tube agglutination (CA) and card agglutination tests, that utilize relatively crude antigens are widely used in the United States.[69,71,72] Use of ELISA systems, radioimmunoassay and Dot-ELISA for antibody detection has also been reported.[73,74]

In our laboratory we routinely use a Dot-ELISA system where formalin-treated CA antigen dotted onto nitrocellulose discs is reacted with test serum and the antigen–antibody complexes, detected with enzyme conjugated Protein-A. The test possesses extremely high specificity but lacks the sensitivity of IFA by being able to only detect IgG_2 antibodies. Purified *A. marginale* polypeptides of defined molecular weight have been used as antigens in the Dot-ELISA. A 38 kDa *A. marginale* antigen has given excellent results with near 100% sensitivity and specificity. Two other polypeptides of 41 and 105 kDa were also found to be suitable antigens for the Dot-ELISA. An IgM response was detected as early as 4 days, which persisted through 28 days postinfection. The specific IgG response which appeared on day 16 postinfection was detectable throughout the experimental period of 150 days in all infected animals.[75]

DNA probes derived from *A. centrale* have been used in hybridization assays to diagnose *A. centrale* and *A. marginale* infections in cattle and in tick midgut tissue.[76] A 2 k fragment from within the gene coding for a surface protein of *A. marginale* was used as a probe to detect the parasite in infected erythrocytes and tissues of adult *Dermacentor spp.* ticks infected as adults or nymphs.[77] A RNA probe developed from a fragment of the gene coding for a surface protein was able to detect infections in carrier cattle with parasitemias as low as 0.000025%, thus making it several times more sensitive than light microscopy.[78]

Treatment and Control

Chemotherapy

Several chemotherapeutic agents have been used to cure anaplasmosis but only the tetracycline compounds and imidocarb are currently in use. The latter is not approved for use in U.S.A.[27]

Chlortetracyclines, at doses of 3–10 mg/kg body weight, have been used to eliminate the carrier state. Feeding chlortetracycline at 1 mg/kg body weight for 120 days, or intramuscular administration of tetracycline hydrochloride at a dose rate of 22 mg/kg body weight on 5 consecutive days, or the administration of two doses of a long acting oxytetracycline preparation intramuscularly seven days apart, also eliminated the carrier state.[60,79]

For the treatment of acute anaplasmosis one intramuscular injection of long acting oxytetracycline at the rate of 20 mg/kg was found to be adequate. Imidocarb given at the rate of 4–6 mg/kg body weight over a three day period also eliminated the carrier state.[80]

Vaccination

Immunization of cattle against anaplasmosis has been done by either (a) the use of infected blood containing virulent *A. marginale*, the less virulent *A. centrale*, or the laboratory attenuated *A. marginale* of bovine and ovine origin (premunization), or (b) use of inactivated erythrocyte-derived antigen fortified with adjuvants.

Premunization. This procedure is based on the concept that immunity to anaplasmosis is dependent on the induction of a primary infection and the maintenance of a carrier state for life following recovery. Persistence of a low-grade parasitemia provides a source of constant antigenic stimulation to the host immune system.[16]

Use of virulent A. marginale. Young animals which are relatively resistant to anaplasmosis as well as susceptible cattle introduced into endemic areas are inoculated with blood from a carrier animal or given a standardized inoculum made from high parasitemic blood of a splenectomized animal. Animals are closely monitored clinically and treatment instituted if severe symptoms develop. This method of immunization, if carried out with a local isolate, mimics the situation that prevails in an endemic area where animals become infected naturally and become immune following recovery. The procedure, however, is laborious, expensive and risky.

Premunization with A. centrale. Theiler demonstrated that cattle premunized with *A. centrale* were able to withstand challenge with the virulent *A. marginale*.[81] Since then *A. centrale* has been used in premunization programs in several countries in Asia, Africa and Latin America.[52,82] Reactions ranging from mild to severe have been reported in premunized animals. The degree of protection conferred by premunization with *A. centrale* against *A. marginale* challenge, however, was variable.[33] Antigenic differences exist between *A. centrale* and *A. marginale* and some isolates of *A. centrale* are more virulent than others, which is suggestive of antigenic and biological differences. Such differences among *A. centrale* and the degree of relatedness of the particular isolate of *A. centrale* used in premunization to the virulent strain of *A. marginale* endemic in an area may be responsible for the variable degree of protection.

Use of laboratory-attenuated A. marginale. A laboratory-attenuated *A. marginale* has been developed and utilized to immunize cattle in field and laboratory experiments in U.S.A., Peru, Mexico and Venezuela.[83–86] The isolate used for attenuation, known to be highly virulent and broadly cross protective, was collected from naturally infected animals in Florida.[63] Attenuation was accomplished by (a) exposure to irradiation to induce mutation, (b) selection of a virulent population by serial passage of the irradiated organisms in splenectomized deer (2 passages) and sheep (130 passages). The attenuated *A. marginale* contained in sheep erythrocytes are preserved in liquid nitrogen. The seed material is reactivated in splenectomized calves or sheep for vaccine production. When administered in 1.0 to 2.0 ml doses intramuscularly, the prepatant period in inoculated animals range from 4 to 5 weeks. Although vaccinated animals do not suffer from clinical disease, they develop parasitemias ranging from 0.5 to 8.0% and show a slight decrease in the packed cell volume, usually not exceeding 5–10%.

The attenuated *A. marginale* has been shown to induce strong humoral and cell-mediated immune responses. An antibody response, as measured by the CA and CF tests, can be detected 3 to 4 weeks postvaccination and the specific antibodies persist for 2 to 3 years in the absence of reinfection.[63,86] The leukocyte migration inhibition test became positive 2–4 weeks postvaccination. The attenuation process has, therefore, resulted in the loss of virulence, but not immunogenicity and the organism did not revert to virulence even after 5 to 12 consecutive passages in susceptible cattle.[86] The attenuated *A. marginale* could not infect ticks. Attempts to transmit the attenuated organism by natural tick feeding or inoculation of cattle with tick tissue homogenates were unsuccessful.

Widespread use of this vaccine did not occur, primarily due to the requirement of a cold-chain. Recently, we were able to preserve the organism and retain the viability of the parasite by lyophilization. The efficacy of the lyophilized vaccine, which contains 5.0×10^8 *A. marginale* infected erythrocytes per dose, was confirmed in vaccination and challenge experiments.[87]

Inactivated A. marginale *vaccines*. Several inactivated vaccines consisting of either the whole organism or fractions isolated from initial bodies supplemented with a variety of adjuvants have been used for immunization.[27,88] Vaccination with inactivated immunogens has several obvious advantages over premunization. In a successful killed vaccine, the immunogen has to be presented in a manner that would stimulate both humoral and cell-mediated immunity and the *A. marginale* isolate used for antigen preparation must be able to induce broad cross-protection. The use of a local isolate or the combination of two or more isolates may help in achieving this objective.

Presently, two killed vaccines are commercially available in the U.S.A. One vaccine, Anaplaz®, (Fort Dodge Laboratories, Fort Dodge, Iowa) is a lyophilized preparation of lyzed erythrocytes obtained from the blood of *A. marginale* infected animals collected at peak parasitemia. Lyophilized material is reconstituted in an oil adjuvant and two doses of the vaccine are administered subcutaneously at 4–19 week intervals. An annual booster injection is recommended. This vaccine induces partial protection against heterologous challenge. Although the vaccine reduced the severity of clinical disease following challenge, the animals developed a parasitemia, anemia and suffered weight loss.[63] This vaccine has been shown to induce antibodies against bovine blood group antigens, which in turn cause neonatal isoerythrolysis (NI) in calves ingesting colostrum from vaccinated dams.[89] Alterations in the vaccination program have been recommended by the manufacturer to reduce the incidence of NI.

Another vaccine recently made available commercially (AM-VAX™), contains purified initial bodies of the Florida isolate of *A. marginale* and is devoid of erythrocyte components that contain blood group antigens. Furthermore, the cattle utilized for vaccine production are screened for blood groups in order to select animals with less common blood groups. No confirmed reports are available of this vaccine causing NI.

Several other killed vaccines consisting of isolated *A. marginale* initial bodies have been used in laboratory and field studies.[90,91] Immunization of cattle with surface proteins isolated from purified initial bodies has also induced protection against homologous and heterologous challenge.[64,92]

Vector Control

Control of ticks or blood-sucking insects which transmit *A. marginale* is difficult to achieve with cattle in open ranches and farms. Dipping or systematic spraying of insecticides and insect repellents is not discouraged, although the cost of acaricides and the likelihood of development of acaricide resistance by the vectors and the disturbance to the enzootic stability are potential drawbacks of such control programs.

References

1. RISTIC, M. and KRIER, J.P. 1974. Manual of determinative bacteriology. In: *Family Anaplasmataceae*. p. 906. BUCHANAN, R.E. and GIBBONS, N.E. (Eds), Williams and Wilkins, Baltimore, MD.
2. SMITH, T. and KILBORNE, F.L. 1893. Investigations into the nature, causation, and prevention of Texas or southern cattle fever. *U.S. Dept. Agr., Bur. Animal Ind. Bull.* **1:** 1–301.
3. KOLLE, W. 1898. Uber einen neuen pathogenen Parasiten im Blute der Rinder in Südafrika. *Z. Hyg.* **27:** 45–48.
4. DSCHUNKOWSKY, E. and LUHS, J. 1904. Die Piroplasmosen der Rinder. *Centr. Bakteriol. Parasitenk.* **35:** 486–492.
5. LIGNIÉRES, J. 1914. L'anaplasmose bovine en Argentine. Contribution à l'étude de cette maladie. *Centr. Bakt. Parasitenk.* **74:** 133–162.
6. THEILER, A. 1910. *Anaplasma marginale.* The marginal points in the blood of cattle suffering from a specific disease. In: Report of the Government Veterinary Bacteriologist 1908–1909, pp. 6–64. THEILER, A. (Ed.), Transvaal Department of Agriculture, Transvaal, South Africa.
7. ANON, 1982. Priorities in biotechnology research for international development. National Research Council, National Academy Press. Washington, D.C., 1–9.
8. GOODGER, W.J., CARPENTER, T. and REIMANN, H. 1979. Estimation of economic loss associated with anaplasmosis in California beef cattle. *J.A.V.M.A.* **174:** 1333–1335.
9. MCCALLON, B.R. 1973. Prevalence and economic aspects of anaplasmosis. In: *Proceedings 6th National Anaplasmosis Conference* pp. 1–3. JONES, E.W. (Ed.), Heritage Press, Stillwater, Okla.
10. PINO, J.A. 1981. The neglected diseases of livestock. In: *Babesiosis* pp. 545–554. RISTIC, M. and KRIER, J.P. (Eds), Academic Press, New York.
11. RISTIC, M. and KRIER, J.P. 1963. Anaplasmosis. XV. Morphologic and chemical properties of the antigen used in the capillary tube agglutination test. *Am. J. vet. Res.* **24:** 985–992.
12. SENITZER, D.G., DIMOPOULLUS, G.T., BRINKLEY, B.R. and MANDEL, N. 1972. Deoxyribonucleic acid of *Anaplasma marginale*. *J. Bact.* **109:** 434–436.
13. RISTIC, M. and WATARACH, A.M. 1961. Studies in Anaplasmosis. II. Electron microscopy of *Anaplasma marginale* in deer. *Am. J. vet. Res.* **22:** 109–116.
14. RISTIC, M. 1968. Anaplasmosis. In: *Infectious Blood Diseases of Man and Animals,* pp. 478–542. WEINMAN, D. and RISTIC, M. (Eds). Academic Press, New York.
15. AMERAULT, T.E., ROBY, T.O. and SEALOCK, R.L. 1975. Ultrastructure of *Anaplasma marginale* after freeze fracture. *Am. J. vet. Res.* **36:** 1515–1519.
16. RISTIC, M. 1960. Anaplasmosis. *Adv. vet. Sci.* **6:** 111–192.

17. KESSLER, R.H., RISTIC, M., SELLS, D.M. and CARSON, C.A. 1979. *In vitro* cultivation of *Anaplasma marginale*: Growth pattern and morphologic appearance. *Am. J. vet. Res.* **40:** 1767–1773.
18. KESSLER, R.H. and RISTIC, M. 1979. *In vitro* cultivation of *Anaplasma marginale*: Invasion of and development of noninfected erythrocytes. *Am. J. vet. Res.* **40:** 1777–1780.
19. MARBLE, D.W. and HANKS, M.A. 1972. A tissue culture method for *Anaplasma marginale*. *Cornell Vet.* **62:** 196–205.
20. MARBLE, D.W. and HANKS, M.A. 1973. Bone marrow cell culture. In: *Proceedings 6th National Anaplasmosis Conference*. pp. 49–54. JONES, E.W. (Ed.), Heritage Press, Stillwater, Okla.
21. SAMISH, M., PIPANO, E. and HANA, B. 1988. Cultivation of *Anaplasma marginale* from cattle in a *Dermacentor* cell line. *Am. J. vet. Res.* **49:** 254–256.
22. HIDALGO, R.J., PALMER, G.H., JONES, E.W., BROWN, J.E. and AINSWORTH, A.J. 1989. Infectivity and antigenicity of *Anaplasma marginale* from tick cell culture. *Am. J. vet. Res.* **50:** 2033–2036.
23. SCHROEDER, W.F. and RISTIC, M. 1965. Anaplasmosis. XVIII. An analysis of autoantigens in infected and normal bovine erythrocytes. *Am. J. vet. Res.* **26:** 679–682.
24. SCHROEDER, W.F. and RISTIC, M. 1968. Blood serum factors associated with erythrophagocytosis in calves with anaplasmosis. *Am. J. vet. Res.* **29:** 1991–1995.
25. AMERAULT, T.E. and ROBY, T.O. 1964. An exoantigen of *Anaplasma marginale* in serum and erythrocytes of cattle with acute anaplasmosis. *Am. J. vet. Res.* **25:** 1642–1647.
26. AMERAULT, T.E. and ROBY, T.O. 1967. Preparation and characterization of a soluble *Anaplasma marginale* antigen. *Am. J. vet. Res.* **28:** 1067–1072.
27. RISTIC, M. 1977. Bovine anaplasmosis. In: *Parasitic Protozoa,* Vol. IV., pp. 235–249. KRIER, J.P. (Ed.), Academic Press, New York.
28. PALMER, G.H. and MCGUIRE, T.C. 1984. Immune serum against *Anaplasma marginale* initial bodies neutralizes infectivity for cattle. *J. Immun.* **133:** 1010–1015.
29. PALMER, G.H., BARBET, A.F., DAVIS, W.C. and MCGUIRE, T.C. 1986. Immunization with an isolate-common surface protein protects cattle against anaplasmosis. *Science* **231:** 1299–1302.
30. BARBET, A.F., PALMER, G.H., MYLER, P.J. and MCGUIRE, T.C. 1987. Characterization of an immunoprotective protein complex of *Anaplasma marginale* by cloning and expression of the gene coding for polypeptide AM 105L. *Infect. Immun.* **55:** 2428–2435.
31. LEGG, J. 1936. Anaplasmosis cross-immunity tests between *Anaplasma centrale* (South Africa) and *Anaplasma marginale* (Australia). *Aust. vet. J.* **12:** 230–235.
32. KUTTLER, K.L. 1967. Serological relationship of *Anaplasma marginale* and *Anaplasma centrale* as measured by the complement-fixation and capillary tube agglutination tests. *Res. vet. Sci.* **8:** 207–211.
33. KUTTLER, K.L. 1967. Study of the immunological relationship of *Anaplasma marginale* and *Anaplasma centrale*. *Res. vet. Sci.* **8:** 467–471.
34. MCGUIRE, T.C., PALMER, G.H., GOFF, W.L., JOHNSON, M.I. and DAVIS, W.C. 1984. Common and isolate-restricted antigens of *Anaplasma marginale* detected with monoclonal antibodies. *Infect. Immun.* **45:** 697–700.
35. PALMER, G.H., KOCAN, K.M., BARRON, S.J., HAIR, J.A., BARBET, A.F., DAVIS, W.C. and MCGUIRE, T.C. 1985. Presence of common antigens including major

surface protein epitopes, between the cattle (intraerythrocytic) and tick stages of *Anaplasma marginale*. *Infect. Immun.* **50:** 881–886.

36. PALMER, G.H., BARBET, A.F., MUSOKE, A.J., KATENDE, J.M., RURANGIRWA, F., STIKAP, V., PIPANO, E., DAVIS, W.C. and MCGUIRE, T.C. 1988. Recognition of conserved surface protein epitopes on *Anaplasma centrale* and *Anaplasma marginale* isolates from Israel, Kenya and the United States. *Int. J. Parasit.* **18:** 33–38.
37. PALMER, G.H., OBERLE, S.M., BARBET, A.F., DAVIS, W.C., GOFF, W.L. and MCGUIRE, T.C. 1988. Immunization with a 36-kilodalton surface protein induces protection against homologous and heterologous *Anaplasma marginale* challenge. *Infect. Immun.* **56:** 1526–1531.
38. CORRIER, D.E. and GUZMAN, S. 1977. The effect of natural exposure to *Anaplasma* and *Babesia* infections on native calves in an endemic area of Colombia. *Trop. Anim. Health Prod.* **9:** 47–51.
39. EWING S.A. 1982. Transmission of *Anaplasma marginale* by arthropods. In: *Proceedings 7th National Anaplasmosis Conference,* pp. 395–423. HIDALGO, R.J. and JONES, E.W. (Eds), Mississippi State University Press, State College.
40. KOCAN, K.M., EWING, S.A., OBERST, R.D., HOLBERT, D., HSU, K.C. and HAIR, J.A. 1981. Ultrastructure of *Anaplasma marginale* (Theiler) in *Dermacentor variabilis* (Say) and associated immunolabelling studies. In: *Proceedings 7th National Anaplasmosis Conference,* pp. 125–165. Mississippi State University Press, State College.
41. SMITH, R.D., LEVY, M.G., KUHLENSCHMIDT, M.S., ADAMS, J.H., RZECHULA, D.L., HARDT, T.A. and KOCAN, K.M. 1986. Isolate of *Anaplasma marginale* not transmitted by ticks. *Am. J. vet. Res.* **47:** 127–129.
42. FRIEDHOFF, K.T. and RISTIC, M. 1966. Anaplasmosis. XIX. A preliminary study of *Anaplasma marginale* in *Dermacentor andersoni* (Stiles) by fluorescent antibody technique. *Am. J. vet. Res.* **27:** 643–646.
43. KOCAN, K.M., YELLIN, T.N., EWING, S.A., HAIR, J.A. and BARRON, S.J. 1984. Morphology of colonies of *Anaplasma marginale* in nymphal *Dermacentor andersoni*. *Am. J. vet. Res.* **45:** 1434–1440.
44. KOCAN, K.M., YELLIN, T.N., CLAYPOOL, P.L., BARRON, S.J., EWING, S.A. and HAIR, J.A. 1990. Development and infectivity of *Anaplasma marginale* in *Dermacentor andersoni* nymphs. *Am. J. vet. Res.* **51:** 1292–1294.
45. KOCAN, K.M., WICKWIRE, K.B., EWING, S.A., HAIR, J.A. and BARRON, S.J. 1988. Preliminary studies of the development of *Anaplasma marginale* in salivary glands of adult, feeding *Dermacentor andersoni* ticks. *Am. J. vet. Res.* **49:** 1010–1013.
46. HAWKINS, J.A., LOVE, J.N. and HIDALGO, R.J. 1981. Mechanical transmission of anaplasmosis by tabanids. *Proc. 7th National Anaplasmosis Conference*, pp. 453–462. HIDALGO, R.J. and JONES, E.W. (Eds), Mississippi State University Press, State College.
47. KOCAN, K.M., STILLER, D., GOFF, W.L., EDWARDS, W., WICKWIRE, K.B., STICH, W., YELLIN, T.N., EWING, S.A., PALMER, G.H., BARRON, S.J., HAIR, J.A. and MCGUIRE, T.C. 1989. A review of the developmental cycle of *Anaplasma marginale* in *Dermacentor spp.* ticks. In: *Proceedings 8th National Vet. Hemoparasite Dis. Conf.* 129–149.
48. RISTIC, M. 1960. Studies of anaplasmosis. I. Filtration of the causative agent. *Am. J. vet. Res.* **21:** 890–894.
49. YSERN-CALDENTEY, M., ADAMS-BURTON, C.R., HART, L.T., LAINE, R.A. 1989. Interaction of *A. marginale* with the bovine erythrocyte surface. In: *Proceedings 8th National Vet. Hemoparasite Dis. Conf.* 49–63.

50. Blouin, E.F., Blankemeyer, J.T. and Kocan, K.M 1990. Changes in bovine erythrocyte membrane potential during infection with *Anaplasma marginale*. *Conf. Res. Workers in Anim. Dis.*, Chicago, p. 25.
51. Rao, P.J. and Ristic, M. 1963. Serum sialic acid levels in experimental anaplasmosis. *Proc. Soc. exp. Biol. Med.* 447–452.
52. Ranatunge, P. and Wanduragala, L. 1972. Reactions and hematology in imported jersey cattle premunized in Ceylon. *Br. vet. J.* **128:** 9–18.
53. Swift, L.A. 1981. Anaplasmosis: Effect on reproduction. In: *Proceedings 7th National Anaplasmosis Conference*, pp. 45–55. Hidalgo, R.J and Jones, E.W. (Eds), Mississippi State University Press, State College.
54. Christensen, J.F. 1963. Diseases of cattle, 2nd ed. *Am. vet. Publ.* 655–665.
55. Boynton, W.H. 1932. Further observations on anaplasmosis. *Cornell Vet.* **22:** 10–28.
56. Ristic, M. and Sippel, W.L. 1958. Effect of cortisone on the mechanism of *Anaplasma* immunity in experimentally infected calves. II. Studies of pathological changes. *Am. J. vet. Res.* **19:** 44–50.
57. Rees, C.W. and Hale, M.W. 1936. Morphological and chemical studies of the blood of cattle in health and during anaplasmosis. *J. agric. Res.* **53:** 477–492.
58. Dimopoullos, G.T. and Beddell, D.M. 1962. Studies of bovine erythrocytes in anaplasmosis. II. Role of chemical and physical changes in erythrocytes in the mechanism of anemia in splenectomized calves. *Am. J. vet. Res.* **23:** 813–820.
59. Krier, J.P. and Ristic, M. 1963. Anaplasmosis. XI. Immunoserologic characteristics of the parasite present in the blood of calves infected with the Oregon strain of *Anaplasma marginale*. *Am. J. vet. Res.* **24:** 688–702.
60. Roby, T.O., Amerault, T.E., Mazzola, V., Rose, J.E. and Ilemobade, A. 1974. Immunity in bovine anaplasmosis after elimination of *Anaplasma marginale* infections with imidocarb. *Am. J. vet. Res.* **35:** 993–995.
61. Magonigle, R.A. and Newby, T.J. 1984. Response of cattle upon reexposure to *Anaplasma marginale* after elimination of chronic carrier infections. *Am. J. vet. Res.* **45:** 695–697.
62. Brock, W.E., Kliewer, I.O. and Pearson, C.C. 1965. A vaccine for anaplasmosis. *J.A.V.M.A.* **147:** 948–951.
63. Kuttler, K.L., Zaugg, J.L. and Johnson, L.W. 1984. Serologic and clinical responses of premunized, vaccinated and previously infected cattle to challenge exposure by two different *Anaplasma marginale* isolates. *Am. J. vet. Res.* 2223–2226.
64. Tebele, N., McGuire, T.C. and Palmer, G.H. 1991. Induction of protective immunity by using *Anaplasma marginale* initial body membranes. *Infect. Immun.* **59:** 3199–3204.
65. Ristic, M., Lykins, J.D., and Morris, H.R. 1972. Anaplasmosis: opsonins and hemagglutinins in etiology of anemia. *Exp Parasit.* **31:** 2–12.
66. Buening, G.M. 1973. Cell-mediated immune responses in calves with anaplasmosis. *Am. J. vet. Res.* **34:** 757–763.
67. Ristic, M. and Carson, C.A. 1977. Methods of immunoprophylaxis against bovine anaplasmosis with emphasis on use of the attenuated *Anaplasma marginale* vaccine. In: *Immunity to Blood Parasites of Animals and Man.* pp. 151–188. Miller, L.H., Pino, J.A. and McKelvey, J.J. (Eds). Plenum Press, New York.
68. Gainer, J.H. 1961. Demonstration of *Anaplasma marginale* with the fluorescent dye, acridine orange; Comparisons with the complement fixation test and Wright's stain. *Am. J. vet. Res.* **22:** 882–886.

69. RISTIC, M. 1962. A capillary tube-agglutination test for anaplasmosis—A preliminary report. *J.A.V.M.A.* **141:** 588–594.
70. MONTENEGRO-JAMES, S., JAMES, M.A. and RISTIC, M. 1985. Modified indirect fluorescent antibody test for the serodiagnosis of *Anaplasma marginale* infections in cattle. *Am. J. vet. Res.* **46:** 2401–2403.
71. FRANKLIN, T.E., HECK, F.C. and HUFF, J.W. 1963. Anaplasmosis—complement fixation antigen production. *Am. J. vet. Res.* **24:** 483–487.
72. AMERAULT, T.E. and ROBY, T.O. 1968. A rapid agglutination test for bovine anaplasmosis. *J.A.V.M.A.* **153:** 1828–1834.
73. BARRY, D.N., PARKER, R.J., DEVOS, A.J., DUNSTER, P. and RODWELL, B.J. 1986. A microplate enzyme-linked immunosorbent assay for measuring antibody to *Anaplasma marginale* in cattle. *Aust. vet. J.* **63:** 73–79.
74. SCHUNTNER, C.A. and LEATCH, G. 1988. Radioimmunoassay for *Anaplasma marginale* antibodies in cattle. *Am. J. vet. Res.* **49:** 504–507.
75. MA, S.J. 1991. An immunodominant peptide-based dot enzyme linked immunosorbent assay for anaplasmosis. M.S. thesis. University of Illinois, Urbana-Champaign.
76. VISSER, E.S. and AMBROSIO, R.E. 1987. DNA probes for the detection of *Anaplasma centrale* and *Anaplasma marginale*. *Onderstepoort J. vet. Res.* **54:** 623–627.
77. GOFF, W., BARBET, A., STILLER, D., PALMER, G., KNOWLES, D., KOCAN, K., GORHAM, J. and MCGUIRE, T. 1988. Detection of *Anaplasma marginale*-infected tick vectors by using a cloned DNA probe. *Proc. natn. Acad. Sci. U.S.A.*, **85:** 919–923.
78. ERIKS, I.S., PALMER, G.H., MCGUIRE, T.C., ALLRED, D.R. and BARBET, A.F. 1989. Detection and Quantitation of *Anaplasma marginale* in carrier cattle by using a nucleic acid probe. *J. clin. Microbiol.* **27**(2): 279–284.
79. RICHEY, E.J., BROCK, W.E. and KLIEWER, I.O. 1978. The effect of feeding low levels of chlortetracycline for extended periods on the carrier state of anaplasmosis. *Bovine Pract.* **11:** 73–75.
80. KUTTLER, K.L. 1971. Promising therapeutic agents for the elimination of *Anaplasma marginale* in the carrier animal. *Proc. 75th Ann. Mtg. of U.S. Anim. Hlth. Ass.* 92–98.
81. THEILER, A. 1912. Gall sickness of imported cattle and the protective inoculation against this disease. *Agr. J. Union. S. Africa.* **3:** 1–11.
82. CALLOW, L.L. and DALGLIESH, R.J. 1980. Ticks and tick-borne diseases. In: *Proceedings Annual Conference, Australian Veterinary Association.* pp. 4–8. JOHNSTON, L.A.Y. and COOPER, M.G. (Eds), Sydney.
83. RISTIC, M., SIBINOVIC, S. and WELTER, C.J. 1968. An attenuated *Anaplasma marginale* vaccine. *Proc. U.S. Livestock Sanit. Ass.* **72:** 56–69.
84. LORA, C.A. and KOECHLIN, A. 1969. An attenuated *Anaplasma marginale* vaccine in Peru. *Am. J. vet. Res.* **30:** 1993–1998.
85. OSORNO, M.B., SOLANA, P.M., PEREZ, J.M. and LOPEZ, T.R. 1975. Study of an attenuated *Anaplasma marginale* vaccine in Mexico—Natural challenge of immunity in an enzootic area. *Am. J. vet. Res.* **34:** 631–633.
86. WELTER, C.J. and RISTIC, M. 1969. Laboratory and field trials with the attenuated *Anaplasma marginale* vaccine. *Proc. 72nd Ann. Mtg. U.S. Livestock Sanit. Assoc.* **72:** 122–130.
87. RISTIC, M. and WANDURAGALA, L. 1991. Modified-live *Anaplasma marginale* vaccine, ANAVIV™. *Proc. 95th Ann. Mtg. U.S. Anim. Hlth. Assoc.* 220–226.
88. PALMER, G.H. 1989. Anaplasma vaccines. In: *Veterinary Protozoan and*

Hemoparasite Vaccines, pp. 2–29. WRIGHT, I.G. (Ed), 2–29, CRC Press, Boca Raton, Florida.

89. DENNIS, R.A., O'HARA, P.J., YOUNG, M.F. and DORRIS, K.D. 1970. Neonatal isoerythrolytic anemia and icterus of calves. *J.A.V.M.A.* **156:** 1861–1869.
90. HART, L., SWANN, A.I., LARSON, A.D., FAGET, V. and MCCORKLE-SHIRLEY, S. 1981. Use of *Anaplasma marginale* devoid of host cell antigen as a vaccine for anaplasmosis. In: *Proceedings 7th National Anaplasmosis Conference,* pp. 495–504.
91. MONTENEGRO-JAMES, S., JAMES, M.A., TORO BENITEZ, M., LEON, E., BACK, B.K. and GUILLEN, A.T. 1990. Efficacy of purified *Anaplasma marginale* initial bodies as a vaccine against anaplasmosis. *Parasit. Res.* **77:** 93–101.
92. PALMER, G.H., BARBET, A.F., CANTOR, G.H. and MCGUIRE, T.C. 1989. Immunization of cattle with the MSP-1 surface protein complex induces protection against a structurally variant *Anaplasma marginale* isolate. *Infect. Immun.* **57:** 3666–3669.

4

Haemobartonellosis

A. S. NASH AND P. A. BOBADE

Introduction

Haemobartonellosis results from infection of mammalian erythrocytes by rickettsial organisms belonging to the genus *Haemobartonella*. Three species of *Haemobartonella* are currently recognized, namely *H. felis* in cats, *H. canis* in dogs and *H. muris* which infects rats, mice and hamsters.[1] An organism designated *H. bovis* has been observed in cattle,[2,3] but the exact classification of this and other organisms such as *H. muris musculi* and *H. tyzerri*,[2] earlier classified as belonging to the genus *Haemobartonella*, remains in doubt.[1] Discussion of these organisms and *H. muris* are beyond the scope of this book.

Feline infectious anemia associated with *H. felis*, was first reported from South Africa in 1942.[4] Small eperythrocytic bodies were observed in blood smears obtained from an anemic cat at necropsy. The name *Eperythrozoon felis* was proposed for the organism. Between 1946 and 1947, a similar organism was observed in the blood of cats in Leningrad and tentatively named *Bartonella felis*.[5] In 1953, an infectious anemia of cats was described in the United States.[6] The causative organisms were small round bodies attached to the erythrocytes, considered to be either *Eperythrozoon* or *Haemobartonella*, or possibly a mixtue of both. In 1955, the organism was named *Haemobartonella felis*.[7] For a long time there was disagreement between authors with regard to the nomenclature. While British and Australian authors favored the name *Eperythrozoon felis*,[8–10] American, Canadian, and other workers[11–13] preferred *Haemobartonella felis*. However, the organism is now universally called *H. felis* since the organisms recognized in different countries are morphologically similar and cause the same disease in infected cats.

H. felis has been reported as the cause of feline infectious anemia worldwide and for a long time it was considered the most common cause of anemia in cats.[14] *H. felis* on its own, or concurrently with other diseases, has been associated with 23–56% of feline anemias in different surveys.[11,15]

Haemobartonellosis of dogs has been reported less frequently than feline haemobartonellosis. It was first recognized in splenectomized dogs in Germany in 1928.[16] The causative organism was designated *Bartonella canis*. However, unlike organisms in the family Bartonellaceae, the organism neither has a cell wall nor grows in culture media, and therefore it was later classified as *Haemobartonella canis*.[1,17] Older literature on *H. canis* has been reviewed elsewhere.[2]

H. canis infection has been reported in all continents. The organism does not usually cause disease in healthy dogs. However severe anemia has been associated with *H. canis* infection in splenectomized dogs, dogs with concurrent diseases, and those that have been immunocompromized through immunosuppressive drug therapy or in other ways.[17,18] Isolated cases of anemia due to *H. canis* infection have been reported,[19–23] but the authenticity of the cases has been questioned.[17]

Causative Agent

Haemobartonellae are Gram-negative, nonacid fast erythrocytic parasites belonging to the family Anaplasmataceae and order *Rickettsiales*. They are coccoid, rod-shaped and, occasionally, ring-shaped organisms which may appear singly, in pairs or groups, in shallow or deep indentations on the erythrocytic surface and sometimes in vacuoles within the erythrocyte.[1] They are firmly attached on the erythrocyte and rarely found in the plasma. They stain well with Romanowsky-type stains but poorly with many other aniline dyes. They divide by binary fission, but have not been cultured on artificial media. *In vitro* cultivation of *H. felis* and *H. canis* has been claimed,[12,24] but the results have not been reproducible. *Haemobartonella* can be preserved indefinitely in 10% dimethyl sulfoxide when stored in liquid nitrogen.[1] Whole blood from cats infected with *H. felis* has remained infective following both storage in liquid nitrogen and being frozen for two weeks.[6,25]

Haemobartonella organisms contain both deoxyribonucleic acid (DNA) and ribonucleic acid (RNA).[26,27] There are no reports of antigenic studies of *Haemobartonella*, so it is not known if antigenic variation occurs within the species.

Morphology

H. felis

H. felis is pleomorphic, appearing as small irregularly round dots, short rods, coccoids and rings when observed with light microscopy.[5,28] Cocci and short rods occur more frequently.[1,29] The coccoid forms may occur singly, paired and sometimes as short chains of three or more. Rarely, coccoid forms are aggregated or arranged in a circle within the periphery of the erythrocyte. The coccoid form measures 0.1–1.7 μ in diameter; the ring form, approximately 1.0 μ; while the rods are 0.2–0.5 μ by 0.8–1.5 μ.[5,29,30] A discoid form of the organism has been described and this is thought to be a vegetative form.[31]

It has been suggested that the relative frequency of the different forms observed with light microscopy might be influenced by the nature of the blood film.[28] While rings and rod-shaped organisms are observed more frequently in thin blood films or in the feathered edge of thick blood films, nearly all *H. felis* organisms appear coccoid in thick blood films or thick areas of thin films.

In blood films stained with Romanowsky-type stains, *H. felis* stains light or deep purple with a tinge of blue or red depending on the stain.[5,29,31] With toluidine blue, the organism stains deep purple while erythrocytes stain blue.[32] The organism also stains with acridine orange.[26,33,34] When illuminated with ultraviolet light the acridine orange stained organism fluoresces a bright yellow colour with an orange tinge, against a yellow–green background.

The pleomorphic and epicellular nature of *H. felis* has been confirmed by transmission and scanning electron microscopic examination. Rods, rings, coccoid, conical and discoid shaped forms of the organism have been observed.[31,35–38] The coccoid and discoid forms vary in diameter from 0.2–0.6 μ.[17,31]

All forms of the organism are surrounded by a single membrane. The cytoplasm consists of electron-dense granules of varying size and density. There is no evidence of cytoplasmic organelles although the presence of microtubules beneath the surrounding membrane has been reported.[35] Electron-lucent areas (vacuoles) have been observed in both round and rod-shaped organisms[35,37] but it is not clear whether these are true vacuoles or invaginations from the surface membrane of the organism.

H. felis organisms attach to the host erythrocytic membrane by intermittent contact points and are partially buried in indented areas of the erythrocytes, with a substantial portion projecting beyond the erythrocytic surface.[31,35,36] Smudging of the erythrocytic membrane in contact with the organism has been reported.[37] In addition shallow, smooth-edged pock-marks, thought to be lesions produced by adherence of the organism to the erythrocyte, have been observed.[36] However, complete erosion of the erythrocytic membranes has not been documented.[17] Sometimes organisms attach to

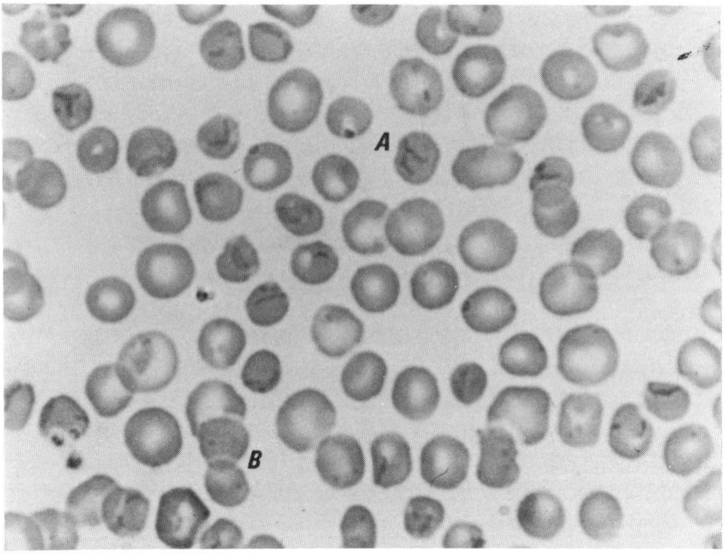

FIG. 4.1. *H. canis* chain (A) and single parasites (B) in canine erythrocytes. (Modified Wrights stain; × 1000).

more than one erythrocyte, resulting in joining of adjacent erythrocytes by an intervening series of organisms.[37]

H. canis

H. canis is similar to *H. felis* in many respects. It is pleomorphic, occurring as small dots, cocci, rings or rods; the coccoid form being observed most frequently. Unlike *H. felis*, the organism commonly forms single or branching chains, measuring up to 5.0 μ, which extend across the surface of the affected erythrocyte. However, individual organisms may also be observed,[17,39,40] (Fig. 4.1). With light microscopy, the coccoid form measures 0.2 to 1.0 μ in diameter; the ring form 0.4 to 3.0 μ while the rods may be 3.0 to 6.0 μ or more in length.[20,41,42]

Ultrastructural studies have confirmed the pleomorphic nature of the organism. Coccoid, rod, and ring forms have been described; with the organism occurring singly, in small groups, or in chains on the erythrocytic surface.[3,41,43,44] With electron microscopy, the coccoid form measures 0.2–1.4 μ in diameter while the rods are 0.3–3.2 μ long.[40.43]

The organism has a single trilaminar membrane. The cytoplasm consists mainly of small, dense, granular, ribosomal-like material and, less frequently, fine filamentous material.[40]

The organism is situated epicellularly in folds or indented areas on the surface of erythrocytes. At some points it may adhere so closely to the erythrocytic membrane that no clear separation is visible between the membranes of the organism and the erythrocyte. However, erosion or penetration of the erythrocytic membrane does not occur.[3,40,43,44] Chains of organisms can occur in grooves or deep infolding, producing marked distortion of the erythrocyte.[40,41,44]

Epidemiology

Geographic distribution

Reported cases of canine and feline haemobartonellosis indicate that both diseases occur worldwide. They have been reported in Africa, North and South America, Asia, Australia and Europe.

Hosts

H. felis. The host range of any *Haemobartonella* species is restricted to a given species of animal and closely related host species.[1] Thus *H. felis* has been reported mainly in domestic cats. A *Haemobartonella*-like organism has been reported in association with anemia in three exotic felidae; a tiger cat (*Leopardus pardinoides*), an ocelot (*Leopardus pardalis*), and a fishing cat (*Prinonailurus viverrinus*).[45] *H. felis* is not infective to rats, mice, swine, cattle, sheep or dogs.[46,47]

All breeds of domestic cats are susceptible to *H. felis* infection. Though one report suggested a relatively greater risk of infection in male cats and all cats of mixed breed,[48] other studies have shown no significant differences between different breeds or between sexes.[29,49] The risk for *H. felis* infection increases with age, peaking at 4 to 6.5 years.[29,48]

H. canis. Naturally occurring *H. canis* infection has been reported only in dogs although experimental subclinical infection of cats with *H. canis* has been reported.[2]

H. canis infection has been encountered in a variety of dog breeds, in both sexes and in dogs aged from six weeks to more than ten years; though most of the reported cases have been in adult dogs aged 2–10 years. There are no reports of studies of risk factors for *H. canis* infection.

Transmission

H. felis. The mode of natural transmission of *H. felis* has not been established. Transmission by blood sucking arthropods such as fleas, ticks and lice has been suggested,[17,29,50] but this has not been confirmed experimentally. While the infection can be transmitted from experimentally infected queens to their newborn offspring in the absence of arthropod vectors,[17,25] it is not known if such transmission occurs *in utero*, during parturition, through milk or during nursing.

Intrauterine transmission from infected queens to kittens has been proposed, following the findings of *H. felis* in kittens less than a day old.[9] Spread of the infection via cat bites has also been suggested.[51]

H. felis has been transmitted experimentally by intraperitoneal and intravenous injection, and oral administration, of infected blood.[5,47] Filtered serum, urine and saliva of carrier cats, and of those with clinical disease, have not been infective.[17,46]

A carrier state occurs in recovered cats and in those with latent infections. Such carrier cats may act as reservoirs of infection and iatrogenic transmission can occur from these to uninfected cats.[46,47]

H. canis. Dissemination by the brown dog tick, *Rhipicephalus sanguineus* is considered to be the major mode of natural transmission of *H. canis*.[52.53] Transovarial and trans-stadial transmission of the infection has been demonstrated in this tick.[54] Thus the tick may serve as a vector and reservoir of infection. There are unconfirmed suggestions that fleas, mosquitoes, lice or flies might be alternative vectors,[53] but transmission by them has not been demonstrated. In two cases there was indirect evidence of *in utero* transmission.[55]

Experimentally, *H. canis* has been transmitted by intravenous infection and oral administration of infected blood.[17,41,44] Clinically normal dogs can act as carriers, so iatrogenic transmission of the infection can occur via blood transfusion. However, the recipient must be splenectomized or severely immunocompromized before clinical disease can occur.[52] It has not been possible to transmit the infection to puppies through maternal milk.[17]

Pathogenesis

H. felis

The prepatent period of *H. felis* in experimentally infected cats varies widely. It is neither affected by the route of infection nor by the presence or absence of the spleen.[47] The prepatent period following intraperitoneal injection of infected blood has varied from two to sixty-nine days,[47,56] and with intravenous injection from two to twenty-three days.[25,47,57] Intact cats infected orally had prepatent periods of thirteen to thirty-one days while in splenectomized cats, the period varied from twenty-two to fifty-one days.[47]

The site of localization of the parasite during the prepatent period is unknown. One probable site is the bone marrow, where the parasite has been observed on immature erythrocytes.[11] In the peripheral circulation, the parasite is seen on mature erythrocytes and does not seem to have affinity for immature erythrocytes.[8] On the erythrocyte, *H. felis* multiplies by binary fission or a form of budding.[31,35,36]

Following the appearance of *H. felis* in the peripheral circulation, parasitemia increases to a peak within 1–5 days and then declines rapidly. Thereafter the parasite appears in discrete parasitemic episodes. All parasites can disappear from the peripheral circulation in a synchronized manner within 2 h or less.[25,58] Thus between parasitemic episodes, parasites are rarely seen in the peripheral circulation. They may remain absent from the peripheral circulation for variable periods of time which in some cases may be up to 10 days or more.[15] Moreover, when the parasites are present in the peripheral circulation, there is a fluctuating degree of parasitema.

Disappearance of the parasite has been partly explained by different studies.[37,38,59,60] Following one study, it was suggested that binding of adjacent erythrocytes by common *H. felis* organisms enhances sequestration of the erythrocytes in narrow vascular spaces.[37] This sequestration potentiates the phagocytosis of such erythrocytes by macrophages of the reticuloendothelial system, a view supported by the finding of free parasites in macrophages in the lung and spleen.

Other studies[38,59,60] showed that sequestration of parasitized erythrocytes occurs in the spleen, where the parasite is detached from the erythrocyte by reticular cells without causing rupture of the host cell. The main mode in which this is done is by phagocytosis following adhesion of the parasites located on the erythrocytes to extended processes of cordal macrophages. A less frequent mode of parasite removal is by a process called pitting, in which the host cell is not destroyed. The parasite is pitted from the erythrocyte when the parasite passes between reticular cells or when the parasitized erythrocyte passes among cytoplasmic processes of the reticular cells in the splenic cord. Once the parasite is removed, the erythrocyte may be returned to circulation. This phenomenon probably explains fluctuations in the hematocrit which commonly occur in cats infected wth *H. felis*.[25,58] A rapid decrease in the hematocrit followed by an increase occurs in association with the respective appearance and disappearance of the parasite from the circulation. The decrease in the hematocrit is associated with splenic sequestration of parasitized erythrocytes while the increase occurs with the return of parasite-free erythrocytes into circulation.[59] The synchronized disappearance of the parasite has not been explained.

Anemia occurs commonly in feline haemobartonellosis but its

pathogenesis is not fully understood. Erythrophagocytosis by macrophages in the spleen, liver, lungs and bone marrow and, to a lesser extent, low levels of intravascular hemolysis, have been suggested as the causes of the anemia.[17,37,59] Hemolysis is thought to occur as a direct result of injury to the erythrocytes by the parasite, or indirectly from local ionic imbalances that result from the infection.[36] Increased erythrocytic osmotic fragility may also contribute to hemolysis. Erythrocytic fragility has been shown to increase progressively with the appearance of *H. felis* in circulation, probably as a result of membrane lipid loss, and erythrocytic fragility does not return to normal during the course of the disease, even when the parasite disappears from circulation.[58,61] This has been attributed to the return into circulation of formerly parasitized erythrocytes after removal of the parasite in the spleen. Frequent parasitemic episodes appear to result in progressive erythrocyte damage and shortened erythrocyte life span.[13]

The role of immune mechanisms in the pathogenesis of the anemia is not fully understood. Positive direct Coombs' test results and autoagglutination at both 37°C and 4°C have been reported in *H. felis* infected cats,[17,58,62] suggesting that immune mechanisms may be involved in the hemolysis that occurs following *H. felis* infection. Cold agglutinins belonging to the IgM class have been detected in *H. felis* infected cats but the significance of this is unknown.[62] Also involvement of antierythrocyte antibodies in the hemolytic process has been suggested, but not conclusively proved.[17.62]

The role of immunosuppression in the pathogenesis of *H. felis* infection has received much attention. *H. felis* has been described as unique among the genus *Haemobartonella* because it is the only species that produces patent parasitemia and anemia in nonsplenectomized animals under field conditions.[1] However the organism is probably an opportunist, like the other members of the genus, creating a secondary problem in immunocompromized cats. Many cats are asymptomatic carriers of *H. felis*, and infection can remain latent for long periods until some immunosuppressive event such as concurrent disease, pregnancy, surgery, or poisoning disturbs the immune balance between the host and parasite.[51,63] Efforts to prove this hypothesis experimentally have failed. Relapses of clinical disease could not be induced in chronically infected cats by treatment with immunosuppressive drugs, experimental abscess production or splenectomy.[64] However, it has been shown in naturally occurring infection that the presence of concurrent disease plays a significant role in the pathogenesis of feline haemobartonellosis.[49,65] Also a high degree of association has been reported between *H. felis* and feline leukemia virus (FeLV) infections.[29,49,65,66] Cats with FeLV infection may be more susceptible to *H. felis* infection or, as has been demonstrated experimentally, *H. felis* infection may increase susceptibility of cats to FeLV.[67]

H. canis

Unlike *H. felis*, little is known about the pathogenesis of *H. canis* infection. *H. canis* is an opportunist and is seldom pathogenic for nonsplenectomized healthy dogs.[53]

The prepatent period following intravenous inoculation of infected blood varies from one to 33 days or more.[17,68,69] In tick transmitted experimental infections, the prepatent period varied from 13 to 22 days.[54]

After an initial appearance in the peripheral circulation, the parasite may rapidly increase in numbers and reach a peak in about two days.[42] Thereafter the parasitemia fluctuates, with distinct parasitemic episodes and the parasite may periodically disappear from the circulation for a few days between episodes.[17,42] The mechanism responsible for the periodic disappearance of the parasite is unknown as this phenomenon has been observed in splenectomized dogs.

Anemia may develop rapidly in association with nearly constant parasitemia in some cases of *H. canis* infection. In others, the anemia develops more gradually over a period of one to two months as a result of repetitive parasitemic episodes.[17,53] The pathogenesis of the anemia is unknown but reports of icterus in some cases of *H. canis* infection indicate the hemolysis may be contributory.[18,55,70] Also, marked deformity of heavily parasitized erythrocytes has been observed[44] and these are prone to early sequestration by macrophages in the spleen and liver.

Immune mediated extravascular hemolysis has been suggested as a cause of anemia.[53] Coombs' positive hemolytic anemia has been reported in a dog with *H. canis* infection.[27]

The presence of a normal spleen protects against the development of clinical disease in dogs infected with *H. canis*[53] and such dogs remain asymptomatic carriers. Prevalence of latent infections has been reported to vary from 8 to over 50%.[17,69] Latent infections can be activated by splenectomy. Clinically significant infections in nonsplenectomized dogs have occurred concurrently with *Ehrlichia, Babesia,* bacterial and viral infections; neoplasia and other immunosuppressive diseases.[17,52] Spontaneous cases may occur following immunosuppressive drug therapy.[18,53] A few cases of clinical haemobartonellosis have been reported in previously healthy nonsplenectomized dogs.[19–23,71] Apart from doubts about the authenticity of these cases,[17] the clinical signs and hemograms suggest the presence of other diseases.

Clinical Disease

H. felis

Many of the reports with descriptions of clinical feline haemobartonellosis were publised before the effects of the association between *H. felis* infection and concurrent clinical conditions or infections were studied. More recent studies have shown that this association significantly affects the course of the disease produced by *H. felis*.[65,67]

The prevalence of *H. felis* infection in selected cat populations has varied from 0 to 28%, depending on whether the cats were ill or not. Infection is more prevalent in ill cats than healthy cats.[15,49] Not all infected cats develop clinical illness. Most cats with uncomplicated *H. felis* infection do not become ill. Among cats with concurrent diseases, the morbidity may be as high as 67–100%.[15.65] The morbidity in reported outbreaks has ranged from 60–100%.[9,10,72]

Feline haemobartonellosis is usually a disease of individual cats although in multicat households, infection may spread from one cat to another, leading to an occasional outbreak.[10,15,72]

The clinical status of an infected cat depends on previous body condition, and the presence and stage of concurrent diseases. Uncomplicated *H. felis* infection is usually subclinical or causes mild disease which is characterized by a mild regenerative anemia.[8,65,67] The cats are usually bright and alert.

Clinical feline haemobartonellosis usually occurs in cats with concurrent diseases.[15,65] It is characterized in most cases by a gradual onset during which cats show nonspecific signs of illness such as depression, lethargy, weakness and progressive weight loss. This may last for 2 to 4 or more weeks. In a few cases, the onset of clinical disease may be marked by sudden collapse and prostration.[63,65] Such cases are usually seen when the progressive anemia, which has probably been developing for some time, reaches a crisis stage. These cats are very pale, with cold extremities and rapidly become moribund.[15]

Anorexia, or various degrees of inappetence, are observed in cats with haemobartonellosis. In a few cases it may be accompanied by halitosis.

Pyrexia is an inconsistent feature of feline haemobartonellosis and when it does occur, it is usually in association with concurrent bacterial or viral infection, or autoimmune disease.[15] Moribund cats often have a subnormal rectal temperature.

Anemia is the most outstanding feature of feline haemobartonellosis. It usually develops gradually and the cat may lose a considerable amount of body weight but still remain bright and alert. In some other cases, however, anemia develops rapidly, causing a sudden drop in the hematocrit. This occurs commonly in cats wth concurrent FeLV infection. Such cats are usually in good bodily condition but have a high level of *H. felis* parasitemia.[15] Mild to moderate icterus and bilirubinuria occur occasionally in cats with concurrent FeLV infection.

The severity of clinical signs often depends on the degree of anemia. The anemia is characterized by moderate to severe pallor of the mucous membranes, skin and sclera. Usually there is tachycardia and the pulse may be feeble. Severely anemic cats may have hemic murmurs.[15,65,73] Tachypnoea or dyspnoea may be observed in some cats at rest and such cats may become cyanotic or collapse after slight exertion. In one unusual case, a cat with concurrent *H. felis* and FeLV infections developed neurologic signs, characterized by periodic convulsions, circling, and champing of the jaws as a result of anemic cerebral anoxia.[15] The convulsions became more frequent as the disease progressed.

Splenomegaly, hepatomegaly, lymph node enlargement and dehydration, though widely reported, seem to occur only in cats with concurrent FeLV infection.[65]

It is difficult to assess the mortality due to *H. felis* infection because many infected cats die from concurrent illnesses rather than anemia caused by *H. felis* infection. Reported mortality (including euthanasia) among all infected cats ranges from 0 to 75%.[10,47,48,65] Among cats with apparently uncomplicated infection, the mortality rate has varied from 0 to 33%, while in those with concurrent diseases it has ranged from 56 to 100%.[11,65] Mortality in experimentally induced disease has varied from about 12 to 35%.[25,46]

H. canis

Information regarding the prevalence of *H. canis* infection in dog populations is scanty. Estimates of latent infections range from 8 to over 50%.[53] There are no reports of outbreaks of the infection.

Most infected dogs do not develop clinical disease. The development of clinical disease is affected by splenectomy, presence of splenic disease, concurrent infections with viruses, bacteria or other hemoparasites, neoplasia, or immunosuppression caused by disease or drugs.[18,52] Thus canine haemobartonellosis is essentially a disease of the splenectomized or immunocompromized individual dog. In an experimental study, two out of three splenectomized dogs developed clinical illness following inoculation of infective blood while nonsplenectomized dogs remained healthy.[70]

Clinical signs that have been described in naturally occurring and experimental infections include listlessness, anorexia, variable pyrexia, anemia and icterus.[18,69,70,74]

Anemia is the most consistent finding. It is usually mild to moderate, and clinical signs are not usually observed until the hematocrit drops below 20%.[52] Icterus occurs infrequently and is usually mild. Splenomegaly, hepatomegaly and lymph node enlargement are variable.

Even though there have been fatalities associated with canine haemobartonellosis,[19,27] most dogs recover following treatment.

Hematology

H. felis

Feline haemobartonellosis is characterized by a regenerative anemia. The degree of anemia depends on the stage of the disease and also influences the magnitude of regenerative response.[15,65] Anemia is more severe in cats with concurrent *H. felis* and FeLV infections than in *H. felis* infected FeLV-free cats.

The hematocrit fluctuates over time. It declines as the parasitemia increases and may increase dramatically following the disappearance of the parasites from circulation.[25,46]

During the early stages of the disease, the anemia may be nonregenerative and thus be normocytic and normochromic. However, as the anemia becomes more severe, it becomes macrocytic and often hypochromic.[65] There is reticulocytosis and the number of reticulocytes in circulation may be as high as 85–91% of the erythrocytes.[15,57] Varying degrees of anisocytosis and polychromasia occur. Occasional poikilocytosis may be observed in cats with concurrent FeLV infection.

Erythrocytes containing Howell–Jolly bodies are more numerous than usual and may be present in more than half of the erythrocytes in some cases. Nucleated erythrocytes may also be present, being numerous in severely anemic animals.

Total and differential leukocyte counts are variable. There may be an increase in the number of neutrophils and platelets as part of the bone marrow response.[5] In some cats with concurrent FeLV infection, myeloid precursors and some bizarre leukocytes are found in circulation.[15] Erythrophagocytosis by mononuclear cells, or rarely by neutrophils, has been observed shortly after the initial parasitemia.[58]

The bone marrow myeloid: erythroid ratios are normal during the early stages of the disease but decrease as erythropoiesis increases in response to the anemia.[25]

Increased erythrocytic sedimentation rates and erythrocyte osmotic fragility have been reported. Autoagglutination and positive direct Coombs' test have also been reported.[17,58,62] The Coombs' test becomes positive within a week of the initial parasitemia.

H. canis

The anemias in canine and feline haemobartonellosis are similar in many respects. In the early stages of canine haemobartonellosis, the anemia is mild and nonregenerative. However, because the hematocrit usually has to fall below 20% before clinical signs are observed, a regenerative anemia is observed in most naturally occurring cases.[52] The anemia is characterized by anisocytosis, reticulocytosis and polychromasia. There is an increased number of erythrocytes with Howell–Jolly bodies, nucleated erythrocytes, target cells and leptocytes. Macrocytosis may not be present when the dog is first examined because it requires more time to develop. Spherocytosis and positive Coombs' test results have been reported.[27]

Changes in the leukogram are not consistent and this is because most cases are probably accompanied by overt or subclinical concurrent diseases.

Clinical Chemistry

H. felis

Plasma protein concentrations are usually normal but may be moderately elevated during the acute phase of the disease.[25]

Hyperbilirubinemia may occur in some cats during the acute phase of the disease but this is not consistently observed.[3] When there is icterus due to severe hemolysis, the urine may contain traces of bile.[11] Hemoglobinuria is rare.

H. canis

Biochemical abnormalities are rare in canine haemobartonellosis and only occur where there is severe anemia or concurrent disease. Bilirubinemia, hemoglobinemia and hemoglobinuria are usually not observed. However, significant bilirubinuria may occur.[52]

Pathology

H. felis

There are no specific or pathognomonic pathologic findings in feline haemobartonellosis. Cats with concurrent FeLV infection develop more pronounced lesions than those with *H. felis* infection alone.[65]

The tissues are usually pale and, in a few cases, icteric. The blood is watery and there may be transudates in the thoracic and abdominal cavities in severely anemic cats. Evidence of moderate to severe weight loss is observed in more than half of the cases.[15,17]

The liver is often pale, yellow, or mottled without any evidence of biliary obstruction. Hepatomegaly is rare. Splenomegaly and lymph node enlargment have been reported,[5,17] but these occur mostly in cats with concurrent FeLV infection.[65] The bone marrow is red in most cases.

Histologic findings in the liver include fatty change, centrilobular congestion, and centrilobular degeneration as a result of hypoxia. In cats with concurrent FeLV, there may be hemosiderosis, or evidence of extramedullary hemopoiesis in the liver. In the spleen, there is passive congestion, extramedullary hemopoiesis, follicular hyperplasia, erythrophagocytosis, and hemosiderosis.[11,15,17] Occasionally, reactive lymphoid hyperplasia may occur in the lymph nodes.

Erythroid hyperplasia is the most common finding in the bone marrow, although in cats with FeLV infection, there may be myeloid hyperplasia or myelofibrosis.

In rare cases, lesions of cerebral anoxia, including ischemia of the neurons, may be present.

H. canis

Reports of pathologic findings in primary canine haemobartonellosis are few. The macroscopic findings include pallor of the tissues, generalized icterus and splenomegaly. The blood appears thin and the bone marrow is red and gelatinous.[17,27,55]

Histologic findings include hemosiderosis in the liver and hyperplasia of the reticuloendothelial system.

Immunity

Little is known about immune responses in feline and canine haemobartonellosis. In the cat, antibodies against *H. felis* have been found in infected animals.[5] Despite this, it seems that clinically recovered cats are unable to eliminate the parasite from the blood and may remain chronically infected for a long time.[15,64] These cats seem to be in an equilibrium whereby replication of the parasite is balanced by phagocytosis. It is not known if recovered cats are resistant to reinfection.

Antierythrocytic antibody has been reported in a dog with *H. canis* infection.[27] However, nothing is known about humoral or cell-mediated immunity to the infection.

Diagnosis

There are no specific or pathognomonic clinical or pathological findings for feline or canine haemobartonellosis. Definitive diagnosis of infection requires the demonstration of parasitized erythrocytes.

H. felis

Histochemical methods that have been used in the demonstration of the organism by light microscopy include toluidine blue[32] and the Romanowsky staining procedures (Giemsa, Wright, Leishman and May–Grunwald–Giemsa).[5,34] The toluidine blue method is unreliable in detecting the parasite. The films tend to stain lightly and few parasites are detectable, even in samples with a high parasitemia.[15]

Descriptions of the Romanowsky procedures are available elsewhere.[3,5,75] The May–Grunwald–Giemsa method is the most efficient of these methods.[34] It reveals more parasites per microscopic field and leaves fewer stain deposits on the film. However, it is more complex and takes longer to perform than the other techniques. We use a modification of the May–Grunwald–Giemsa procedure earlier described[75] as follows: Freshly made blood films are air-dried and fixed in methanol for 10 min. They are then stained in a coplin jar containing May–Grunwald stain, freshly diluted with an equal volume of phosphate buffer, pH 6.8, for 10 min. The films are rinsed briefly in phosphate buffer, pH 6.8, and transferred to a jar containing Giemsa stain, freshly diluted with nine volumes of phosphate buffer, pH 6.5 for 15 min. The films are rinsed in phosphate buffer as before and stained in another jar of Giemsa stain for 15 min. The films are then differentiated in buffer, pH 6.8, for 3–5 min, rinsed in 3 or 4 changes of distilled water and air dried.

With the Romanowsky staining procedures, the reagents readily precipitate and leave stain deposits which may be difficult to differentiate from the parasite. Therefore attention to detail is necessary to avoid artefacts. Glass slides must be clean and grease-free, so are best washed and left in acid–alcohol until needed. The stain solutions should be filtered daily with ashless filter paper. Slides may be stained, horizontally inverted over a shallow trough, or vertically in a jar, and the reagents should not be allowed to dry out. Where an automatic stainer is used, the plate should be cleaned with alcohol and lint-free soft tissue just before staining the films.

Acridine orange staining is more efficient than the Romanowsky staining procedures for detecting *H. felis*,[5,34,76] but requires ultraviolet microscopy. The parasites are readily detected and can be distinguished from Howell–Jolly bodies. The method described by Small[33] is easier to use and requires little blood. Microcapillary blood from the pinna can be used. However the blood films need to be fixed for 24 h. Acridine orange solution is unstable, so fresh solutions should be made from a 0.1% solution which is stable at 4°C for up to four weeks.

A major problem in the detection of *H. felis* is the cyclical parasitemia. Therefore, blood smears from a cat should be examined on consecutive days for at least 10–14 days before the cat can be regarded as being free of the infection.

H. felis organisms are removed from the erythrocytes by chelating agents like ethylene diamine tetra acetic acid (EDTA). Thus in blood samples stored in EDTA, the number of erythrocytes with *H. felis* decreases with time, and in some cases the parasite may disappear from the erythrocytes as quickly as 3 h after storage.[15] Therefore, films should be made from freshly drawn blood to enhance detection of the parasite.

H. felis must be differentiated from *Cytauxzoon felis* and *Babesia felis* which are also erythrocytic parasites that cause anemia in cats. Both are protozoa, with cytoplasm and intracytoplasmic chromatin or nuclear material.

Feline haemobartonellosis can be diagnosed by the indirect fluorescent antibody test.[5] This test is as efficient as acridine orange staining and is useful for diagnosis in the absence of a parasitemia.

Attempts at serodiagnosis of *H. felis* using Coombs' test lacked specificity and sensitivity.[77] Moreover, efforts that have been made to develop an enzyme-linked immunosorbent assay (ELISA)[76] have been unsuccessful.

H. canis

Romanowsky staining procedures are the only methods that have been used for the demonstration of *H. canis*.[43,44] The parasite tends to form chains of organisms across the erythrocytic surface, although single parasites may also be present. At times parasites are so few that they may be difficult to detect, especially in poorly prepared blood films. Therefore, as for *H. felis*, attention to details in the preparation and staining of blood films is necessary.

There are no serologic tests for detecting *H. canis* infection.

Treatment

The goal in the treatment of haemobartonellosis is to eliminate the parasite and restore the erythrocytic parameters to normal values. To achieve this, specific drug therapy against the parasite and, where necessary, supportive measures are employed.

H. felis

Various antimicrobial agents have been used in attempts to eliminate *H. felis* but there are no reports of satisfactorily controlled evaluations of these agents. Results have been variable.

Oxytetracycline has been widely used and it is presently the drug of choice. Tetracycline is the second choice. These are given orally at doses of 25 and 22 mg/kg, respectively, three times daily for two to three weeks.[5,15,17,53]

Chloramphenicol at a dose of 10 to 15 mg/kg, up to a maximum of 50 mg/cat, twice a day for 10 to 14 days have been found to be effective in about half the cases of *H. felis* infection.[5] An initial loading dose of 100 mg may be advantageous. This drug often causes erythroid hypoplasia at high doses but at the above dose and duration of treatment, adverse effects are few and mild.[57,78]

Thiacetarsamide sodium injected intravenously at 1.0 to 1.1 mg/kg given on two occasions 48 h apart, has been effective in some cases but not in others.[57,64,79] The drug is no more effective than oxytetracycline, and it may cause toxicity, characterized by depression, vomiting and diarrhoea.[5]

Oxytetracycline, tetracycline, chloramphenicol and thiacetarsamide sodium do not completely eliminate *H. felis* from infected cats though clincal recovery may occur.[15,17,57] Thus recovered animals may remain carriers of infection for a long time.

Short term corticosteroid therapy at 1–2 mg/kg orally, daily, has been recommended in conjunction with tetracycline. The purpose of this is to reduce immune mediated hemolysis and inhibit erythrophagocytosis.[5,17] However opinions differ as to the beneficial effects of this.[5,57]

The most beneficial supportive measure is blood transfusion. Cats with hematocrit levels below 15% usually require transfusion. A single transfusion of 50–60 ml of fresh whole blood usually suffices in FeLV-free cats. Anemic FeLV-positive cats are likely to benefit only transiently from blood transfusions.[15,65]

Other beneficial supportive therapy includes administration of B-complex vitamins and a high protein diet to aid erythropoiesis. Hematinics are not indicated. Administration of parenteral glucose has been recommended in moribund cats since hypoglycemia has been observed in such cases.[17] The need for fluid therapy must be carefully evaluated because the subsequent hemodilution will exacerbate existing anemia.

The long term prognosis for FeLV-free cats that recover from haemobartonellosis is good if there are no severe complicating diseases.[15,65] Although these cats may have the latent infection for a long time, most of them remain healthy, with very low parasitemias. FeLV-positive cats with concurrent haemobartonellosis have a poor long term prognosis. Some may recover from haemobartonellosis but many eventually develop FeLV-related diseases, recrudescence of *H. felis* parasitemia, severe anemia and death.

H. canis

Very little has been done to evaluate therapy for canine haemobartonellosis.[68,69] Antimicrobial agents which may have been effective in treating canine haemobartonellosis are oxytetracycline, orally at 40 mg/kg twice daily for 9 to 14 days; chloramphenicol intravenously at 22 mg/kg for nine days; and thiacetarsamide intravenously at 0.22 ml/kg of a 10% solution for 9 days.[69,74] Oxytetracycline has been most widely used and it is probably the drug of choice.

Therapy with corticosteroids to reduce immune mediated hemolysis has been recommended.[74] The dose should be decreased gradually as the hematocrit rises. Blood transfusion is indicated in dogs with severe anemia.

The long term prognosis for uncomplicated canine haemobartonellosis is good. Recrudescence of clinical disease in recovered dogs has not been reported. However, low parasitemias have been detected in some cases a few months after recovery.[69,74] Thus recovered dogs may have latent infections.

Control

Haemobartonellosis can be prevented by eliminating blood sucking arthropod vectors from dogs and cats. Ticks transmit *H. canis*[54] while fleas are suspected to be vectors of *H. felis*.[17,29] Avoidance of areas where these vectors are abundant and treatment of the animals with topical parasiticides will reduce, if not eliminate, the arthropod vectors.

To prevent iatrogenic transmission of haemobartonellosis through blood transfusion, donor animals should be splenectomized. Their blood should be checked on consecutive days for at least 4–6 weeks after splenectomy and thereafter, periodically for *Haemobartonella* infection.

References

1. Ristic, M. and Kreier, J.P. 1984. Family III. Anaplasmataceae. In: *Bergey's Manual of Systematic Bacteriology*. Vol. 1, 9th edn, pp. 719–729. Kreig, N.R. and Holt, J.G. (Eds). Williams and Wilkins, Baltimore/London.
2. Kreier, J.P. and Ristic, M. 1968. Haemobartonellosis, Eperythrozoonosis, Grahamellosis and Ehrlichiosis. In: *Infectious Blood Diseases of Man and Animals*. Vol. 2, pp. 387–472. Weinmann, D. and Ristic, M. (Eds), Academic Press, New York.
3. Jain, N.C. 1986. *Schalm's Veterinary Hematology,* 4th edn., pp. 602–608. Lea and Febiger, Philadelphia.
4. Clark, R. 1942. *Eperythrozoon felis* (Sp. Nov.) in a cat. *J.S. Afr. vet. Med. Assoc.* **13:** 15–17.
5. Small, E. and Ristic, M. 1987. Haemobartonellosis. In: *Diseases of the Cat: Medicine and Surgery,* pp. 301–308. Holzworth, J. (Ed.), W.B. Saunders Company, Philadelphia.
6. Flint, J.C. and Moss, L.C., 1953. Infectious anaemia in cats. *J. Am. vet. Med. Ass.* **122:** 45–48.
7. Flint, J.C. and McKelvie, D.H. 1955. Feline infectious anaemia—Diagnosis and treatment. *Proc. Am. vet. Med. Ass.* **92:** 240–242.
8. Seamer, JC. and Douglas, S.W. 1959. A new blood parasite of British cats. *Vet. Rec.* **71:** 405–408.
9. Harbutt, P.R. 1963. A clinical appraisal of feline infectious anaemia and its transmission under natural conditions. *Aust. vet. J.* **39:** 401–404.
10. Bedford, P.G.C. 1970. Feline infectious anaemia in the London area. *Vet. Rec.* **87:** 305–310.
11. Holzworth, J. 1956. Anemia in the cat. *J. Am. vet. Med. Ass.* **128:** 471–488.
12. Balazs, T., Robinson, J., Grey, D. and Grice, H.C. 1961. Feline haemobartonellosis—A case report. *Can. J. comp. Med. Vet. Sci.* **25:** 220–222.
13. Maede, Y. 1975. Studies on feline haemobartonellosis IV. Lifespan of erythrocytes of cats infected with *Haemobartonella felis*. *Jap. J. Vet. Sci.* **37:** 269–272.
14. Hathaway, J.E. 1976. Feline anaemia. *Vet. clin. North Am.* **6:** 495–510.
15. Bobade, P.A. 1980. Anaemia in the cat with particular reference to infection with *Haemobartonella felis*. M.V.M. Thesis, University of Glasgow.
16. Kikuth, W. 1928. Uber einen neuen anamieereger *Bartonella canis,* nov spec. *Klin. Wochenschr.* **7:** 1729–1730.
17. Harvey, J.W. 1984. Haemobartonellosis. In: *Clinical Microbiology and Infectious Diseases of the Dog and Cat,* pp. 576–587. Greene, C.E. (Ed.), W.B. Saunders Company, Philadelphia.
18. Handcock, W.J. 1989. Clinical haemobartonellosis associated with use of corticosteroid. *Vet. Rec.* **125:** 585.
19. North, D.C. 1978. Fatal haemobartonellosis in a non-splenectomised dog—a case report. *J. Small Anim. Pract.* **19:** 769–773.
20. West, H.J. 1979. Haemobartonellosis in the dog. *J. Small Anim. Pract.* **20:** 543–549.
21. Austerman, J.W. 1979. Haemobartonellosis in a non-splenectomised dog. *Vet. Med. Small Anim. Clin.* **74:** 954.
22. Gretillat, S. 1981. *Haemobartonella canis* (Kikuth, 1928) in the blood of dogs with parvovirus disease. *J. Small Anim. Pract.* **22:** 647–653.
23. Ingle, R.T. 1946. Bartonella infection in a dog. *North Am. Vet.* **27:** 501.
24. Bellocq, B. and Lacroze, R. 1955. *Rev. Corps Vet. Armee* **4:** 156 (cited by Kreier, J.P. and Ristic, M. 1968).[2]

25. HARVEY, J.W. and GASKIN, J.M. 1977. Experimental feline haemobartonellosis. *J. Am. Anim. Hosp. Ass.* **13:** 28–38.
26. SMALL, E. and RISTIC, M. 1967. Morphologic features of *Haemobartonella felis*. *Am. J. vet. Res.* **28:** 845–851.
27. BUNDZA, A., LUMSDEN, J.H., MCSHERRY, B.J., VALLI, V.E.O. and JANZEN, E.A. 1976. Haemobartonellosis in a dog in association with Coombs' positive anaemia. *Can. vet. J.* **17:** 267–270.
28. HARVEY, J.W. 1977. Feline hematology. *Proc. 44th Annual Meeting, Am. Anim. Hosp. Assoc.* 75–79.
29. NASH, A.S. and BOBADE, P.A. 1986. *Haemobartonella felis* infection in cats from the Glasgow area. *Vet. Rec.* **119:** 373–375.
30. BUTT, M.T. 1990. Diagnosing erythrocyte parasitic diseases in cats. *Compend. Contin. Ed. Pract. Vet.* **12:** 628–638.
31. MAEDE, Y. and SONODA, M. 1975. Studies on feline haemobartonellosis III. Scanning electron microscopy of *Haemobartonella felis*. *Jap. J. vet. Sci.* **37:** 209–211.
32. WILKINSON, G.T. 1969. Feline infectious anaemia. *Vet. Rec.* **84:** 331–333.
33. SMALL, E. 1971. Feline infectious anaemia. In: *Current Veterinary Therapy IV. Small Animal Practice,* p. 681. KIRK, R.W. (Ed.), W.B. Saunders Company, Philadelphia.
34. BOBADE, P.A. and NASH, A.S. 1987. A comparative study of the efficiency of acridine orange and some Romanowsky staining procedures in the demonstration of *Haemobartonella felis* in feline blood. *Vet. Parasitol.* **26:** 169–172.
35. DEMAREE, R.S. JR and NESSMITH, W.B. 1972. Ultrastructure of *Haemobartonella felis* from a naturally infected cat. *Am. J. vet. Res.* **33:** 1303–1308.
36. JAIN, N.C. and KEETON, K.S. 1973. Scanning electron microscopic features of *Haemobartonella felis*. *Am. J. vet. Res.* **34:** 697–700.
37. SIMPSON, C.F., GASKIN, J.M. and HARVEY, J.W. 1978. Ultrastructure of erythrocytes parasitized by *Haemobartonella felis*. *J. Parasit.* **64:** 504–511.
38. MAEDE, Y. and MURATA, H. 1978. Ultrastructural observation on the removal of *Haemobartonella felis* from erythrocytes in the spleen of a cat. *Jap. J. vet. Sci.* **40:** 203–205.
39. BUCKNER, R.G. and EWING, S.A. 1971. Canine haemobartonellosis. In: *Current Veterinary Therapy IV. Small Animal Practice*, p. 680. KIRK, R.W. (Ed.), W.B. Saunders Company, Philadelphia.
40. MCKEE, A.E., ZIEGLER, R.F. and GILES, R.C. 1973. Scanning and transmission electron microscopy of *Haemobartonella canis* and *Eperythrozoon ovis*. *Am. J. vet. Res.* **34:** 1196–1201.
41. VENABLE, J.H. and EWING, S.A. 1968. Fine-structure of *Haemobartonella canis* (Rickettsiales: Bartonellaceae) and its relation to the host erythrocyte. *J. Parasit.* **54:** 259–268.
42. WRIGHT, I.G. 1971. The isolation of *Haemobartonella canis* in association with *Babesia canis* in a splenectomised dog. *Aust. vet. J.* **47:** 157–159.
43. BELLAMY, J.E.C., MACWILLIAMS, P.S. and SEARCY, G.P. 1978. Cold-agglutinin haemolytic anaemia and *Haemobartonella canis* infection in a dog. *J. Am. vet. Med. Ass.* **173:** 397–401.
44. SONODA, M., TAKAHASHI, K., TAMURA, T. and KOIWA, M. 1978. Studies on canine haemobartonellosis I. *Haemobartonella canis* detected in the blood of dogs inoculated with *Babesia gibsoni*. *Jap. J. vet. Sci.* **40:** 335–341.
45. KRAFT, W. 1974. Haemobartonellose/Eperythrozoonose bei tigerkatze, ozelot und fischkatze. *Kleintierpraxis* **19:** 267–269.

46. SPLITTER, E.J., CASTRO, E.R. and KANAWYER, W.L. 1956. Feline infectious anaemia. *Vet. Med.* **51:** 17–22.
47. FLINT, J.C., ROEPKE, M.H. and JENSEN, R. 1959. Feline infectious anaemia II. Experimental cases. *Am. J. vet. Res.* **20:** 33–40.
48. HAYES, H.M. and PRIESTER, W.A. 1973. Feline infectious anaemia. Risk by age, sex and breed; prior disease; seasonal occurrence; mortality. *J. Small Anim. Pract.* **14:** 797–804.
49. GRINDEM, C.B., CORBETT, W.T. and TOMKINS, M.T. 1990. Risk factors for *Haemobartonella felis* infection in cats. *J. Am. vet. Med. Ass.* **196:** 96–99.
50. EDWARDS, F.B. 1960. A new blood parasite in British cats. *Vet. Rec.* **72:** 439.
51. FLINT, J.C., ROEPKE, M.H. and JENSEN, R. 1958. Feline infectious anaemia I. Clinical aspects. *Am. J. vet. Res.* **19:** 164–168.
52. HIBLER, S.C., HOSKINS, J.D. and GREENE, C.E. 1986. Rickettsial infection in dogs Part III. Salmon disease complex and haemobartonellosis. *Compend. Contin. Ed. Pract. Vet.* **8:** 251–257.
53. MACWILLIAMS, P.S. 1987. Erythrocytic Rickettsia and Protozoa of the dog and cat. *Vet. clin. North Am. Small Anim. Pract.* **17:** 1443–1461.
54. SENEVIRATNA, P., WEERASINGHE, N. and ARIYADASA, S. 1973. Transmission of *Haemobartonella canis* by the dog tick, *Rhipicephalus sanguineus. Res. vet. Sci.* **14:** 112–114.
55. KRAKOWKA, S. 1977. Transplacentally acquired microbial and parasitic diseases of dogs. *J. Am. vet. Med. Assoc.* **171:** 750–753.
56. SCHWARTZMAN, R.M. and BESCH, E.D. 1958. Feline infectious anaemia. *Vet. Med.* **53:** 494–500.
57. WATSON, A.D.J., FARROW, B.R.H. and HOSKIN. L.P. 1978. Some observations on treating cats infected with *Haemobartonella felis. Aust. vet. Pract.* **8:** 129–132.
58. MAEDE, Y. and HATA, R. 1975. Studies on feline haemobartonellosis II. The mechanism of anemia produced by infection with *Haemobartonella felis. Jap. J. vet. Sci.* **37:** 49–54.
59. MAEDE, Y. 1978. Studies on feline haemobartonellosis V. Role of the spleen in cats infected with *Haemobartonella felis. Jap. J. vet. Sci.* **40:** 141–146.
60. MAEDE, Y. 1979. Sequestration and phagocytosis of *Haemobartonella felis* in the spleen. *Am. J. vet. Res.* **40:** 691–695.
61. MAEDE, Y. 1980. Studies on feline haemobartonellosis VI. Changes of erythrocyte lipids concentration and their relation to osmotic fragility. *Jap. J. vet. Sci.* **42:** 281–288.
62. ZULTY, J.C. and KOCIBA, G.J. 1990. Cold agglutinins in cats with haemobartonellosis. *J. Am. vet. Med. Ass.* **196:** 907–910.
63. WALTNER-TOEWS, D. 1981. Organophosphate poisoning and hemobartonellosis in a cat. *Med. vet. Pract.* **62:** 48.
64. HARVEY, J.W. and GASKIN, J.M. 1978. Feline haemobartonellosis: Attempts to induce relapses of clinical disease in chronically infected cats. *J. Am. Anim. Hosp. Ass.* **14:** 453–456.
65. BOBADE, P.A., NASH, A.S. and ROGERSON, P. 1988. Feline haemobartonellosis: Clinical, haematological and pathological studies in natural infections, and the relationship to infection with feline leukaemia virus. *Vet. Rec.* **122:** 32–36.
66. PRIESTER, W.A. and HAYES, H.M. 1973. Feline leukemia after feline infectious anemia. *J. natn. Cancer Inst.* **51:** 289–291.
67. KOCIBA, G.J., WEISER, M.G. and OLSEN, R.G. 1983. Enhanced susceptibility to feline leukemia virus in cats with *Haemobartonella felis* infection. *Leuk. Rev. Int.* **1:** 88–89.

68. Buckner, R.G. and Ewing, S.A. 1967. Experimental treatment of canine ehrlichiosis and haemobartonellosis. *J. Am. vet. Med. Ass.* **150:** 1524–1530.
69. Pryor, W.H. Jr and Bradbury, R.P. 1975. *Haemobartonella canis* infection in research dogs. *Lab. Anim. Sci.* **25:** 566–569.
70. Seino, M., Sonoda, M., Takahashi, M., Kurosawa, T. and Koiwa, M. 1984. Studies on canine haemobartonellosis I. Clinical observations on dogs inoculated with *Haemobartonella canis*. *J. College of Dairying,* Hokkaido, Japan **10:** 399–412.
71. Biondini, J., Lopes, Z., Viana, F.A.B. and Araujo, T. 1983. Diagnostico laboratorial de *Haemobartonella canis* em Belo Horizonte, MG. *Arq. Bras. Med. vet. Zoot.* **35:** 743–744.
72. Ojeda, J.D. and Skewes, H.R. 1978. Haemobartonellosis felina. Comunicacion de un brote y su tratamiento. *Vet. Mex.* **9:** 55–60.
73. Fisher, E.W., Toth, S. and Collier, W.O. 1983. Anaemia in a litter of Siamese kittens. *J. Small Anim. Pract.* **24:** 215–219.
74. Middleton, D.J., Moore, A.S. and Medhurst, C.L. 1982. Haemobartonellosis in a dog. *Aust. vet. J.* **59:** 29–31.
75. Archer, R.K. 1977. Technical methods. In: *Comparative Clinical Haematology*, pp. 537–610. Archer, R.K. and Jeffcott, L.B. (Eds), Blackwell Scientific Publications, Oxford.
76. Turner, C.M.R., Bloxham, P.A., Cox, F.E.G. and Turner, C.B. 1986. Unreliable diagnosis of *Haemobartonella felis*. *Vet. Rec.* **119:** 534–535.
77. Sheriff, D. 1974. Feline infectious anaemia. *Vet. Rec.* **94:** 385.
78. Watson, A.D.J. 1991. Chloramphenicol 2. Clinical pharmacology in dogs and cats. *Aust. vet. J.* **68:** 2–5.
79. Sauerwein, G. and Grabner, A. 1982. Zur behandlung der Haemobartonellose der katze mit thioacetarsamid—natrium (Caparsolate). *Kleintierpraxis* **27:** 323–328.

5

Eperythrozoonoses

G. R. SCOTT AND Z. WOLDEHIWET

Introduction

In the first decade of the 20th century Barton[1] and other pioneer observers of pleomorphic organisms in or on erythrocytes of man and animals assumed that the parasites were protozoa. Most other workers at that time did not believe that the bodies were live. With time four genera were identified and were classified as rickettsias, despite growth of three of them in cell-free media.[2] The fourth genus, *Eperythrozoon,* is herein discussed.

Eperythrozoon coccoides was first observed independently in the blood of splenectomized mice by Schilling[3] in Germany and Dinger[4] in the Netherlands. Since then similar organisms have been described as parasitizing erythrocytes of man and several domestic and wild species of animals;[5] most were detected fortuitously complicating severely stressed animals. Three, *Ep. ovis, Ep. suis* and *Ep. wenyonii,* however, are pathogenic in their own right in sheep, pigs and cattle respectively. Three nonpathogenic species of domestic animals are *Ep. parvum* in pigs and *Ep. teganodes* and *Ep. tuomii* in cattle.

Causative Agent

Background

Hindsight indicates that Doyle[6] in 1932 was the first to recognize pathogenic eperythrozoons parasitizing the blood of domestic animals when he described a rickettsia-like or anaplasmosis-like disease in pigs. He did not identify the parasite. Neitz and his colleagues,[7] two years later, identified a parasite in sheep associated with erythrocytes as an eperythrozoon; it emerged when a splenectomized sheep was injected with blood from a sheep with clinical signs of heartwater. Four days later in the heartwater prepatent period ring-shaped bodies were observed in blood smears. At first they were dismissed as artefacts but their number increased daily. Three normal sheep subinoculated with blood became parasitemic seven days later, but did not develop heartwater. Neitz and his colleagues[7] commented that they had observed similar organisms previously on many occasions but had failed to appreciate their significance.

In a brief addendum to their published paper Neitz recorded that he and Quinlan had found a species of eperythrozoon in splenectomized calves at Onderstepoort. In the same year Adler and Ellenbogen[8] described in splenectomized cattle blood a similar organism which they named *Ep. wenyonii*. Nearly 30 years later Hoyte[8] described a new species, *Ep. teganodes,* in the plasma of splenectomized calves and Uilenberg[9] detected a small eperythrozoon that exclusively parasitized thrombocytes which he named *Ep. tuomii*.

Doyle's observation of an anaplasmosis-like disease of pigs was confirmed in the early 1930s by Adler and Ellenbogen[10] and Dicke[11] but it was not until 1950 that Splitter[12] identified the pathogenic erythroparasite as *Ep. suis* and the nonpathogenic parasite as *Ep. parvum*.

Classification

The name *Eperythrozoon,* coined by the first observers, has protozoal connotations but subsequently it was shown that the organisms were prokaryotes and not eukaryotes. Although they are now recognized as Gram-negative bacteria, the generic name persists. They are difficult to differentiate by light microscopy from species of *Haemobartonella*. For example, *H. bovis*[13] has the morphology of *Ep. wenyonii*[14] and *H. felis* has been known as *Ep. felis*.[15] Two characteristics of eperythrozoa as seen by light microscopy allegedly help to distinguish them from haemobartonellas, *viz.*, their frequent free presence in plasma and their tendency to occur as ring forms.[5] Currently both are classified in the order 1: Rickettsiales; Family III, Anaplasmataceae. Haemobartonellas, however are placed in genus III and eperythrozoa in genus IV.[16] Nevertheless Zwart and colleagues[17] have suggested that the name "Eperythrozoon" be dropped and the name "Haemobartonella" be accepted if only because *Ep. tuomii* is not eperythrocytic.

Morphology

The pathogenic eperythrozoa are either eperythrocytic, nesting in depressions in the cell surface (Fig. 5.1), or free in the plasma. They

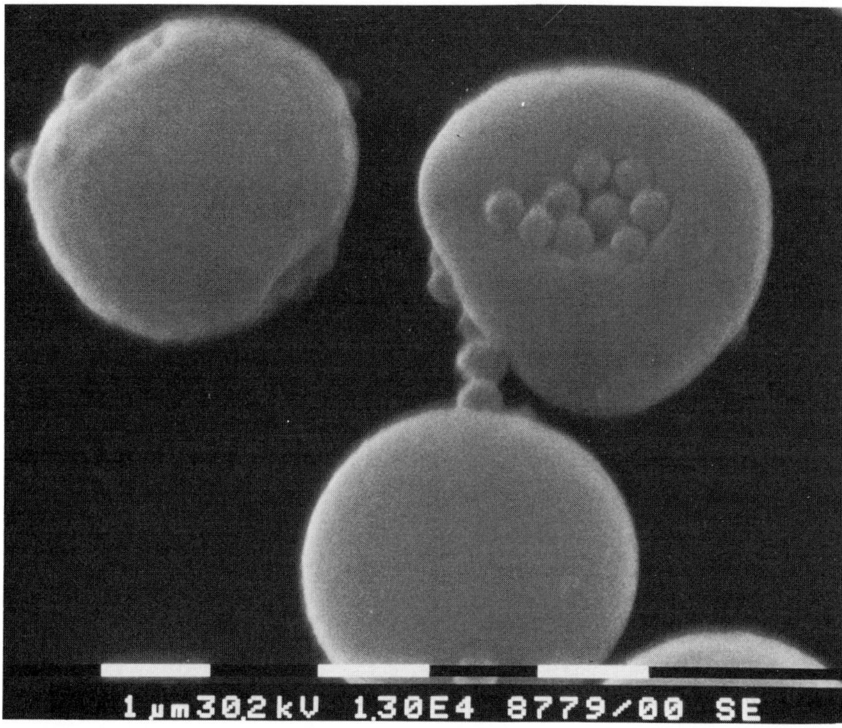

FIG. 5.1. Epi-erythrocytic *Eperythrozoon ovis* nesting in a depression on the surface of an erythrocyte.

are very pleomorphic, the common shapes being cocci, bacilliforms, comma-shapes, rings and irregular complex bodies.[7] The proportions of the different shapes vary with the severity of the parasitemia. In *Ep. ovis* infections, for example, single cocci predominated in light and moderate parasitemias whereas the irregular complex forms predominated in severe parasitemias.[18] Chains were only observed in severe parasitemias. In wet preparations observed by phase-contrast microscopy eperythrozoa appeared as dark spheres.[19]

The plasticity of the shapes of eperythrozoa is reflected in the variation in the estimates of their size. Diameters of cocci and bacilliforms range from 400 to 2500 mm.[5] However, they have no rigid cell walls and, therefore, may pass through most bacteria-retaining filters.[16]

Staining Characteristics

Although eperythrozoa are Gram-negative they are more often stained with the Giemsa modification of Romanowsky's stain which colors them light blue to pinkish-blue (Fig. 5.2). If the parasitemia is light, scarce eperythrozoa are more easily detected by fluorescent microscopy of acaridine-orange stained blood smears which reveals them as greenish-orange spots on the surfaces of the erythrocytes.[18]

Ultrastructure

Scanning electron microscopy of infected erythrocytes reveals irregular cocci, chains of cocci and bacilliforms on the surfaces of the erythrocytes (Fig. 5.3) and clusters of cocci in depressions of the host cell surface (Fig. 5.1). Both large and tiny cocci are evident either lying in surface depressions or protruding from the large cocci.[18] Pospischil and Hoffman[19] called it binary fission whereas Gulland and her colleagues[18] called it budding.

Transmission electron microscopy of ultra-thin sections reveals irregular wall-less cocci bound by a single unit membrane. There is no nucleus or organelles but the cytoplasm contains aggregates of electron-dense ribosomal-like material and delicate filaments in an electron-lucid substance.[20,21] Ring forms have an electron-lucent area within the cytoplasm.[21] Some cocci appear to be attached to the plasmalemma of the erythrocytes eroding the cells at the point of attachment.[20,21] Others seem to be entering into or emerging from the cell[18] but there is no clear evidence of intracytoplasmic vacuoles.[19]

Physico-Chemical Properties

The physico-chemical properties of eperythrozoa have been meagerly studied. Peters and Wigand[22] carried out extensive cytochemical studies of *Ep. coccoides*, a common eperythrozoon of mice, and concluded that the organisms were rich in nucleic acids. Using nucleases they identified both RNA and DNA. Lipids are also present; when *Ep. coccoides* was treated with lipid solvents infectivity was destroyed.[25]

Eperythrozoa in heparinized or EDTA-treated blood samples retain their infectivity at −70°C for up to three months when cryopreserved with 10% glycerol[24] and for longer periods in liquid nitrogen in the presence of 10% dimethyl sulphoxide.[25] *Ep. suis*, purified from infected blood by differential centrifugation with Tween-20, retains its infectivity but not when treated with EDTA although the yield is higher in the presence of EDTA.[26]

Cultural Characteristics

Eperythrozoa do not grow in cell-free media. However, *Ep. coccoides* has been propagated in embryonated hen eggs.[27]

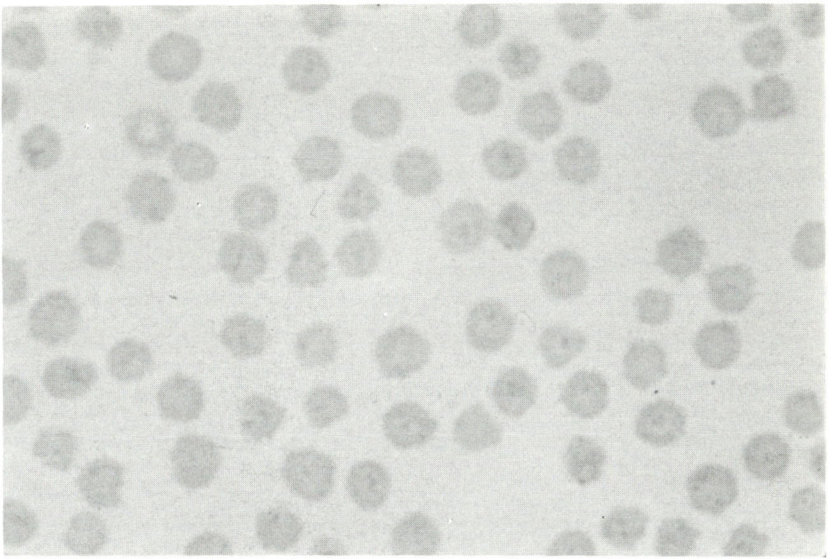

FIG. 5.2. Giemsa-stained blood of *Eperythrozoon ovis*.

Antigenicity

Eperythrozoa infecting domestic animals stimulate the production of antibodies within 1–2 weeks of infection that reach peak titres in 5–6 weeks and thereafter decline. *Ep. suis* antibodies measured by indirect hemagglutination disappear in 2–3 months but reappear if the pig relapses.[28] On the other hand, *Ep. ovis* antibodies detected by indirect immunofluorescence in the sera of infected goats were present for at least 15 months.[29] Hung and Lloyd[30] suggested that the antibodies might have a protective role because the initial increases in antibodies coincided with a fall in the primary parasitemias. Moreover they noted that parasitemias in sheep were lower in the presence of passively transferred hyperimmune serum.

Other tests used to detect eperythrozoan antibodies are complement fixation[30,31] and ELISA.[31] The most sensitive appears to be a modified immunofluorescent assay developed by Nicholls and Veale[24] with which titres as high as 1/50,000 were observed.

Detailed studies on antigenic relationships or differences between species or within species have not been done. Kreier and Ristic[19] record strong evidence of shared antigens between *Ep. ovis* and *Ep. wenyonii* and weak links between *Ep. ovis* and *Anaplasma marginale*. In contrast cattle infected with *Ep. tuomii* have no immunity to *Ep. teganodes*.[9] Moreover *Ep. wenyonii* and *Ep. tuomii* do not cross-react in immunofluorescent assays.[32]

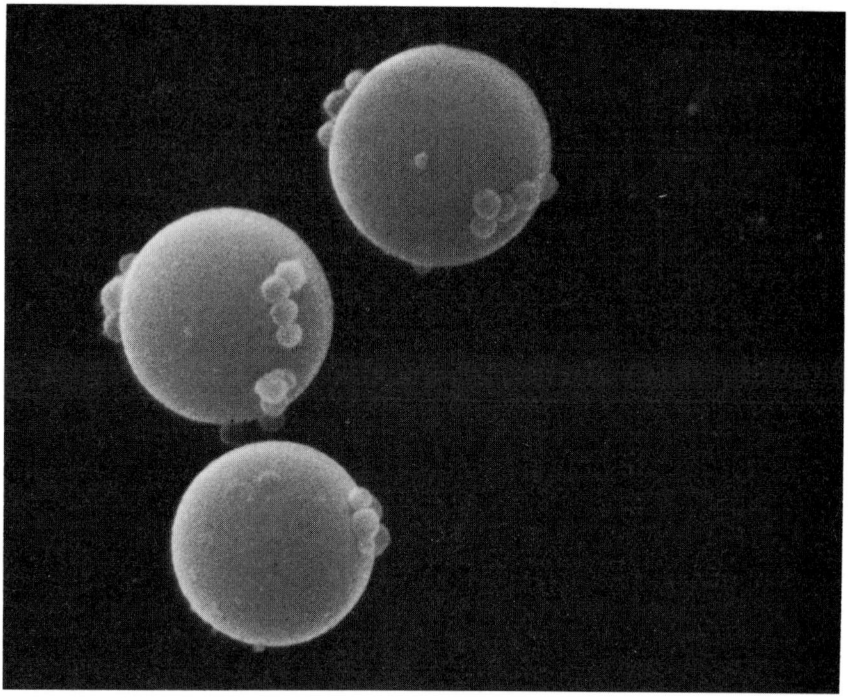

FIG. 5.3. Chain of eperythrozoon cocci.

Epidemiology

Geographical Distribution

The three pathogenic eperythroza of domestic animals, *Ep. ovis*, *Ep. wenyonii* and *Ep. suis*, occur on all continents with the fewest sightings from Asia. *Ep. ovis* is particularly prevalent in sheep in Australia[33] and *Ep. suis* infections are widespread in midwestern U.S.A.[34] and southern Germany.[35]

Transmission

Any injection of a drop of blood from a parasitemic animal into a susceptible animal will initiate infection;[36] consequently blood-sucking arthropods are frequently incriminated in the spread of infection. For example, in temperate areas transmission of *Ep. ovis* is attributed to stable flies (*Stomoxys calcitrans*) and keds (*Malophagus ovinus*)[37] and in the tropics and subtropics by mosquitoes (*Aedes camptorhynchus*),[38] *Anopheles annulipes*[39] and *Culex annulurostris*[30] and by ticks (*Haemaphysalis plumbeum* and *Rhipicephalus bursa*).[40]

Mason and Statham[33] demonstrated that the minimal *Ep. ovis* infective dose was equivalent to one parasitized erythrocyte. They further calculated that a mosquito transfers 1 to 2 erythrocytes and a stable fly about 400 erythrocytes following an interrupted meal on a sheep with an erythrocyte count of 10^{10} per ml and concluded that the stable fly was potentially a more effective vector.

Transmission of *Ep. suis* is seasonal, being more common in summer and autumn when biting diptera are active.[5] The pig louse (*Haematopinus suis*) has been implicated in the transmission of *Ep. suis* within a piggery.[36]

Maintenance of eperythrozoa in a flock or herd, however, is more plausibly linked to transplacental infection which has been demonstrated with *Ep. suis* in pigs[41] and with *Ep. ovis* in sheep.[42]

Natural Host Range

The natural hosts of *Ep. ovis* are goats and sheep but the prevalence in goats is much lower than in sheep; for example, Mason and his colleagues[13] conducted a serological survey in Tasmania and found that only one of 600 goat sera had antibodies to *Ep. ovis* whereas 550 out of 1224 sheep sera were positive. They subsequently showed that goats and sheep were equally susceptible to experimental challenge and concluded that the explanation of the different prevalence rates lay in vector preference and the failure of goats to develop a sustained parasitemia.[44]

Ep. suis occurs in domestic pigs,[45] feral pigs[46] and captive peccaries (*Tayassu tajacu*). *Ep. wenyonii* appears to be host specific.[48]

Sheep of all ages and breeds are susceptible to infection with *Ep. ovis*,[49] but detailed studies of age-related innate resistance have yet to be published. Overt disease, however, is more common in lambs,[50] heifers[51] and piglets[6] than in adult sheep, cattle and pigs.

Experimental Host Range

Only a few trivial transmission trials have been attempted. *Ep. ovis* has been observed in infected blesbok (*Damalisus albifrons*)[49] and eland (*Taurotragus oryx*)[52] but attempts to infect cattle, dogs, guinea pigs and rabbits failed.[53] Kreier and Ristic[20] succeeded in infecting a splenectomized calf from which they successfully infected a splenectomized goat, a splenectomized fallow deer (*Dama virginiana*) and two intact sheep producing clinical signs typical of eperythrozoonosis. In contrast, they were unable to infect a splenectomized goat or a splenectomized fallow deer by injecting *Ep. wenyonii*-infected blood. Similary Neitz[54] was unable to infect splenectomized sheep with *Ep.*

wenyonii. Subsequently the sheep proved to be susceptible to *Ep. ovis*. When *Ep. suis*-infected blood was inoculated into rats (species not named) patent parasitemias developed that persisted for more than 12 months.[55]

Carrier State

The durations of the primary patent parasitemias vary enormously; for example, Gulland and her colleagues[25] found in some sheep the primary parasitemia was self-limiting in 20–90 days, but in others a continuous initial parasitemia was evident for more than 300 days. Many infected animals have intermittent relapse parasitemias.[55] Recovered animals probably remain permanent carriers[12] and Daddow[56] claimed a record for an *Ep. ovis*-infected sheep of ten and a half years.

In the past the carrier state was revealed by the stress of an intercurrent disease such as babesiosis,[57] by splenectomy,[12] by subinoculating blood into splenectomized antibody-free recipient animals[58] or by the injection of betamethasone.[25] *Ep. suis*-carriers have been identified by having IHA antibodies which are IgM immunoglobulins.[28] A molecular approach detected *Ep. suis*-carriers by using a DNA probe in whole-organism DNA hybridization.[59]

Pathogenesis

Most eperythrozoal infections are clinically inapparent and are discovered accidently.[58] When and why disease occurs in individual animals is poorly understood although it has long been known that the spleen plays a crucial role;[60] for example, clinical signs of disease and higher and longer parasitemias are much more likely to occur in infected splenectomized animals than in intact animals.[48] Similarly other stressors potentiate carrier animals precipitating latent parasitemias and clinical signs.[25]

When eperythrozoa are injected intravenously into a susceptible host they disappear. The length of the prepatent period, which ranges from 1–4 weeks, is inversely related to the number of parasites injected.[61] The primary target cells of *Ep. ovis* are in the bone marrow, where the organism multiples before it appears in the peripheral blood.[62] When the parasitemia becomes patent multiplication continues on the surfaces of erythrocytes by budding of small forms from larger forms producing, with time, deformations of the surfaces of the erythrocytes.[18,34] Hung and Lloyd[63] observed in *Ep. ovis* infections phagocytosis of parasitized and nonparasitized erythrocytes by cordal reticular cells in the spleen. Lymph node endothelial cells and probably sinusoidal endothelial cells in the liver have a similar function.[19]

Doyle[6] reported spontaneous agglutination of erythrocytes collected from piglets infected with *Ep. suis* and his observations have been frequently confirmed. Krier and Ristic[5] suggested and Hoffmann and colleagues[60] demonstrated that antierythrocyte antibodies were responsible. The antibodies were firmly attached to the surfaces of the erythrocytes and proved to be "cold" agglutinins. Hoffmann's group[60] therefore concluded that disease, when manifested, was the result of an acquired autoimmune hemolytic anemia, the primary clinical signs of icterus and anemia being due to a rapid resorption and degradation of erythrocytes in lymph nodes, liver and spleen. Other clinical signs in pigs infected with *Ep. suis* such as cyanosis and partial ear necrosis caused by agglutinated erythrocytes blocking blood vessels, are characteristic of cold antibody anemias.[60]

Clinical Signs

Disease in pigs may be very severe and fatal and is manifested by different age-related syndromes.[36] Disease in lambs is milder and limited to a vague ill-thrift syndrome.[64] In cattle infections are even milder, producing, in the absence of a stressor, only slight anemia.[54] In all species the clinical picture is often complicated by other concurrent infections.

Prepatent Periods

Prepatent periods vary with the numbers of organisms injected but, on average, they last for one week in intact sheep injected with *Ep. ovis*[61] and three weeks in intact cattle injected with *Ep. wenyonii*.[54] *Ep. suis* organisms, injected into intact pigs, apparently rarely induced parasitemias,[65] but in splenectomized pigs parasitemias are evident in 2–5 days.[45]

Ill-Thrift Lambs and Weaners

The onset of clinical signs in lambs infected with *Ep. ovis* is insidious. The lambs appear to grow well until they are two to three months old but, thereafter, their growth is retarded and they become smaller than healthy lambs of the same age and are slower to reach sexual maturity.[66] Wool production is reduced and there is a marked decrease in exercise tolerance.[67] The lambs develop pot-bellies and become emaciated and anemic.[66] There is no hemoglobinemia.[68]

Affected lambs are more susceptible to other diseases and more affected by nutritional deficiences.[66]

Flocks in Africa[69] and Australia[39,43] have seropositive prevalence rates that range from 36 to 51%. The prevalence of patent parasitemias were much lower at 3%.[69] Case mortality rates are cited as being between 2 and 6%.[70]

Bovine Eperythrozoonosis

Frank clinical disease is rare in cattle infected with *Ep. wenyonii* and occurs only after stress. For example, Poole and his associates[71] in England investigated a herd of 46 cows that had been turned out of their winter quarters onto pasture. Eighteen animals were visibly sick; being lethargic, febrile, reluctant to move and diarrhoeic. Examinations revealed a macrocytic, normochromic anemia and five were still parasitemic. Similarly Smith and his colleagues[51] investigated a disease outbreak in Colorado in which 10 out of 100 newly calved heifers had transient fevers and rough coats, secreted less milk and developed edema of the teats and lower limbs. Subsequently there was a loss of weight and failure to breed. The clinical signs correlated with massive numbers of *Ep. wenyonii* and resolved with the reduction and disappearance of the parasites. In contrast, the response to the stress of splenectomy in naturally infected calves was relatively mild, being manifested six weeks after splenectomy by 11 day long parasitemias followed only by slight anemias.[54]

Porcine Eperythrozoonosis

Smith[36] recognized four age-related syndromes in pigs infected with *Ep. suis*. In newborn pigs the clinical signs are skin pallor and mild icterus, that in uncomplicated infections, resolve within a week.[72] In very cold weather cyanosis and gangrenous necrosis of the ears may occur.[19] By the time the piglets are weaned they are recognized as being members of an uneven group.

The classic syndrome of ictero-anemia, now rarely seen, occurs in stressed feeder or store pigs 4–5 days after the onset of parasitemia.[12] The pigs, at first, are depressed and inappetant and have high fevers and go on to develop acute anemias as the fever regresses. They become weaker and gaunt and are constipated with bile-streaked faeces. The pallid mucous membranes turn icteric. Death is preceded by subnormal rectal temperatures and supervenes in less than seven days of the onset of illness. Repeated relapses of decreasing severity are common in recovering animals. In the past morbidity rates in classic ictero-anemia were estimated to range between 10 and 60% and mortalities might reach 90%.[73]

Ep. suis infections of sows produces two syndromes, one acute and one chronic.[72] Acute cases have high fevers ranging from 40.0°C to 41.7°C, are anorectic and may show mammary and vulvar edema. Cases occur immediately postpartum. The milk flow is depressed and maternal behavior is subnormal. Recovery without treatment occurs in 2–3 days.[36]

Chronic cases are very difficult to diagnose. They tend to be in poor condition, are pale and may be icteric. Their breeding performance is subnormal. Death from secondary infection is common.[72]

Dual Infections

Concurrent infections of eperythrozoa and other pathogens are usually mutually antagonistic but may enhance synergetically the pathogenicities of each. When, for example, *Ep. suis* was injected into pigs with patent *Ep. parvum* parasitemias the pathogenic *Ep. suis* rapidly displaced the nonpathogenic *Ep. parvum.*[45] Mixed infections of *Ep. suis* and *Babesia trautmannii* delayed the *babesia* parasitemia and depressed the peak parasitemias of both parasites. Similarly *Ep. wenyonii* in cattle inhibited the development of *Babesia bigemina*[75] and *Anaplasma marginale*, provided that the eperythrozoon was established first, otherwise the anaplasma inhibited the eperythrozoon.[76] *Ehrilichia (Cytoecetes) phagocytophila* injected into sheep with patent *Ep. ovis* parasitemias rapidly cleared the eperythrozoon from the blood.[61]

Synergism was postulated by Beveridge and his colleagues[77] to explain summer deaths among weaner sheep in Australia. They thought that nematodes were the predisposing cause and *Ep. ovis* anemia the precipitating factor. Similarly in sows chronically infected with *Ep. suis* sacroptic manage flourished.[73] Clinical signs were more pronounced and lasted longer in sheep infected concurrently with *Ep. ovis* and *Listeria monocytogenes* but listeria antibody titers were depressed.[78]

Pathology

Hematology

The initial hematological changes are parasitism on the surfaces of the erythrocytes together with falls in PCV, total erythrocytes and hemoglobin.[12] Thereafter as the parasitemia lessens there is a gradual development of an autoimmune hemolytic anemia.[68] Erythrocytes spontaneously agglutinate.[6] Infected erythrocytes have an increased fragility and a greater tendency to lyze.[64] There is active erythropoesis manifested by basophilic stippling of immature cells.[12] Changes in leucocyte numbers are not significant.[12] Platelets, however, are depleted giving prolonged prothrombin times.[79]

Clinical Pathology

All three pathogenic eperythrozoa of domestic animals induce similar metabolic changes but the degree differs being most marked in frank clinical cases of ictero-anemia in pigs. Early in the parasitemia hypoglycemia,[80] acidosis[81] and moderate bilirubinemia[34] are evident. Simultaneously blood lactic acid and pyruvic acid levels increase while glycogen levels in liver and muscles fall.[82] Parasitized erythrocytes utilize more glucose than normal cells[14,83] and the eperythrozoon itself causes glycolysis faster than the gluconeogenic pathways can cope with.[80,83] A sequel is high concentrations of magnesium in plasma, serum and erythrocytes.[84] The parasite also interferes with the maintenance of glutathione that is necessary for the preservation of the function and structure of erythrocytes, thus enhancing molecular denaturation.[84]

Gross Pathology

Uncomplicated deaths are rare in sheep and even rarer in cattle infected with eperythrozoa whereas acute deaths in pigs affected with the ictero-anemia syndrome of *Ep. suis* are well documented. Doyle,[6] for instance, recorded generalized icterus throughout the body fat and tissues. The blood was thin with yellow plasma and frequently erythrocytes spontaneously agglutinated. Occasionally hydropericardium, hydrothorax and ascites with yellow fluid were observed. In addition, Kreier and Ristic[5] reported lung edema. Livers were yellow and the gall-bladders were full of thick gelatinous yellow bile. Spleens and kidneys were enlarged and soft. The contents of the intestine, and even the stomach, were streaked in yellow bile pigments. Splitter[12] reported that the gross pathology of infected splenectomized pigs that died was similar but more exaggerated.

In lambs infected with *Ep. ovis* and killed sequentially[61] or six weeks after infection[85] the notable change was enlargement of the spleen, the cut surface of which revealed easily visible large, swollen Malpighian corpuscles. The hemolymph nodes were also enlarged but all other organs appeared normal.[86] Neitz[49] observed a hydropericardium together with a gelatinous infiltration of the subcutaneous tissues of the ventral neck.

Histopathology

The principal microscopic changes in dead pigs infected with *Ep. suis* were in the liver and spleen.[12,60] In the liver they ranged from mild fatty degeneration to marked atrophy and necrosis of central hepatic cells. Lymphocytic infiltration was widespread. Reticulo-endothelial cells in liver, spleen and lymph nodes were hypertrophied and filled with hemosiderin deposits and erythro-phagocytotic debris. Kidneys exhibited parenchymatous degeneration only.[12] Erythropoiesis in the bone marrow was active.[60]

Microscopic changes in sheep were fewer, affecting the spleen, liver and kidneys. Lymphoid hyperplasia enlarged the Malpighian corpuscles of the spleen.[61,86] Hemosiderin deposits were seen in the splenic red pulp phagocytes, in the cells of the proximal convoluted tubules in the kidney cortex and within the parenchymal and Kupffer cells of the liver.[61,86,87] The eperythrozoon itself is difficult to find in tissue sections.

Diagnosis

Apart from the classic ictero-anemia syndrome in weaner pigs eperythrozoa are seldom suspected on the basis of clinical signs. Even though *Ep. ovis* is an important contributory factor in the ill-thrift syndrome in lambs, confirmation of its presence is often difficult. Moreover *Ep. ovis* outbreaks may occur in apparently healthy and well-nourished sheep.[64,88] A major pitfall in a field diagnosis is the frequency with which infected animals mask the presence of eperythrozoa by the clinical signs of exacerbated conditions.[34]

The cornerstone of the diagnosis of eperythrozoonosis is the demonstration of epi-erythrocytic parasites in Giemsa-stained blood films.[34] If parasitemias are light staining with acaridine-orange is more effective than Giemsa.[18] *But* a diagnosis cannot be based solely on the identification of an eperythrozoon;[89] other supplementary tests are essential, e.g. spontaneous erythrocyte agglutination[6] or subinoculation of heparinized blood into splenectomized susceptible animals.[12,36,90] The detection of rising antibody titers in paired serum samples supports a provisional diagnosis, the tests commonly employed being an indirect (passive) hemagglutination,[91] indirect immunofluorescence[69] and enzyme-linked immunosorbent assay.[92]

Operative cell-mediated immune mechanisms will confirm the presence of potentially pathogenic levels of eperythrozoa; for instance, persistent suppression of the uptake of [^{3}H]-thymidine by peripheral blood lymphocytes incubated *in vitro* with mitogens is correlated with initial massive parasitemias and increased blastogenic responses of lymphocytes incubated with lipopolysaccharide precedes hyperglobinemia and high titers of cold agglutinins.[34]

The development of *Ep. suis* DNA probes has significantly enhanced the probability of detecting *Ep. suis* in parasitized pigs.[59,93] In particular, the recombinant DNA probe derived from *Ep. suis* clone KSU-2 has such a high specificity that it should not only aid diagnosis, but should enable the prevalence of *Ep. suis* infection to be determined, the pathogenesis to be studied and the selection of safer specific drugs to be made.[93]

Treatment

Before the advent of antibiotics arsenical formulations were used to treat eperythrozoon parasitemias; for example, Neitz[54] cleared *Ep. ovis* from the blood within 24 hours with "Neosalvarsan" but they reappeared 16 days later. Higher doses cleared the blood in 15 min but the sheep still relapsed. Antimony–arsenic compounds also abated parasitemias and higher doses allegedly sterilized the infection.[54] Similarly Sheriff[94] found that "Spirotrypan Forte", a sulphur-containing arsenobenzene, reliably cleared *Ep. ovis* parasitemias despite some toxicity. Hung[95] also abated *Ep. ovis* parasitemias in sheep with imidocarb dipropionate but they recrudesced within 2–4 weeks. Sheriff[94] queried the value of treating sheep because they became susceptible to reinfection.

Arsenic formulations have also been used to treat pigs with *Ep. suis*-induced illness. However, adding arsanilic acid to pig feed had no effect on the course of *Ep. suis* infection.[96] Korean workers[55] compared the effect of feeding "Roxarsone" for 6 days to pigs infected with *Ep. suis* with intramuscular injection of oxytetracycline at the rate of 3 mg/kg body weight for 10 days; both abated clinical signs but only "Roxarsone" eliminated the eperythrozoon. Other antibiotics behaved like oxytetracycline and reduced the numbers of *Ep. suis* but did not sterilize.[96]

Control

Any attempts to control *Ep. suis* in herds must begin first with the control of sarcoptic mange, lice and helminths.[72] Traditionally ictero-anemia in the U.S.A. is controlled by adding arsenicals, particularly arsanilic acid, to the feed or water.[36] Different dosage regimens are used for different droves but it is essential that the schedules be intermittent to lessen the risk of arsenic poisoning.[72] Other feed additives are aureomycin[73] and chlortetracycline.[97]

Iatrogenic transmission is averted by good hygienic practice in handling syringes, needles and surgical instruments.[36]

References

1. Barton, A.L. 1909. Descripción de elemantos endoglobulares hallados en los enfermos de fiebre verrucosa. *Cron. Med.* **26:** 7–10.
2. O'Leary, W. 1989. *Practical Handbook of Microbiology*, pp. 182–184. CRC Press, Boca Raton.
3. Schilling, V. 1928. *Eperythrozoon coccoides*, eine neue durch Splenectomie aktivierbare Dauerinfektion der weissen Maus. *Klin. Wschr.* **7:** 1854–1855.
4. Dinger, J.G. 1929. Näheras über des *Eperythrozoon coccoides. Zentbl. Bakt. Parasitkde.* Abt. I. Orig. **113:** 503–509.
5. Kreier, J.P. and Ristic, M. 1968. Haemobartonellosis and related diseases. In: *Infectious Blood Diseases of Man and Animals. Diseases caused by Protista. Volume II. "The Pathogens, The Infections and the Consequences"*, p. 425. Weinman, D. and Ristic, M. (Eds), Academic Press, New York.
6. Doyle, L.P. 1932. A rickettsia-like or anaplasmosis-like disease in swine. *J. Am. Vet. Med. Assoc.* **81,** 668–671.
7. Neitz, W.O., Alexander, R.A. and Du Toit, P.J. 1934. *Eperythrozoon ovis* (sp. nov.) infection in sheep. *Onderstepoort J. Vet. Sci.* **3:** 263–269.
8. Hoyte, H.M.D. 1962. *Eperythrozoon teganodes* sp. nov. (Rickettsiales) parasitic in cattle. *Parasitology.* **52:** 527–532.
9. Uilenberg, G. 1967. *Eperythrozoon tuomii* n. sp. (Rickettsiales), troisième espèce d'Eperythrozoon des bovins à Madagascar. *Rev. Elev. Méd Vét. Pays Trop.* **20:** 563–569.
10. Adler, S. and Ellenbogen, V. 1934. A note on two new blood parasites of cattle: *Eperythrozoon* and *Bartonella. J. comp. Path.* **47:** 219–221.
11. Dicke, W.E. 1934. Anaplasmosis-like disease in swine. *Vet. Med.* **29:** 288.
12. Splitter, E.J. 1950. *Eperythrozoon suis*, the etiologic agent of ictero-anemia or an anaplasmosis-like disease in swine. *Am. J. Vet. Res.* **11:** 324–330.
13. Simpson, C.F. and Love, J.N. 1970. Fine structure of *Haemobartonella bovis* in blood and liver of splenectomized calves. *Am. J. Vet. Res.* **31:** 225–231.
14. Love, J.N., Wilson, R.P., McEwen, E.G. and Wiygul, G. 1977. Metabolism of [^{14}C] glucose in haemobartonella-like infected erythrocytes in splenectomized calves. *Am. J. Vet. Res.* **38:** 739–741.
15. Harbutt, P.R. 1963. A clinical appraisal of feline infectious anaemia and its transmission under natural conditions. *Aust. Vet. J.* **39:** 4101–4104.
16. Kreier, J.P. and Ristic, M. 1984. *Genus IV.* Eperythrozoon *Schilling 1928.* In: *Bergey's Manual of Systemic Bacteriology*, Vol. 1, pp. 726–729. Krieg, N.R. and Ristic, M. (Eds), Williams and Wilkins, Baltimore.
17. Zwart, D., Leeflang, P. and Vorstenbosch, C.J.A.H.V.V. 1969. Studies on an eperythrozoon associated with bovine thrombocytes. *Zentbl. Bakt. Parasitkde. Infekt. Hyg.* **210:** 82–102.
18. Gulland, F.M., Doxey, D.L. and Scott, G.R. 1987. Changing morphology of *Eperythrozoon ovis. Res. Vet. Sci.* **43:** 88–91.
19. Pospischil, A. and Hoffman, R. 1982. *Eperythrozoon suis* in naturally infected pigs: a light and electron microscope study. *Vet. Path.* **19:** 651–657.
20. Kreier, J.P. and Ristic, M. 1963. Morphologic, antigen and pathogenic characteristics of *Eperythrozoon ovis* and *Eperythrozoon wenyonii. Am. J. Vet. Res.* **24:** 488–500.
21. McKee, A.E., Ziegler, R.F. and Giles, R.C. 1973. Scanning and transmission

electron microscopy of *Haemobartonella canis* and *Eperythrozoon ovis*. *Am. J. Vet. Res.* **34:** 1196–1201.
22. PETERS, D. and WIGAND, R. 1955. *Bartonellaceae*. *Bact. Rev.* **19:** 150–155.
23. STANSLY, P.G. and NEILSON, C.F. 1966. Sedimentation of *Eperythrozoon coccoides*. *Proc. Soc. exp. Biol. Med.* **121:** 363–365.
24. NICHOLLS, T. and VEALE, P. 1986. A modified indirect immunofluorescent assay for the detection of antibody to *Eperythrozoon ovis* in sheep. *Aust. Vet. J.* **63:** 157–159.
25. GULLAND, F.M., DOXEY, D.L. and SCOTT, G.R. 1987. The effects of *Eperythrozoon ovis* in sheep. *Res. Vet. Sci.* **43:** 85–87.
26. HALL, S.M., CIPRIANO, J.A., SCHONEWEIS, D.A., SMITH, J.E. and FENWICK, B.W. 1988. Isolation of infective and non-infective *Eperythrozoon suis* bodies from the whole blood of infected swine. *Vet. Rec.* **123:** 25, 651.
27. SEAMER, J. 1959. The propagation and preservation of *Eperythrozoon coccoides*. *J. gen. Microbiol.* **21:** 244–251.
28. BALJER, G., HEINRITZI, K. and WIELER, L. 1989. Demonstration of *Eperythrozoon suis* in experimentally and naturally infected pigs by indirect haemagglutination. *J. Vet. Med. B.* **36:** 417–423.
29. MASON, R.W., CORBOULD, A. and STATHAM, P. 1989. Experimental *Eperythrozoon ovis* infection in goats. *Aust. Vet. J.* **66:** 221–222.
30. DADDOW, K.N. 1980. *Culex annulirostris* as a vector of *Eperythrozoon ovis* infection in sheep. *Vet. Microbiol.* **7:** 313–317.
31. SCHULLER, W., HEINRITZI, K., AL NUKTHA, S., KOLBL, S. and SCHUH, M. 1990. Serologische Verlaufruntersuchungen mittels KBR und ELISA zum Nacheseis von Antikorpern gegen die *Eperythrozoon-suis-Infektion* des Schweines. *Berl. Münch. Tierärztl. Wschr.* **103:** 9–12.
32. TUOMI, J. and TANSKANEN, R. 1980. Antigenic non-relationship of two bovine eperythrozoa demonstrated by the immunofluorescent method. *Acta vet scand.* **21:** 699–701.
33. MASON, R.W. and STATHAM, P. 1991. The determination of the level of *Eperythrozoon ovis* parasitaemia in clinically infected sheep and its significance to the spread of infection. *Aust. Vet. J.* **68:** 115–116.
34. ZACHARY, J.F. and SMITH, A.R. 1985. Experimental porcine eperythrozoonosis: T-lymphocyte suppression and misdirected immune responses. *Am. J. Vet. Res.* **46:** 821–830.
35. HOFFMANN, H. 1984. Symptomatologie und Diagnostik der Eperythrozoonose in Ferkelerzeugerbetrieben. *Tierärztl. Umsch.* **39:** 474–479.
36. SMITH, A.R. 1986. Porcine eperythrozoonosis. In: *Current Veterinary Therapy 2: Food Animal Practice,* pp. 626–628. HOWARD J.L. (Ed), Saunders, Philadelphia.
37. OVERÄS, J. 1969. Studies on *Eperythrozoon ovis*—infection in sheep *Acta vet. scand. (Suppl.)* 148 pp.
38. HOWARD, G.W. 1975. The experimental transmission of *Eperythrozoon ovis* by mosquitoes. *Parasitology* **71:** xxxiii.
39. NICHOLLS, T.J. and VEALE, P.I. 1986. The prevalence of *Eperythrozoon ovis* infection in weaner and adult sheep in north-eastern Victoria. *Aust. Vet. J.* **63:** 118–120.
40. NIKOL'SKII, S.N. and SLIPCHENKO, S.N. 1969. [Experimental transmission of *Eperythrozoon ovis* by the ticks *Hyalomma plumbeum* and *Rhipicephalus bursa*]. *Veterinariya, Moscow* **(5):** 46; Abstr. *Vet. Bull.* **40:** 15 (1970).
41. BERRIER, H.H. and GAUGE, R.E. 1954. Eperythrozoonosis transmitted *in utero* from carrier sows to their pigs. *J. Am. Vet. Med. Assoc.* **124:** 98–100.

42. GRETILLAT, S. and GEVREY, J. 1983. Note préliminaire sur l'anémie infectieuse des agneux à *Eperythrozoon ovis* (Neitz, Alexander et Du Toit, 1934) en France. *Rev. Méd Vét.* **134:** 399–405.
43. MASON, R.W., CORBOULD, A. and STATHAM, P. 1989. A serological survey of *Eperythrozoon ovis* in goats and sheep in Tasmania. *Aust. Vet. J.* **66:** 122–123.
44. MASON, R.W. and STATHAM, P. 1991. The determination of the level of *Eperythrozoon ovis* parasitaemia in chronically infected sheep and its significance to the spread of infection. *Aust. Vet. J.* **68:** 115–116.
45. SPLITTER, E.J. 1950. *Eperythrozoon suis* n. sp. and *Eperythrozoon parvum* n. sp., two new blood parasites of swine. *Science* **111:** 513–514.
46. SMITH, H.M., DAVIDSON, W.R., NETTLES, V.F. and GERRISH, R.R. 1982. Parasitisms among wild swine in south-eastern United States. *J. Am. Vet. Med. Assoc.* **181:** 1281–1284.
47. HANNON, P.G., LOCHMILLER, R.L., MELLEN, J.W., CRAIG, T.M. and GRANT W.E. 1985. Eperythrozoon in captive juvenile collared peccaries in Texas. *J. Wildlife Dis.* **21:** 439–440.
48. WEINMAN, D. 1944. Infectious anaemia due to bartonella and related red cell parasites. *Trans. Phil. Soc.* **33:** 243–250.
49. NEITZ, W.O. 1968. *Eperythrozoon ovis* infection. *Bull. Off. Int. Epiz.* **70:** 373–378.
50. DADDOW, K.N. 1979. *Eperythrozoon ovis*—a cause of anaemia, reduced production and decreased exercise tolerance in sheep. *Aust. Vet. J.* **55:** 433–434.
51. SMITH, J.A., THRALL, M.A., SMITH, J.L., SALMAN, M.D., CHING, S.V. and COLLINS, J.K. 1990. *Eperythrozoon wenyonii* infection in dairy cattle. *J. Am. Vet. Med. Assoc.* **196:** 1244–1250.
52. ENIGK, K. 1942. Cited by Neitz (49).
53. NEITZ, W.O. 1937. Eperythrozoonosis in sheep. *Onderstepoort J. Vet. Sci.* **9:** 9–30.
54. NEITZ, W.O. 1940. Eperythrozoonosis in cattle. *Onderstepoort J. Vet. Sci.* **14:** 9–24.
55. RIM, B.M., KIM, J.C.S. and HAN, D.S. 1984. Porcine eperythrozoonosis-like disease in Korea: epidemiological observations. *Kor. J. Vet. Res.* **24:** 237–244.
56. DADDOW, K.N. 1981. The duration of the carrier state of *Eperythrozoon ovis* infection in sheep. *Aust. Vet. J.* **57:** 49.
57. HUSSEIN, H.S. 1976. The effect of a concurrent *Eperythrozoon coccoides* infection on the development of *Babesia microti* and *B. hylomysci* in mice. *Sudan J. Vet. Sci. Anim. Husb.* **17:** 53–59.
58. GOTHE, R. and KREIER, J.P. 1977. *Aegyptionella, Eperythrozoon,* and *Haemobartonella.* In: *Parasitic Protozoa. IV. Babesia, Theileria, Myxosporida, Microsporida, Bartonellaceae, Anaplasmataceae, Ehrlichia, and Pneumocystis,* pp. 263–294. KREIER J.P. (Ed.), Academic Press, New York.
59. OBERST, R.D., HALL, S.M. and SCHONEWEIS, D.A. 1990. Detection of *Eperythrozoon suis* DNA from swine blood by whole-organism DNA hybridizations. *Vet. Microbiol.* **24:** 127–134.
60. HOFFMANN, R., SCHMID, D.O. and HOFFMANN-FEZER, G. 1981. Erythrocyte antibodies in porcine eperythrozoonosis. *Vet. Immun. Immunopath.* **2:** 111–119.
61. FOGGIE, A. and NISBET, D.I. 1964. Studies on eperythrozoon infection in sheep. *J. comp. Path.* **74:** 45–61.
62. INADA, I., ICHIJO, S., SARASHINA, T. and OSAME, S. 1985. Studies on eperythrozoonosis in sheep—clinical, hematological and electromicroscopic findings in cases experimentally infected with *E. ovis*. *Res. Bull. Obhiro Univ.* **14:** 195–209.

63. HUNG, A.L. and LLOYD, S. 1989. Role of the spleen and rosette-formation response in experimental *Eperythrozoon ovis* infection. *Vet. Parasit.* **32:** 119–126.
64. SHERIFF, D., CLAPP, K.H. and REID, M.A. 1966. *Eperythrozoon ovis* infection in South Australia. *Aust. Vet. J.* **42:** 169–176.
65. MOLLWEIDE, G. 1984. Klinish-hematologische und serologisch–immunologische Untersuchungen bei der Eperythrozoonose des Schweines. Inaug. Diss. Univ. Münch. 119pp. *Abstr. Vet. Bull.* **56:** 93 (1986).
66. BURROUGHS, G.W. 1988. The significance of *Eperythrozoon ovis* in ill-thrift in sheep in the Eastern Cape coastal areas of South Africa. *J. S. Afr. Vet. Assoc.* **59:** 195–199.
67. DADDOW, K.N. 1979. *Eperythrozoon ovis*—cause of anaemia, reduced production and decreased exercise tolerance in sheep. *Aust. Vet. J.* **55:** 433–434.
68. SHERIFF, D. 1978. The pathology of *E. ovis*. *Aust. Vet. J.* **26:** 315.
69. ILEMOBADE, A.A. and BLOTKAMP, C. 1978. *Eperythrozoon ovis*. II. Prevalence studies in sheep in Nigeria using the indirect immunofluorescent antibody test. *Tropenmed. Parasit.* **29:** 311–314.
70. HUNGERFORD, T.G. 1975. *Diseases of Livestock,* 8th edn. pp. 149–151. McGraw-Hill, Sydney.
71. POOLE, D.B.R., CUTLER, R.S., KELLEY, W.R. and COLLINS, J.D. 1976. *Eperythrozoon wenyonii* anaemia in cattle. *Vet. Rec.* **99:** 481.
72. HENRY, S.C. 1979. Clinical observations on eperythrozoonosis. *J. Am. Vet. Med. Assoc.* **174:** 601–603.
73. ANTHONY, H.D., KELLEY, D.C., NELSON, D.L. and TWIEHAUS, M.J. 1962. Suppressing eperythrozoon infection in swine. *Vet. Med.* **57:** 702–703.
74. DIPEOLU, O.O., OTESILE, E.B., FAGBEMI, B.O. and ADETUNJI, A. 1983. Pathogenicity of *Eperythrozoon suis* alone and when mixed with *Babesia trautmannii* in experimentally infected pigs. *Vet. Parasitol.* **13:** 127–134.
75. HOYTE, H.M.D. 1961. Initial development of infections with *Babesia bigemina*. *J. Protozool.* **8:** 462–466.
76. FOOTE, L.E., LEVY, H.E., TORBERY, B.J. and OGLESBY, W.T. 1957. Interference between anaplasmosis and eperythrozoonosis in splenectomized cattle. *Am. J. Vet. Res.* **18:** 556–559.
77. BEVERIDGE, I., BROWN, T.H., FITZSIMONS, S.M., FORD, G.E., JUDSON, G.J., MARTIN, R.R. and MILLER, D.W. 1985. Mortality in weaner sheep in South Australia under different regimes of anthelmintic treatment. *Aust. J. Agric. Res.* **36:** 857–865.
78. GRØNSTØL, H. and ØVERÅS, J. 1980. Listeriosis in sheep: *Eperythrozoon ovis* infection used as a model to study predisposing factors. *Acta vet. scand.* **21:** 523–532.
79. PLANK, G. and HEINRITZI, K. 1990. Disseminierte intravasale Gerinnung bei der Eperythrozoonose des Schweiner. *Berl. Münch tierärztl. Wschr.* **103:** 13–18.
80. SUTTON, R.H. 1976. *Eperythrozoon ovis*: The difference in carbohydrate metabolism between infected and uninfected sheep erythrocytes. *Aust. J. exp. Biol. Med.* **54:** 449–458.
81. HEINRITZI, K., PETERANDERL, W. and PLANK, G. 1990. *Eperythrozoon-Infektion* beim Schwein: Einfluss auf Saure-Basen-Haushalt sowie Glucose-, Lactat-und Pyruvatgehalt des venosen Blutes. *Dtsch. Tierärztl. Wschr.* **97:** 31–34.
82. ZWART, D., SCHOTMAN, A.J.H. and STRAVER, A.J.M. 1970. Metabolic changes during eperythrozoon infection in cattle. *Res. Vet. Sci.* **11:** 105–111.
83. SMITH, J.E., CIPRIANO, J.E. and HALL, S.M. 1990. *In vitro* and *in vivo* glucose consumption in swine eperythrozoonosis. *J. Vet. Med. B.* **37:** 587–592.

84. Brown, J.E., Hildalgo, R.J., Jones, E.W. and Boyle, C.R. 1986. Blood magnesium values in healthy cattle and in cattle affected with anaplasmosis and eperythrozoonosis. *Am. J. Vet. Res.* **47:** 158–162.
85. Sutton, R.H. 1979. Effect of *Eperythrozoon ovis* infection on the reduction potential of sheep erythrocytes. *Vet Parasitol.* **5:** 11–15.
86. Sutton, R.H. 1978. Observations on the pathology of *Eperythrozoon ovis* infection in sheep. *N.Z. Vet. J.* **26:** 229–230.
87. Sutton, R.H. 1979. The pathology of *Ep. ovis*. *N.Z. Vet. J.* **27:** 18.
88. Nicholls, T.J., Veale, P.I. and Overend, D. 1989. The effect of artificial *Eperythrozoon ovis* infection on the growth rate of stressed and non-stressed sheep. *Aust. Vet. J.* **66:** 184–185.
89. Hoffman, H. 1984. Symtomatologie und Diagnostik der Eperythrozoonose in Ferkelerzeugerbetrichen. *Tierärztl. Umsch.* **39:** 474–479.
90. Bugnowski, H., Horsche, F., Muller, D., Sattler, H.G. and Zepezauer, V. 1989. Reproduktion der Eperythrozoonose des Schweines mittels Tierversuchs nach Splenektomie. *Arch. exp. Vet. Med.* **43:** 391–403.
91. Finerty, J.F., Hidalgo, R.J. and Dimopoullos, G.T. 1969. A passive hemagglutination procedure for the detection of *Eperythrozoon* infections in calves. *Am. J. Vet. Res.* **30:** 43–45.
92. Lang, F.M., Ferrier, G.R. and Nicholls, T.J. 1987. Detection of antibodies to *Eperythrozoon ovis* by the use of an enzyme-linked immunosorbent assay. *Res. Vet. Sci.* **43:** 249–252.
93. Oberst, R.D., Hall, S.M., Jasso, R.A., Arndt, T. and Wen, L. 1990. Recombinant DNA probe detecting *Eperythrozoon suis* in swine blood. *Am. J. Vet. Res.* **51:** 1760–1764.
94. Sheriff, D. 1973. The effect of Spirotypan on *Eperythrozoon ovis* in sheep. *Vet. Rec.* **93:** 288–289.
95. Hung, A.L. 1986. Chemotherapeutic efficacy of imidocarb dipropionate on experimental *Eperythrozoon ovis* infection in sheep. *Trop. Anim. Hlth. Prod.* **18:** 97–102.
96. Halfmann, S. 1983. Hematologisch–therapeutische Untersuchungen bei der Eperythrozoonose des Schweines. *Inaug. Diss. Univ. Münch.* 165 pp. *Abst. Vet. Bull.* **54:** 745 (1984).
97. Rosenkrans, C., Jr, Zinn, G.M. and Jesse, G.W. 1984. Chlortetracycline as a treatment against the effects of eperythrozoonosis on poor productivity. *Proc. Int. Pig. Vet. Soc. Congr. Ghent.* **8:** 21.

6

Coxiellosis (Q fever)

Z. WOLDEHIWET AND I. D. AITKEN

Introduction

Since its first description as a febrile disease among workers in a meat plant in Brisbane, Australia[1] Q fever has been associated with animals but it was regarded as causing little or no clinical disease in domestic animals themselves.[2,3,4,5,6] In man, the clinical pattern of the disease, the modes of transmission and the course of the illness are well described.[7] At the time of the first description of the disease in man, American workers had isolated from ticks a rickettsial organism pathogenic to guinea pigs which they named *Rickettsia diaporica*.[8] The Nine Mile isolate is now one of the well-characterized strains of *Coxiella burnetti*. Shortly after the isolation of the Nine Mile strain, Dyer,[9] established that *R. diaporica* was pathogenic to man producing a disease similar to that described as Q fever by Australian workers.[10] Subsequently, the organism was isolated from a wide range of free-living and domestic animals, thus highlighting their importance in the epidemiology of the disease.

However, little information was obtained about the importance of the organism as a cause of disease in animals. Despite the earlier reports of respiratory disease due to *C. burnetii* in sheep, goats and cattle,[11,12,13] the only clinical disease of domestic animals attributable to *C. burnetii* is that of abortion in sheep, goats and cows.[2,3]

This chapter briefly describes the organism and its importance in animal health. The significance to public health is covered in Chapter 21.

Etiology

Classification

The causative agent of Q fever *Coxiella burnetii,* is a nonmotile obligate intracellular organism wich completes its life cycle within the phagosomes of infected cells. The organism is classified in the family Rickettsiaceae, tribe *Rickettsieae*, but differs significantly from members of the tribe which cause typhus, spotted or scrub type fevers in man in its physiology and its composition.[14] Unlike the other members of the tribe *Rickettsieae*, it is highly resistant to adverse physical and chemical agents, is characterized by the presence of small structures similar to endospores[15] and undergoes phase variation. Furthermore, the organism completes its life cycle within phagolysosomes and its DNA base composition is different from that of members of the genus *Rickettsia* and *Rochalimaea*.

C. burnetii is similar to the ehrlichiae in that it remains within the phagosomes after internalization and that all stages of its development are accomplished within the phagosomes[16] (Fig. 6.1). Recent phylogenetic studies on selected members of the family Rickettsiaceae indicated that *C. burnetii* appears to bear no relationship whatever to other members of its tribe but is distantly related to *Legionella*.[17]

Staining Characteristics

The organisms do not always stain well with the Gram method and slight modifications of the Gram stain may result in Gram-positive

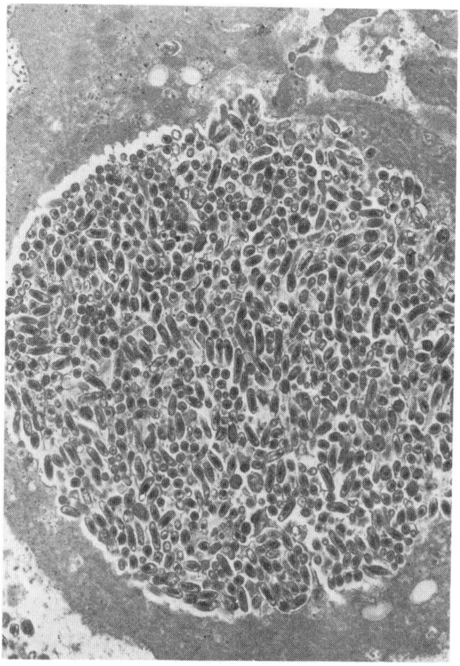

FIG. 6.1. An intracytoplasmic vacuole in an ovine chorionic epithelial cell packed with *Coxiella burnetii* (× 12,000).

reactions,[18] but on the basis of their ultrastructure and chemical composition, they are regarded as Gram-negative bacteria. They appear as purple pleomorphic coccobacilli when stained with the Gimenez and/or the Macchiavello methods.[19] McCaul and Williams[15] found that up to 10% of cells may be acid-fast and some cells exhibited staining features of endospores as demonstrated by the Dorner spore-staining procedures.

Morphology and Ultrastructure

Coxiellae are highly pleomorphic coccobacilli. The most common form of the organism is that of a rod-shaped, small bacterium about 250 nm wide and 500–1250 nm long.

At least three morphological variants of *C. burnetii* have been described. These are the terminal large cell variants (LCVs), the small cell variants (SCVs) and the dense intracellular structures within the LCVs regarded by some workers as endospores. The pleomorphism of the organism has been explained as reflecting the developmental cycle.[15,20] Some workers have used density gradient centrifugation to separate these cell variants with some success.[20,21]

The ultrastructure and chemical composition of *C. burnetii* are similar to those of Gram-negative bacteria. The organisms contain an electron dense structure surrounded by a two-layered membrane[22] containing a peptidoglycan structure with muramic acid[23] and a lipopolysaccharide (LPS) complex.[24,25] The composition of the peptidoglycan has been shown to be similar to that found in the members of the family Enterobacteriaceae.[26]

Apart from the morphological variants, *C. burnetii* has two antigenic phases.[27] Phase I and phase II have cell coats with significantly different antigenic compositions. The two phases differ in their pathogenic and immunogenic properties.[28] They are morphologically similar but phase I variants have higher densities than those of phase II.[29]

Growth and Cultural Characteristics

C. burnetii does not grow in artificial media. The organism was successfully cultivated in the yolk sacs of embryonated hens' eggs as early as 1938[8] and this method of cultivation is still widely used to obtain large numbers of *C. burnetii*. The organism also has been cultivated in primary cells and several cell lines, including Vero cells and a number of macrophage-like cell lines. Embryonated eggs, and susceptible cell lines, have been used to study the methods of entry and multiplication of the parasite. After inoculation into the yolk sacs of embryonated hens' eggs, *C. burnetii* multiplies rapidly in the yolk sac membranes but to a lesser extent in the chorioallantoic membrane, allantoamnion, amniotic fluid and in the intestines and other parts of the embryo.[30,31]

The organisms are believed to enter host cells by a process of phagocytosis.[32] After entry, the organism multiplies within clearly delineated vacuoles.[32–34] Intracellular survival, particularly within professional phagocytes, may be aided by the organism's ability to contend with the host cell's production of superoxide anions by blocking oxidative metabolism and generating its own superoxide-degrading enzymes.[35] Certain cell lines may become persistently infected with *C. burnetii*[36,37] and have been used as models for studying the possible mechanisms by which the organism stays latent in infected animals.[36] *C. burnetii* maintains its pleomorphism during its multiplication in vacuoles *in vitro*.[38–40] The main mode of multiplication is believed to be by binary fission[20] but other complicated forms of replication and a developmental cycle have been proposed to explain the varied morphology of the organism.[15,19] For example, McCaul and Williams[15] observed that while cell division by binary fission occurred in both the SCVs and LCVs, some LCVs were observed to undergo concurrent binary transverse fission with unequal cell division characterized by endospore formation.

Methods of obtaining cell-free *C. burnetii* have enabled several workers to investigate the metabolism of the organism. It was demonstrated that *C. burnetii* produces low levels of CO_2 from pyruvates and glutamates.[41] More recent evidence suggests that the transport, catabolism and incorporation of both glucose and glutamate are stimulated by the concentration of hydrogen ions, indicating that the metabolic processes of *C. burnetii* are pH-dependent.[42]

The organism is now regarded as acidophilic because it prefers the low pH environment of the phagolysosome[42] and its capacity to survive harsh environmental factors is explained by the fact that it lacks metabolic activity at high pH.[43] This low pH environment favors its multiplication and the endosporic small forms may be designed for this purpose.

Molecular Biology of *C. burnetii*

The DNA of *C. burnetii* is 1.04×10^9 daltons.[44] This compares well with genome sizes of the other members of the tribe *Rickettsieae*[45,46] and with *Chlamydia psittaci*.[47] However, the base composition of the DNA is different to other rickettsiae.[44,48] The guanine plus cytosine

(G+C) content of the DNA of *C. burnetii* is 42.7% compared to 29.0% in *Rickettsia prowazekii* and *R. mooseri* and 39.3% in *Rochalimaea quintana*.[45] O'Rouke *et al.*[49] found no differences in the endonuclease cleavage patterns of different strains of *C. burnetii* that could be attributed to phase changes but cleavage patterns could be used to differentiate isolates. At least three plasmids, ranging from 36 to 45 kilobases, have been isolated from strains of *C. burnetii*.[50] For example, plasmid QpHI was isolated from both antigenic phases of the Nine Mile strain and another plasmid, QpRS, was isolated from other strains recovered from cases of endocarditis in man.[51,52] Both phase I and phase II may harbor plasmids[50] but whether phase variation is mediated by plasmids has not been elucidated. However, Samuel *et al.*[52] suggested that the strains of *C. burnetii* which cause various diseases may have specific virulence determinants. This is based on their findings that while most isolates of *C. burnetii* from acute Q fever contained the plasmid QpH1, another plasmid QpRS was common to *C. burnetii* isolates from cases of human endocarditis and caprine abortions.

Phase Variation and Antigenic Composition

C. burnetii undergoes antigenic phase variation when serially passaged in embryonated hen's eggs.[27,53] Such phase variants differ in their biological and immunological properties. Guinea pigs immunized with dead *C. burnetii*, that had been serially passaged through embryonated eggs, rapidly produced aggultinating and complement-fixing antibodies to these egg-adapted strains (phase II). In contrast, when inoculated with *C. burnetii* isolated from animals (phase I) guinea pigs initially produced anti-phase II antibodies and anti-phase I antibodies later. This antigenic variation is host-dependent. *C. burnetii* is present in its phase I form in nature and laboratory animals but repeated passage of phase I organisms in embryonated eggs results in its conversion to phase II. Phase II organisms are less virulent than phase I. How these antigenic changes occur is not well-established but there are several phenomena which may be responsible. Baca[54] suggested that gene expression of the organism may be influenced by the environment of the host, resulting in the expression or the suppression of the phase characteristics of the parasite or it could be due to the simple host lysosomal enzymatic modification of the cell surfaces of *C. burnetii*. Kordova[55] thought that repeated mutations may be responsible for phase variation. The two phases are morphologically indistinguishable but there is some evidence to suggest that phase I variants have a higher density (1.33 g/cm^3) than phase II (1.22 g/cm^3).[29] The two phases also exhibit quantitative and qualitative differences in their carbohydrate and LPS composition.

Both the lipopolysaccharide (LPS) and the surface proteins elicit antibody response. The LPS antigenic component of *C. burnetii* was demonstrated in phase I by Baca and Paretsky.[24,25] It is now established that the endotoxic LPS is also present in phase II.[56,57] Several workers have reported that the LPS obtained from phase I and phase II are antigenic[56,58,59] but that the two LPSs were chemically and immunologically distinct.[59,60] Some studies on the immunogenic proteins of *C. burnetii* suggest that a number may be phase-specific while others are shared.[61] In contrast, other studies found no differences in the proteins of the two phases.[59] Williams *et al.*[61] produced monoclonal antibodies to differentiate phase I and II. One monoclonal antibody (MabI-1) was specific to phase I variants while another (MabII-1) recognized only phase II. The epitope for MabII-1 was found to be a 25.7 kDa protein while the phase I specific epitope for MabI-1 is LPS. These observations were reinforced by the findings of Hackstadt *et al.*[59] that the differences between the two phases reside in the composition of their polysaccharides. They argued that LPS antigens are probably the major antigens which distinguish the two phases. In contrast, the surface protein antigens of phase I and phase II are shared.[59] The fact that the changes in LPS composition may be responsible for the phase variation suggests the antigenic variation is similar to the smooth to rough (S–R) variation observed in enteric Gram-negative bacteria.[59,61]

Host–Parasite Interactions

C. burnetii accomplishes its entire developmental cycle within phagosomes but the molecular basis of the organism's adherence to susceptible cells and interactions between the host and the organism are not clearly established. There is a difference between the rate of phagocytic uptake of phase I and phase II organisms. Once internalized, mainly by passive pinocytosis, the organism remains within a phagocytic vacuole. Acidification within the vacuole appears to play a major role in the transport of substrates and the growth of the organism.[42,43] While some organisms such as *Toxoplasma gondii* and *Chlamydia* spp., which grow in phagocytic vacuoles, ensure their survival by inhibiting phagosome–lysosome fusion, in cells infected with *C. burnetii* phagosome-lysosome fusion occurs without apparent damage to the organism.[62] It has been suggested that the fusion of lysosomes with the vacuoles containing the organism and the resulting low pH are required for the metabolism of the organism.[42]

Epidemiology

Host Distribution

Although clinical disease is limited largely to man,[6] a wide range of domestic and free-living ungulates are naturally infected.[2,3] The first report of the disease by Derrick[1] among slaughterhouse workers established a clear relationship between the disease and work in slaughter houses. Subsequently, Derrick and other Australian workers showed that several free-living animals carried the organism.[63–66] Thus, Q fever is a zoonosis affecting a very wide range of hosts. Horses, pigs, dogs, cats, camels and buffaloes and wild and domestic birds such as chickens, pigeons, ducks, geese and turkeys can be infected without any clinical signs.[2] *C. burnetii* has been isolated from rabbits, cats,[67,68] squirrels, mice and deer,[69] but cattle, sheep and goats are the most important reservoirs for human infections.[2] Evidence of infection has also been shown in various species of ticks, fleas, mites and flies.[2] Ticks and other arthropods are believed to play an important role in maintaining the organism in nature.[7]

Geographic Distribution

Because *C. burnetii* has not been regarded as affecting the health and production of domestic animals, the geographic distribution of animal coxeillosis is not well established[4,5] but as Q fever is a zoonosis, several serological surveys have been carried out in attempts to establish the association of human infection with infections of domestic and wild animals. Human Q fever has been reported from all parts of the world, except for the Antarctic regions. Serological tests in man and animals suggest that infections are more frequent in tropical than in temperate climates. *C. burnetii* has been reported from over 50 countries in different parts of the world.[7]

Transmission

C. burnetii is unique among the members of the family Rickettsiaceae in its nondependence on arthropod transmission and its remarkable resistance to adverse environmental conditions. That resistance and the presence of small dense cell variants has led some workers to suggest that it has an endospore form.[15] The organism is readily excreted in milk, urine, feces and uterine discharge of affected cattle, sheep, goats and other ungulates, although the period of shedding is shorter in sheep than in cows. *C. burnetii* is present in very high numbers in the amniotic fluid, the placenta and fetal membranes of parturient ewes, goats and cattle.[70–75] People and animals usually become infected by inhaling aerosols generated from infected placentae, body fluids or contaminated dust after desiccation of the primary source. Infection by ingesting infected milk or contaminated food is also possible. The organism can survive in the environment for long periods. For example, it remained in infective aerosols for up to 2 weeks and in infected soil for up to 5 months.[76,77] Because of the organism's extreme resistance to environmental factors, several types of inanimate objects (fomites) may serve as vehicles for its dissemination. They include wool,[78] shoes and other clothing, straws and other material contaminated with animal excreta.[2,79] People may be infected indirectly by handling contaminated straw or manure or by dust from farm vehicles.[80,81] The most likely way in which animals acquire infection is by inhalation of organisms from an infected environment and by ingestion of contaminated pastures, hay, straw, etc. Infection of domestic ruminants is usually seasonal, infection occurring mainly in relation to lambing or calving seasons[82] but *C. burnetii* generated by ticks, and other arthropods, may be a source of infection for domestic animals. Marrie[7] hypothesized that there may be an epidemiological circuit involving ticks, wild rodents, cats and man. He thought that in Nova Scotia ticks infect voles. Cats become infected by eating infected voles and, during parturition, can be a source of human infection. In sheep, there is some experimental evidence to suggest that pregnant animals are more susceptible to infection than nonpregnant ones. For example, Rosati[83] and Carporale *et al.*[84] reported that infected pregnant ewes were able to transmit disease to other healthy pregnant sheep placed in contact with them but not to nonpregnant animals.

Chronically infected cows may shed the organism in their milk and birth secretions for successive years.[85] There is no evidence of the organism being regularly shed from infected animals, shedding being limited to the parturient period in sheep, goats, cows and cats.[68,70,82] Ticks are important for the maintenance of the organism in nature but are not essential vectors for animal or human infection. However, the organism is shed in tick feces which may remain infectious for up to 586 days.[86]

Pathogenesis

The portal of entry is the oropharynx. After primary multiplication in the regional lymph nodes, an ensuing rickettsiamia lasts for 5–7 days and the organism then localizes in the mammary glands and the placenta of pregnant animals.[2] After a nonproductive period, experimental infection is followed by the presence of large numbers of organisms in the placenta and various secretions and excretions of parturient animals.[70] The period of maximum shedding coincides with parturition and for up to 2 weeks thereafter. Infected dairy cows excrete coxiellae in milk for many months[71] but excretion in sheep milk is short lived. The duration of shedding by dairy goats is not known but may match that of cows.[3]

Following experimental infection in sheep, the organism was isolated from the blood, milk and urine and localized in the kidneys, udder and the placenta. Occasional ewes may shed the organism at successive parturitions[87] suggesting that infection is persistent and that pregnancy enhances multiplication of the organism but how and where the organism persists during the nonpregnant period and the mechanisms which initiate its active multiplication in the placenta are not clearly understood. It has been suggested that the immunosuppressive effects of pregnancy may be responsible for the increased multiplication of the organism in the placenta.[88]

Various routes of inoculation have been used to study the pathogenesis of the organism in laboratory animals. Guinea pigs inoculated by aerosol inhalation developed interstitial pneumonia within 5–7 days and the organisms were recovered from the lungs.[89,90] Experimentally infected guinea pigs recovered from the clinical and pathological effects within 2–4 weeks, but in guinea pigs too the organism can cause a nonclinical carrier state. Several workers induced reactivation by exposing recovered guinea pigs to irradiation, treatment with cortisone or cyclophosphamide or by pregnancy.[91,92,93] It is generally thought that the organism persists in fixed macrophages and persistent infections have been established in some macrophage-like cell lines without causing apparent damage to the cells.[62]

The virulence and pathogenic mechanisms of *C. burnetii* are not clearly understood but it is generally accepted that rickettsial factors such as the LPS are important in the pathogenesis of Q fever in man and animals.[24,94] For example, experimental inoculation of guinea pigs with *C. burnetii* LPS causes clinical and pathological changes similar to those caused by experimental infection with viable organisms.[24] Although some strains of the organism may harbor plasmids, it is not yet established whether these plasmids encode any virulence factors. It may be significant, however, that some plasmids were present only in strains of *C. burnetii* isolated from cases of human chronic endocarditis and from aborting goats.[52]

Clinical Disease

There is very little information about the clinical signs of Q fever in domestic animals. Despite the earlier reports of respiratory disease due to *C. burnetii* in sheep, goats and cattle,[11–13] the only clinical disease of domestic animals attributable to *C. burnetii* is abortion in naturally and experimentally infected sheep, goats and cattle.[2] Epidemics of abortions in goats and cattle have occasionally been reported.[2,72] Most observations indicate that affected animals show no clinical signs other than abortion.[4]

Guinea pigs are highly susceptible to experimental infection. Experimental disease in guinea pigs may vary from mild to fatal conditions. Occasional chronic infections have also been reported.

In human infections acquired from cats, the greatest risk of infection follows exposure to still-born kittens,[7] suggesting that infection of cats too may be characterized by abortion and/or stillbirth. The clinical syndrome in man may be atypical febrile reactions with uneventful recovery or more serious manifestations of pneumonia, nephritis, hepatitis, meningitis, chronic endocarditis and other conditions.

No significant pathological lesions have been reported in animals naturally infected with *C. burnetii* but variable degrees of pneumonia, granulomatous hepatitis, granulomata of the bone marrow and chronic endocarditis may be present in human cases.[94] In experimental infections, pneumonia or bronchopneumonia have been reported in monkeys and mice and granulomata of the liver, bone marrow and spleen in guinea pigs.[94]

Immunity

Interaction of *C. burnetii* with the host's immune system is complex and still poorly understood. Of central significance is the organism's ability to grow and multiply within phagolysosomes and its propensity to establish persistent infection. Chronic infections are believed to be a result of immunological reactions and/or defects.[95,96]

Infection with (or vaccination against) *C. burnetii* induces both humoral and cell-mediated immunity. The latter probably effects elimination of the pathogen whereas specific antibodies serve to accelerate the process.

Role of Antibodies

While the experimental data of different sets of authors are conflicting there is, on balance, fair evidence that antibodies do play a role in immunity to coxiella infection. For example, exposure to immune serum rendered *C. burnetii* noninfectious to experimental animals[97] but not to chick embryos.[98] Similarly, some authors found that treatment with immune serum enhanced uptake of *C. burnetii* by macrophages but did not alter intracellular multiplication of the organism whereas others reported that such pretreatment of *C. burnetii* did enhance its killing by naive macrophages.[39,62,99] The effect of immune serum was further tested by its passive transfer to intact and athymic mice before and after challenge with *C. burnetii*.[100] Only when serum was given to intact mice 24 h before infection was clearance of the challenge dose enhanced. No effect was observed when serum was given with or after challenge of intact mice nor at any time in athymic mice. This led the authors to conclude that antibodies enhanced bacterial clearance by accelerating interactions of the inductive phase of the cellular arm of the immune system and activation of macrophages.

The expression of antigens specific to *C. burnetii* in the membranes of infected host cells[101] support the hypothesis that infected cells are detected by the immune system and lyzed by antibody-dependent cellular cytotoxicity (ADCC) by monocytes and other effector cells.[102] Released organisms are then vulnerable to attack by activated macrophages. Because there is greater expression of *C. burnetii* antigens by cells infected with "acute" isolates of the pathogen, the weaker and less immunologically visible expression of antigens by "chronic" strains may be a factor in persistent infections.[101]

Role of T Cells

Cellular immunity plays a central role in the clearance of the organisms from infected animals. Intact mice clear a *C. burnetii* infection within 14 days but the organism persists for at least 60 days in athymic mice, despite the production of antibody.[103] The presence of cellular immune response was demonstrated by *in vitro* tests such as lymphocyte proliferation,[95,104] macrophage migration inhibition[105] and by delayed type hypersensitivity reactions.[106] There is no evidence that cytotoxic T cells are directly involved in the lysis of infected cells but ADCC type reactivity has been demonstrated. It is interesting to note that suppressor T cells were implicated in the generation of the lymphokines which modulate immunosuppression following experimental infection of mice with *C. burnetii*.[95]

Role of Macrophages

Macrophages are important in the defence of the host against infectious agents. However, *C. burnetii* is one of those unusual intracellular rickettsiae capable of growing within macrophages. While the other members of the tribe *Rickettsieae* avoid destruction by macrophages by actively avoiding the lysosomes,[107] *C. burnetii* appears to prosper in the acid environment of the phagolysosomes.[15] It is, therefore, important to know whether or not macrophages play any role in the host's immune responses against *C. burnetii*. Normal resting macrophages appear to have no bactericidal effect on *C. burnetii* but opsonization with immune serum and, more importantly, activation by interferon render them more effective against the organism.[99,108]

Recent studies have shown that recombinant interferon (IFN-j) inhibits the growth of *C. burnetii* in L929 cells and macrophages.[108,109] These findings suggest that the clearance of the organism is probably accomplished by macrophages activated by lymphokines, particularly interferons (IFN-j).

Immunopathology and Immunosuppression

Experimental infection of mice with *C. burnetii* is often characterized by splenomegaly and hepatomegaly and in man adverse local or systemic reactions occur frequently when inactivated whole cell vaccines against *C. burnetii* are given.[110] This immunosuppression has been associated with adherent cells and with other factors such as prostaglandins.[95,111] Koster *et al.*[95] found that chronic infection with *C. burnetii* was characterized by lymphocyte unresponsiveness modulated by antigen-specific T suppressor cells which secrete lymphokines that stimulate the production of prostaglandins by monocytes or other adherent cells. Damrow *et al.*[111] demonstrated suppression of mitogen-induced lymphocyte proliferation in mice vaccinated with formalin-inactivated phase I variants but no such suppression was induced in mice inoculated with a phase II variant. The cells which mediate the immunosuppression are antigen-specific but the unresponsiveness is non-specific.[95] The immunosuppressive and pathological components of phase I whole cell vaccines can be extracted by chloroform-methanol.[112]

It has also been shown that lymphocytes obtained from persons with chronic endocarditis caused by *C. burnetii* do not respond to *C. burnetii* antigens *in vitro*.[96]

Diagnosis

Clinical Signs

In animals, coxiellosis is predominantly an asymptomatic infection[3] but the organism does have pathogenic potential.[6] The commonest expression of disease is late abortion in ruminant animals, particulary sheep and goats, sporadically or as outbreaks.

The birth of weak, nonviable offspring also occurs in infected flocks. However, abortion due to *C. burnetii* is influenced by climate and systems of animal husbandry, occurring more frequently in warm dry areas and when animals are closely herded. Abortion is more common in goats and sheep than in cows[3] but endemic infection in dairy cattle is considered to reduce fertility.[3,113]

Clinical signs in other animals which are susceptible to infection are not well-documented but human infection has been linked to parturient cats which delivered still-born kittens.[3,6,68] In man, the clinical signs are very variable but febrile "flu-like" syndromes in people whose work associates them with animals must raise the possibility of Q fever.

Post-Mortem Findings

Aborted fetuses appear normal but the heavily infected placenta exhibits intercotyledonary leathery thickening and a discolored exudate of variable consistency.[114]

Histopathology

Affected areas of the placenta show accute diffuse inflammatory and suppurative changes in the chorion without vasculitis. Intact infected chorionic epithelial cells have cytoplasmic vacuoles containing large numbers of coxiellae.[114,115]

Laboratory Diagnosis

The organism can be demonstrated in impression smears or histological sections prepared from pathological material, from the placenta and from uterine discharges and other secretions from aborting ewes, goats and cows. The presence of large masses of red-colored coccobacilli in preparations stained with Machiavello or modified Ziehl Neelson stains will indicate a strong presumptive diagnosis but must be differentiated from abortions due to *Chlamydia psittaci* or *Brucella abortus.* Impression smears and histological sections could also be used to demonstrate antigens by direct and indirect immunofluorescence and immunoperoxidase techniques (Fig. 6.2).

The most common way of establishing laboratory diagnosis is by serological means using the complement-fixation (CF) and agglutination tests.[2] In the past, the CF test was the most widely used serological test for the diagnosis of human and animal Q fever, using antigens prepared from infected yolk sacs. Human CF antibodies can

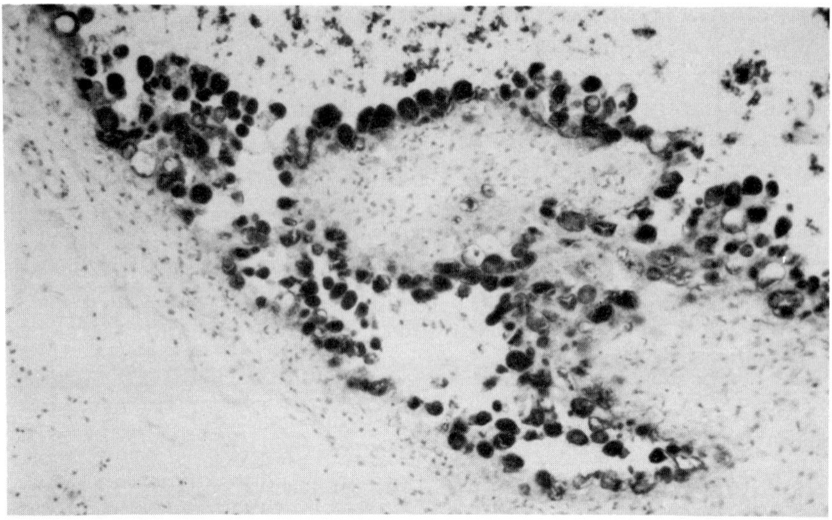

FIG. 6.2. Section of ovine placenta showing *C. burnetii* infection of chorionic epithelial cells by specific immunoperoxidase staining (× 1200). Courtesy of Dr D. Buxton.

be demonstrated at high titers for up to 2 months or longer after infection but the response usually lasts for only two weeks in animals. In infected ruminants, antibodies can be detected in milk whey as well as in serum. CF tests are widely used to differentiate phase I and phase II variants. In recent years, immunofluorescence techniques and the enzyme-linked immunosorbent assay (ELISA) have replaced the CF test in serodiagnosis.

The organism can be isolated by inoculating chick embryos or susceptible cell lines with blood and sputum from human cases and with uterine discharges, placental material and other secretions from animals.

Modern DNA probes and the polymerase chain reaction (PCR) have not yet found wide application but they will probably overtake the other tests soon. Restriction endonuclease digestion of various strains of *C. burnetii* has been used to differentiate new isolates.[49] The presence or lack of plasmids is an additional typing aid.

Treatment and Control

Treatment with antibiotics appears to have limited value in animals but chloramphenicol, lincomycin and tetracyclines have bacteriostatic effects on *C. burnetii* and are, therefore, indicated for human use.

Control measures should include the pasteurization or sterilization of milk to protect susceptible consumers and the removal and destruction of placenta. Materials such as bedding and straw contaminated by birth fluids and other secretions from affected ewes, goats and cows should be similarly destroyed. Alternatively, long term (at least 6 months) composting of bulked bedding and manure, preferably under a surface cover, will substantially reduce the level of contamination. Utensils and vehicles for animal transport must be disinfected and thoroughly washed down, to avoid contamination of the environment. However, the resistance of *C. burnetii* to standard disinfectants must be borne in mind.[116]

When abortions due to *C. burnetii* are enzootic in an area, separation of pregnant ewes, goats and cows should be considered. Vaccination of cattle, sheep and goats may be advocated in endemic areas.[117,118] Vaccine production has been hampered by the phase variation of *C. burnetii* when adapted to grow in embryonated eggs or cell culture systems. The two phases differ in their antigenicity and virulence. In general, vaccines prepared from phase II are less protective than those prepared from phase I[41] but the latter is more virulent and an immunosuppressive component has been demonstrated in whole cell vaccines prepared from phase I variants.[111] Chemical treatment of phase I cells removes undesirable immunosuppressive and reactogenic components leaving a residue from which effective experimental vaccines for animal protection have been prepared.[6,112,119] Refined vaccines containing specific protective epitopes may be expected in the future.

References

1. DERRICK, E.H. (1937. "Q" fever, new fever entity: clinical features, diagnosis and laboratory investigation. *Med. J. Aust.* **2:** 281–299.
2. BABUDIERI, B. 1959. Q fever: A zoonosis. *Adv. Vet. Sci. comp. Med.* **5:** 81–181.
3. LANG, G.H. 1990. Coxiellosis (Q fever) in animals. In: *Q fever, Vol. 1: The Diseases,* pp. 23–48. MARRIE, T.J. (Ed.). CRC Press, Boca Raton, Florida.
4. LOSOS, G.J. 1986. *Infectious Tropical Diseases of Domestic Animals,* pp. 833–848. Longman Scientific and Technical, Essex, U.K.
5. BURGDORFER, W. 1975. Q fever. In: *Diseases Transmitted from Animals to Man,* pp. 387–392. HUBBERT, W.T. and MCCULLOCH, P.R. (Eds). Charles C. Thomas, Springfield, Illinois.
6. AITKEN, I.D. 1989. Clinical aspects and prevention of Q fever in animals. *Eur. J. Epidemiol.* **5:** 420–424.
7. MARRIE, T.J. 1988. Q fever, clinical signs, symptoms and pathophysiology. In: *Biology of Rickettsial Diseases,* Vol. II, pp. 1–16. WALKER, D.G. (Ed.). CRC Press, Boca Raton, Florida.
8. DAVIS, G.E. and COX, H.R. 1938. A filter-passing infectious agent isolated from ticks. I. Isolation from *Dermacentor andersoni,* reactions in animals, and filtration experiments. *Publ. Hlth. Rep.* **53:** 2259–2267.

9. Dyer, R.E. 1938. A filter-passing infectious agent isolated from ticks. IV. Human infection. *Publ. Hlth. Rep.* **53:** 2277–2282.
10. Dyer, R.E. 1939. Similarity of Australian "Q" fever and a disease caused by an infectious agent isolated from ticks in *Publ. Hlth. Rep.* **54:** 1229–1237.
11. Caminopetros, J. 1949. La broncho-pneumonie epidemique fievre Q ou Grippe des Balkans, a *Rickettsia burneti* var *caprina*. Les caracteres particuliers de l'infection animale, *Ann. Inst. Pasteur* **77:** 750–756.
12. Caporale, G. 1950. Nuove ricerche sul ruolo degli animali nella insorgenza della febbre Q nell'uomo. *Atti. Soc. Ital. Sci. Vet.* **4:** 587–601.
13. Payzin, S. 1953. Epidemiological investigations on Q fever in Turkey. *Bull. World Hlth. Ord.* **9:** 553–558.
14. Thompson, H.A. 1986. Relationship of the physiology and composition of *Coxiella burnetii* to the *Coxiella*–host cell interaction. In: *Biology of Rikettsial Diseases,* pp. 51–78. Walker, D.H. (Ed.). CRC Press, Boca Raton, Florida.
15. McCaul, T.F. and Williams, J.C. 1981. Developmental cycle of *Coxiella burnetii*: structure and morphogenesis of vegetative and sporogenic differences. *J. Bacteriol.* **147:** 1063–1076.
16. Baca, O.G. and Paretsky, D. 1983. Q fever and *Coxiella burnetii*: a model for host–parasite interactions. *Microbiol. Rev.* **47:** 127–149.
17. Weisburg, W.B., Dobson, M.E., Samuel, J.E., Dasch, G.A., Mallavia, L.P., Baca, O.G., Mandelco, L., Sechrest, J.E. and Woese, C.R. 1989. Phylogenetic diversity of the rickettsiae. *J. Bacteriol.* **171:** 4202–4206.
18. Gimenez, D.F. 1065. Gram staining of *Coxiella burnetii*. *J. Bacteriol.* **90:** 834–835.
19. Kordova, K. 1959. Filterable particles of *Coxiella burnetii*. *Acta Virol.* **3:** 25–36.
20. Wiebe, M.E., Burton, P.R. and Shankel, D.M. 1972. Isolation and characterization of two cell types of *Coxiella burnetii* phase I. *J. Bacteriol.* **110:** 368–377.
21. Canonica, P.G., Van Zwieten, M.J. and Christmas, W.A. 1972. Purification of large quantities of *Coxiella burnetii* rickettsia by density gradient zonal centrifugation. *Appl. Microbiol.* **23:** 1015–1022.
22. Burton, P.R., Stueckemann, J. and Paretsky, D. 1975. Electron microscopy studies of the limiting layers of the rickettsia *Coxiella burnetii*. *J. Bacteriol.* **122:** 316–324.
23. Jerrels, T.R., Hinrichs, D.J. and Mallavia, L.P. 1974. Cell envelope analysis of *Coxiella burnetii* phase I and phase II. *Can. J. Microbiol.* **20:** 1465–1470.
24. Baca, O.G. and Paretsky, D. 1974a. Some physiological and biochemical effects of *Coxiella burnetii* lipopolysaccharide preparation on guinea pigs. *Infect. Immunol.* **9:** 939–945.
25. Baca, O.G. and Paretsky, D. 1974. Physical characterization of toxic lipopolysaccharide from *Coxiella burnetii*. *Infect. Immunol.* **9:** 959–961.
26. Amano, K.I. and Williams, J.C. 1984. Sensitivity of *Coxiella burnetii* peptidoglycan to lysozyme hydrolysis and correlation of sacculus rigidity with peptidoglycan-associated proteins. *J. Bacteriol.* **160:** 989–993.
27. Stoker, M.G.P. and Fiset, P. 1956. Phase variation of the Nine Mile and other strains of *Rickettsia burnetii*. *Can. J. Microbiol.* **2:** 310–321.
28. Williams, J.C., Peacock, M. and McCaul, T.F. 1981. Immunological and biological characterization of *Coxiella burnetii*, phase I and phase II, separated from host components. *Infect. Immunol.* **32:** 840–851.
29. Hoyer, B.H., Ormsbee, R.A., Fiset, P. and Lackman, D.B. 1963. Differentiation of phase I and phase II *Coxiella burnetii* by equilibrium density gradient sedimentation. *Nature* **197:** 573–574.

30. ORMSBEE, R.A.E. 1952. The growth of *Coxiella burnetii* in embryonated eggs. *J. Bacteriol.* **63:** 73–86.
31. LEYK, W. and SCHEFFER, R. 1975. Multiplication of *Coxiella burnetii* in different tissues and organs of embryonated eggs. *Zentralbl. Baketeriol. Parasitenkd Infektionskr. Hyg. Abt.* **231:** 519–524.
32. BURTON, P.R., KORDOVA, N. and PARETSKY, D. 1971. Electron microscopic studies of the rickettsia *Coxiella burnetii*: entry, lysosomal response, and fate of rickettsial DNA in L-cells. *Can. J. Microbiol.* **17:** 143–158.
33. WEISS, E. and PIETRYK, H.C. 1956. Growth of *Coxiella burnetii* in monolayer cultures of chicken embryo endodermal cells. *J. Bacteriol* **72:** 544–552.
34. BLACKFORD, V.I. 1961. Influence of various metabolites on growth of *Coxiella burnetii* in monolayer cultures of chicken embryo endodermal cells. *J. Bacteriol.* **81:** 747–754.
35. BACA, O.G. 1991. Pathogenesis of rickettsial infections-emphasis on Q fever. In: *Proceedings of the IVth International Symposium on Rickettsioses and Rickettsial Diseases,* pp. 221–231. KAZAR, J. and RAOULT, D. (Eds). Publishing House of Slovak Academy of Sciences, Bratislava.
36. BACA, O.G., ARAGON, A.S., AKPORIAYE, E.T., MARTINEZ, I.L. and WARNER, N.L. 1981. Interaction of *Coxiella burnetii* in several macrophage-like cells lines. In: *Rickettsiae and Rickettsial Diseases,* pp. 91–101. BURGDORFER, W. and ANACKER, R.L. (Eds). Academic Press Inc., New York.
37. BURTON, P.R., STUECKEMANN, J., WELSH, R.M. and PARETSKY, D. 1978. Electron microscopy—Some ultrastructural effects of persistent infection by the rickettsia *Coxiella burnetii* in mouse L cells and green monkey kidney (Vero) cells. *Infect. Immunol.* **21:** 556–566.
38. ROSENBERG, M. and KORDOVA, K. 1960. Study of intra-cellular forms of *Coxiella burnetii* in the electron microscope. *Acta Virol.* **4:** 52–55.
39. KISHIMOTO, R.A. and WALKER, J.S. 1976. Interaction between *Coxiella burnetii* and guinea pig peritoneal macrophages. *Infect. Immunol.* **14:** 416–421.
40. KISHIMOTO, R.A., VELTRI, B.J., SHIRLEY, F.G., CANONICO, P.G. and WALKER, J.S. 1977. Fate of *Coxiella burnetii* in macrophages from immune guinea pigs. *Infect. Immunol.* **15:** 601–607.
40. ORMSBEE, R.A.E. and PEACOCK, M.G. 1964. Metabolic activity in *Coxiella burnetii. J. Bacteriol.* **88:** 1205–1210.
42. HACKSTADT, T. and WILLIAMS, J.C. 1981a. Biochemical stratagem for obligate parasitism of eukaryotic cells by *Coxiella burnetii. Proc. natn. Acad. Sci. U.S.A.* **78:** 3240–3244.
43. HACKSTADT, T. and WILLIAMS, J.C. 1981b. Stability of adenosine 5'-triphosphate pool in *Coxiella burnetii.*: Influence of pH and substrate. *J. Bacteriol.* **148:** 419–425.
44. MYERS, W.F., BACA, O.G. and WISSEMAN, C.L. 1980. Genetic relatedness among the typhus group of rickettsiae. *J. Syst. Bacteriol.* **30:** 143–150.
45. MYERS, W.F. and WISSEMAN, C.L. 1980. Genome size of the rickettsia *Coxiella burnetii. J. Bacteriol.* **144:** 460–461.
46. REGENRY, R.L., TZIANABOS, T., ESPOSITO, J.J. and MCDADE, J.E. 1983. Strain differentiation of epidemic typhus rickettsiae (*Rickettsia prowazekii*) by DNA restriction endonuclease analysis. *Curr. Microbiol.* **8:** 355–358.
47. MCCLENGHAN, M., HERRING, A.J. and AITKEN, I.D. 1984. Comparison of *Chlamydia psittaci* isolated by DNA restriction endonuclease analysis. *Infect. Immunol.* **45:** 384–389.
48. SCHRAMEK, S. 1968. Isolation and characterization of deoxyribonucleic acid from *Coxiella burnetii. Acta Virol.* **12:** 18–22.

49. O'Rourke, A.T., Peacock, M., Samuel, J.E., Frazier, M.E., Natvig, D.O., Mallavia, L.P. and Baca, O. 1985. Genomic analysis of phase I and phase II *Coxiella burnetii* with restriction endonucleases. *J. gen. Microbiol.* **131:** 1543–1546.
50. Sawyer, L.A., Fishbein, D.B. and McDade, J.E. 1987. Q fever: Current concepts. *Rev. Infect. Dis.* **9:** 935–946.
51. Samuel, J.E., Frazier, M.E., Kahn, M.L., Thompson, L.S. and Mallavia, L.P. 1983. Isolation and characterization of a plasmid from phase I *Coxiella burnetii. Infect. Immunol.* **41:** 488–493.
52. Samuel, J.E., Frazier, M.E. and Mallavia, L.P. 1985. Correlation of plasmid type and disease caused by *Coxiella burnetii. Infect. Immunol.* **49:** 775–779.
53. Brezina, R. 1958. Contribution to the study of phase variation in *Coxiella burnetii. Acta Virol.* **2:** 91–102.
54. Baca, O.G. 1988. Surface antigens of *Coxiella burnetii.* In: *Biology of Rickettsial Diseases,* Vol. II, pp. 127–134. Walker, D.H. (Ed.). CRC Press, Boca Raton, Florida.
55. Kordova, N. 1970. *Coxiella burnetii. Acta Virol.* **14:** 78.
56. Baca, O.G., Martinez, I.L., Aragon, A.S. and Klassen, D. 1980. Isolation and partial characterization of lipopolysaccharide from phase II *Coxiella burnetii. Can. J. Microbiol.* **26:** 819–825.
57. Schramek, S. and Brezina, R. 1979. Isolation of endotoxic lipopolysaccharide from phase II *Coxiella burnetii. Acta Virol.* **23:** 349.
58. Schramek, S. and Brezina, R. 1976. Characterization of an endotoxic lipopolysaccharide from *Coxiella burnetii. Acta Virol.* **20:** 152–158.
59. Hackstadt, T., Peacock, M.G., Hitchcock, P.J. and Cole, R.L. 1985. Lipolysaccharide variation in *Coxiella burnetii. Infect. Immunol.* **48:** 359–365.
60. Schramek, S. and Meyer, H. 1982. Different sugar compositions of phase I and phase II cells of *Coxiella burnetii. Infect. Immunol.* **38:** 53–57.
61. Williams, J.C., Johnston, M.R., Peacock, M.G., Thomas, L.A., Stewart, S. and Portis, J.L. 1984. Monoclonal antibodies distinguish phase variants of *Coxiella burnetii. Infect. Immunol.* **43:** 421–428.
62. Akporiaye, E.T., Rowatt, J.D., Aragon, A.A. and Baca, O.G. 1983. Lysosomal response of urine macrophage-like cell line persistently infected with *Coxiella burnetii. Infect. Immunol.* **40:** 1155–1162.
63. Derrick, E.H., Smith, D.J.W., Brown, H.E. and Freeman, M. 1939. The role of the bandicoot in the epidemiology of Q fever: a preliminary study. *Med. J. Aust.* **1:** 150–155.
64. Burnet, F.M., Freeman, M., Derrick, E.H. and Smith, D.J.W. 1939. The search for immunological relationship between Q fever and other rickettsioses. *Med. J. Aust.* **1:** 51–54.
65. Derrick, E.H. and Smith, D.J.W. 1940. Studies in the epidemiology of Q fever. 2. The isolation of three strains of *Rickettsia burnetii* from the bandicoot *Isoodon torosus. Aust. J. exp. Med. Sci.* **18:** 99–102.
66. Freeman, M., Derrick, E.H., Brown, H.E., Smith, D.J.W. and Johnson, D.W. 1940. Studies on the epidemiology of Q fever. 5. Survey of human and animal sera for *Rickettsia burnetii* agglutinins. *Aust. J. exp. Med. Sci.* **18:** 193–200.
67. Marrie, T.J., Schlech, W.F., Williams, J.C. and Yates, L. 1986. Q fever pneumonia associated with exposure to wild rabbits. *Lancet* **i:** 427–429.
68. Kosatsky, T. 1984. Household outbreak of Q fever pneumonia related to parturient cat. *Lancet* **ii:** 1447–1449.
69. Enright, J.B., Franti, C.E., Behymer, D.E., Longhurst, W.M., Dutson,

V.J. and WRIGHT, M.E. 1971. *Coxiella burnetii* in wildlife–livestock environment: Distribution of Q fever in wild mammals. *Am. J. Epidemiol.* **94:** 79–90.
70. ABINANTI, F.R., LENNETTE, E.H., WINN, J.F. and WELSH, H.H. 1953. Q fever studies. XVIII. Presence of *Coxiella burnetii* in the fluids of naturally infected sheep. *Am. J. Hyg.* **58:** 385–388.
71. GRIST, N.R. 1959. The persistence of Q fever infection in a dairy herd. *Vet. Rec.* **71:** 839–841.
72. LUOTO, L. and HUEBNER, R.J. 1950. Q fever in Southern California. IX. Isolation of Q fever organisms from parturient placentas of naturally infected dairy cows. *Publ. Hlth. Rep.* **65:** 541–544.
73. STOKER, M.G.P. and MARMION, B.P. 1955. The spread of Q fever from animals to man: The natural history of a rickettsial disease. *Bull. World Hlth. Org.* **13:** 781–806.
74. STOKER, M.G.P., BROWN, R.D., KETT, F.J.L., COLLINGS, P.C. and MARMION, B.P. 1955. Q fever in Britain. Isolation of *Rickettsia burnetii* from placenta and wool of sheep in an endemic area. *J. Hyg.* **53:** 313–321.
75. WELSH, H.H., LENNETTE, E.H., ABINANTI, F.R. and WINN, J.F. 1983. Q fever in California: IV. Occurrence of *Coxiella burnetii* in the birth fluids of naturally infected sheep. *Am. J. Hyg.* **58:** 385–388.
76. LENNETTE, E.H. and WELSH, H.H. 1951. Q fever in California. X. Recovery of *Coxiella burnetii* from the air of premises harbouring infected goats. *Am. J. Hyg.* **54:** 44–49.
77. WELSH, H.H., LENNETTE, E.H., ABINANTI, F.R. and WINN, J.F. 1958. Airborne transmission of Q fever: the role of parturition in the generation of infective aerosols. *Ann. N.Y. Acad. Sci.* **70:** 528–540.
78. ABINANTI, F.R., LENNETTE, E.H., WINN, J.F. and WELSH, H.H. 1955. Q fever studies. XIX. Presence and epidemiologic significance of *Coxiella burnetii* in sheep wool. *Am. J. Hyg.* **61:** 362–370.
79. HARVEY, M.S., FORBES, G.B. and MARMION, B.P. 1951. An outbreak of Q fever in East Kent. *Lancet* **2:** 1152–1157.
80. MARMION, B.P. and STOKER, M.G.P. 1958. The epidemiology of Q fever in Great Britain, an analysis of the findings and some conclusions. *Br. Med. J.* **2:** 809–816.
81. BENSON, W.W., BROCK, D.W. and MATHER, J. 1963. Serological analysis of penitentiary group using raw milk from an infected herd. *Publ. Hlth. Rep.* **78:** 707–710.
82. ENRIGHT, J.B., LONGHURST, W.M., FRANTI, C.E. 1971. *Coxiella burnetii* in wildlife–livestock environment. Isolation of rickettsiae from sheep and cattle. *Am. J. Epidemiol.* **94:** 72–79.
83. ROSATI, T. 1952. In Seminario sull'epidemiologia della febbre Q in Italia. *Ann. Sanit. Publicn.* **13:** 88–89.
84. CAPORALE, G., MIRRI, A. and ROSATI, T. 1953. La febbre Q quale zoonosi. *Atti. Soc. Ital. Sci. Vet.* **7:** 13–96.
85. BIBERSTEIN, E.L., BEHYMER, D.E., BUSHNELL, R., CRENSHAW, G.L., REINMANN, H.P. and FRANTI, C.E. 1974. A survey of Q fever (*Coxiella burnetii*) in Californian dairy cows: results of field trials. *Am. J. Vet. Res.* **35:** 1577–1582.
86. ORMSBEE, R.A. 1972. In: *Viral and Rickettsial Infections of Man,* 4th edn, pp. 1144–1160. HORSFALL, F.L.J.C. and TAMM, I. (Eds). J. B. Lippincott, Philadelphia.
87. WELSH, H.H., JENSEN, F.W. and LENNETTE, E.H. 1959. Q fever studies. XX. Comparison of four serologic techniques for the detection and measurement of antibody to *Coxiella burnetii* in naturally exposed sheep. *Am. J. Hyg.* **70:** 1–13.

88. Polydorou, K. 1981. Q fever in Cyprus: a short review. *Br. Vet. J.* **137:** 470–477.
89. Kishimoto, R.A. and Burger, G.T. 1977. Appearance of cellular and humoral immunity in guinea pigs after infection with *Coxiella burnetii* administered in small particle aerosole. *Infect. Immunol.* **16:** 518–521.
90. Powanda, M.C., Machotka, S.V. and Kishimoto, R.A. 1978. Metabolic sequelae of respiratory Q fever in the guinea pig. *Proc. Soc. exp. Biol. Med.* **158:** 626.
91. Sidwell, R.W., Thorpe, B.D. and Gebhardt, L.P. 1964a. Studies of latent Q fever infections. I. Effects of whole body X-irradiation upon latently infected guinea pig, white mice and deer mice. *Am. J. Hyg.* **79:** 113–124.
92. Sidwell, R.W., Thorpe, B.D. and Gebhardt, L. P. 1964. Studies of latent Q fever infections. II. Effects of multiple cortisone injections. *Am. J. Hyg.* **79:** 320–327.
93. Johnson, J.W., Eddy, G.A. and Pederson, C.E. 1976. Biologic properties of the M-44 strain of *Coxiella burnetii. J. Infect. Dis.* **133:** 334–338.
94. Walker, D.H. 1988. Pathology of Q fever. In: *Biology of Rickettsial Diseases,* Vol. II, pp. 17–27. Walker, D.H. (Ed.). CRC Press, Boca Raton, Florida.
95. Koster, F.T., Williams, J.C. and Goodwin, J.S. 1985. Cellular immunity in Q fever: modulation of responsiveness by suppressor T cell–monocyte circuit. *J. Immunol.* **135:** 1067–1072.
96. Koster, F.T., Goodwin, J.S. and Williams, J.C. 1985. Selective antigen-specific anergy in patients with Q fever. *J. Infect. Dis.* **152:** 1283–1289.
97. Abinanti, F.R. and Marmion, B.P. 1957. Protective or neutralizing antibody to Q fever. *Am. J. Hyg.* **66:** 173–195.
98. Brezina, R. and Kazar, J. 1965. Study on the antigenic structure of *Coxiella burnetii.* IV. Phagocytosis and opsonization in relation to phases of *C. burnetii. Acta Virol.* **9:** 268–274.
99. Hinrichs, D.J. and Jerrells, T.R. 1976. *In vitro* evaluation of immunity to *Coxiella burnetii. J. Immunol.* **117:** 996–1003.
100. Humphries, R.C. and Hinrichs, D.J. 1981. Role for antibody in *Coxiella burnetii* infection. *Infect. Immunol.* **31:** 641–645.
101. Baca, O.G., Roman, M.J., Samsonoff, W.A., Crissman, H.A. and Hechemy, K.E. 1991. Analysis of *Coxiella burnetii* isolated in cell culture. In: *Proceedings of the IVth International Symposium on Rickettsioses and Rickettsial Diseases,* pp. 221–231. Kazar, J. and Raoult, D. (Eds). Publishing House of the Slovak Academy of Sciences, Bratislava.
102. Koster, F.T., Kirpatrick, T.L., Rowatt, J.D. and Baca, O.G.J.S. 1984. Antibody-dependent cellular cytotoxicity of *Coxiella burnetii* infected J774 macrophage target cells. *Infect. Immunol.* **43:** 253–256.
103. Kishimoto, R.A., Rozmiavek, H. and Larson, E.W. 1978. Experimental Q fever infection in congenitally athymic nude mice. *Infect. Immunol.* **22:** 69–71.
104. Jerrells, T.R., Mallavia, L.P. and Hinrichs, D.J. 1975. Detection of long-term cellular immunity to *Coxiella burnetii* as assayed by lymphocyte transformation. *Infect. Immunol.* **11:** 280–286.
105. Heggers, J.P., Mallavia, L.P. and Hinrichs, D.J. 1974. The cellular immune response to antigens of *Coxiella burnetii. Can. J. Microbiol.* **20:** 657–662.
106. Brezina, R., Pospisil, V. and Schramek, R. 1970. Study of the antigenic structure of *Coxiella burnetii.* VII. Properties of phenol-extracted phase I antigenic components. *Acta Virol.* **14:** 295–301.
107. Weiss, E. 1973. Growth and physiology of rickettsiae. *Bacteriol. Rev.* **37:** 259–283.

108. JERRELS, T.R. 1988. Mechanisms of immunity to Rickettsia species and *Coxiella burnetii*. In: *The Biology of the Rickettsiae*, pp. 79–100. WALKER, D.H. (Ed.). Vol. II. CRC Press, Boca Raton, Florida.
109. TURCO, J., THOMPSON, H.A. and WALKER, H.H. 1984. Interferon-j inhibits the growth of *Coxiella burnetii* in mouse fibroblasts. *Infect. Immunol.* **45:** 781.
110. WILLIAMS, J.C. and CANTRELL, J.L. 1982. Biological and immunological properties of *Coxiella burnetii* vaccines in C57BL/10ScN endotoxin non-responsive mice. *Infect. Immunol.* **35:** 1091–1102.
111. DAMROW, T.A., WILLIAMS, J.C. and WAAG, D.M. 1985. Suppression of *in vitro* lymphocyte proliferation in C57BL/10ScN mice vaccinated with phase I *Coxiella burnetii. Infect. Immunol.* **47:** 149–156.
112. WILLIAMS, J.C., DAMROW, T.A., WAAG, D.M. and AMANO, K. 1986. Characterization of phase I *Coxiella burnetii* chloroform–methanol residue vaccine that induces active immunity against Q fever in C57BL/10ScN mice. *Infect. Immunol.* **51:** 851–858.
113. SCHMEER, N., WIEDA, J., FROST, J.W., HERBST, W., WEISS, R. and KRAUSS, H. 1987. Diagnosis, differential diagnosis and control of bovine Q fever in dairy herd with infertility. *Tierartzl. Umsch.* **42:** 287.
114. PALMER, N.C., KIERSTEAD, M., KEY, D.W., WILLIAMS, J.C., PEACOCK, M.G. and VELLAND, H. 1983. Placentitis and abortion in goats and sheep in Ontario caused by *Coxiella burnetii. Can. Vet. J.* **24:** 60–61.
115. JUBB, K.V.F., KENNEDY, P.C. and PALMER, N. 1985. *Pathology of Domestic Animals*, 3rd edn, Vol. 3, pp. 305–407. Academic Press Inc.
116. SCOTT, G.H. and WILLIAMS, J.C. 1990. Susceptibility of *Coxiella burnetii* to chemical disinfectants. In: Rickettsiology: Current issues and perspectives. HECHEMY, K.E., WALKER, D.H. and MALLAVIA, L.P. (Eds). *Ann. N.Y. Acad. Sci.* **590:** 291–296.
117. LUOTO, L., WINN, J.F. and HUEBNER, R.J. 1952. Q fever in Southern California. XIII. Vaccination of dairy cattle against Q fever. *Am. J. Hyg.* **55:** 190–202.
118. BIBERSTEIN, E.L., REIMANN, H.P., FRANTI, C.E., BEHYMER, D.E., RUPPANNER, R., BUSHNELL, R. and CRENSHAW, G.L. 1977. Vaccination of dairy cattle against Q fever (*Coxiella burnetii*): results of field trials. *Am. J. Vet. Res.* **38:** 189–193.
119. SCHMEER, N., MULLER, P., LANGEL, J., KRAUSS, H., FROST, J.W. and WEIDA, J. 1987. Q fever vaccines for animals. *Zentral. Bakt. Micro. Hyg.* **A267:** 79–88.

7

Rocky Mountain Spotted Fever in Dogs

C. E. GREENE AND E. B. BREITSCHWERDT

Introduction

Rocky Mountain spotted fever (RMSF) is a tickborne, rickettsial disease of the Americas that affects dogs and people. Prior to 1930 it was recognized primarily in the western United States. Overall, the reported prevalence of the human disease appears to have increased since its discovery, with the highest yearly prevalence now being reported from the eastern United States. Presumably, this increase reflects increased recognition and reporting rather than geographic spread of the disease.[1]

Causal Agent

Rickettsia rickettsii, the etiologic agent of RMSF, is an obligate intracellular parasite in the family Rickettsiaceae. Members of the spotted fever group (SFG), such as *R. rickettsii,* are related to the typhus group of rickettsiae but are more distinct from the other genera. Serologically and pathogenically distinct strains of SFG rickettsiae have been described throughout the world.[2–4] Four main SFG species, *R. rickettsii, R. montana, R. rhipicephali* and *R. bellii,* can be isolated from ticks in the United States. *R. rickettsii* is the only SFG rickettsia in the Western Hemisphere known to be pathogenic for people and animals. Pathogenic differences have also been noted between different isolates of *R. rickettsii.* Comparative infectivity studies have indicated that strains do vary in virulence. Nevertheless, some of these differences may reflect susceptibility of different experimental hosts, the handling and passage of various isolates in the laboratory and the amount of inoculum used in various experiments.

Molecular Biology

Members of the genus *Rickettsia* have been shown to contain heat-shock proteins (HSP), common to many pathogenic bacteria, which are thought to have a role in protection against the host's immune system.[5] The presence of immune responses to specific bacterial HSP60 antigen may be an important stimulus for the host response to the organism. Because of similarities of HSP60 to host cell proteins, there is speculation that the immune response to bacterial HSPs may induce autoimmune responses in the course of rickettsial infections.

A number of outer membrane proteins of *R. rickettsii* that have been separated by sodium dodecyl sulfate-polyacrylamide gel electrophoresis (SDS-PAGE) have been shown to react with convalescent antisera from mice, guinea pigs and humans following infection or immunization with SFG rickettsiae. A 17 kDa protein has been found to be unique to the genus *Rickettsia* including typhus and spotted-fever species.[6] The fact that this protein is preserved suggests its beneficial role in survival of these organisms. Immunoelectron microscopy has identified this antigen in the outer membrane fraction and it may play a role in joining the outer membrane with associated lipopolysaccharide complexes.

Organisms of the genus *Rickettsia* also possess outer crystalline surface layer (S-layer) proteins which are found in most other bacteria. Two major polypeptides found in most members of *Rickettsia* play important roles as immunogens and may be responsible for some of the pathogenic features of these organisms.[7] Hypotonic shock solubilizes the high molecular weight, species (serotype)-specific protein antigens (SPAs) from this layer. All of the members in the genus (typhus and spotted fever groups), with the exception of *R. bellii,* have a small SPA (S-SPA) with a size of 115–120 kDa when solubilized with SDS prior to SDS-agar electrophoresis. *R. canada* and all other spotted fever rickettsiae have a second larger SPA (L-SPA) with a size range of 130–200 kDa that varies with the strain and species. Both L- and S-SPAs have low- and high-temperature forms (LT and HT) depending whether room temperature or 40°C is used respectively during their solubilization. Monoclonal antibodies that can react with LT but not HT forms of S-SPA and L-SPA can neutralize rickettsial pathogenicity in laboratory rodents.[8,9]

Differentiation of species of the genus *Rickettsia* has been aided by comparison of their DNA sequences. Analysis of restriction endonuclease digestion of DNA following PCR amplification and hybridization with labelled probes has been used as an alternative to serologic differentiation of the rickettsiae.[10–12] Compared to isolates of eubacterial species, rickettsial isolates within a species have relatively concerned genomic sequences. Results of these studies suggest that several SFG strains worldwide are closely related to *R. rickettsii*.

The genes encoding large and small SPAs of some species of Rickettsia have been cloned, however, the sequences have not yet been completely mapped or compared.[13] Sequencing of the cloned 155 kDa antigen from the "R" strain of *R. rickettsii* is complete.[14] Differentiation of closely-related SFG rickettsiae can be accomplished with PCR using primers that amplify the 155 kDa surface antigen gene of *R. rickettsii*.[10,15] The gene encoding the 17 kDa antigen has also been found to be unique for each species allowing their genetic differentiation and separation of the spotted-fever group from the typhus group rickettsiae.[12]

Epidemiology

Natural Transmission

Ticks become infected by two means. First, horizontal transmission can occur during feeding of noninfected ticks on small mammals, including chipmunks, voles and ground squirrels that have developed sufficient rickettsemia during acute infection. The primary sylvan cycle, which maintains the transmission cycle in nature, occurs between these small rodents and immature (larval and nymphal) tick stages. It is also possible that medium-sized mammals such as racoons, opossums and foxes are additional sources for infecting ticks. Although of minor importance, birds are a means by which infected ticks can be transported into new areas.

Second, ticks can be infected trans-stadially by transovarial passage between generations. *R. rickettsii* initially replicates in the epithelial cells of the tick midgut, enters the hemocoel, and from there spreads to, and multiplies in, other tick tissues, including the salivary glands and ovaries. Ticks must ingest numerous rickettsiae for successful transovarial transmission.

Several factors may explain why RMSF is limited to geographic foci in the Americas. The overall low prevalence of infection in ticks, less than 2% even in areas with a high prevalence of RMSF, suggests that most mammalian hosts of adult ticks, such as dogs, rarely develop rickettsemias of sufficient magnitude and duration to infect large numbers of ticks.[16] Sampling errors also may explain why focal ecologic pockets of infected ticks have been found.

Spread of infection within tick and host populations also appears to be limited by certain factors. Transmission of infection from male to female ticks during mating does not occur.[1] Immature ticks do not usually feed more than once between each stage before moulting. Adult female ticks feed only once; following a bloodmeal, they drop from the dog, deposit eggs, and die. Females with ovarian infection may transmit rickettsiae to as many as 100% of progeny. Adult male ticks may have some importance in spread of RMSF to mammals because they feed intermittently on a succession of hosts in search of female ticks.

Tick immobility and restricted territorial movement of small rodents may be additional factors in limiting the uniform spread of *R. rickettsii* through tick populations. Environmental factors such as low (<50%) humidity, colder temperatures and decreased vegetation further inhibit survival of infected ticks. Resistance to infection with *R. rickettsii* develops in ticks and possible mammalian hosts as a result of infection with the three other common nonpathogenic SFG rickettsiae.

For reasons that are not completely understood, ticks do not usually infect a new host until they have been attached for a minimum of 5 to 20 h. A period of feeding may be needed for the production of infective organisms in the salivary glands. It may also relate to the need of the tick to produce a cement collar around their mouth parts before they begin feeding. Although infections that people acquire from being bitten by ticks require extended attachment, those acquired from contact of mucous membranes with feces or hemolymph from pre-engorged ticks attached to animals do not appear to involve extended contact periods.

Hosts Affected

This disease has been described as a clinical entity in people and dogs. Although cats and other domestic animals can have a seropositive test result for the organism, knowledge concerning the seroprevalence or clinical disease in these animals is minimal.

Geographic Distribution

Deciduous forests, increased humidity and warmer temperatures are factors associated with the high prevalence of RMSF. It is known to occur throughout the contiguous United States with the exception of Maine. It has been reported in western Canada, Mexico, Panama, Costa Rica, Honduras, Nicaragua, Colombia and Brazil.

The natural history and distribution of RMSF in the United States appears to center primarily on the distribution of two ticks,

Dermacentor andersoni and *D. variabilis,* which serve as natural hosts, reservoirs and vectors for *R. rickettsii.*

D. andersoni (the woodtick) is a three-host tick that is found from the Cascades to the Rocky Mountains.[17] It is the principal vector of RMSF in the western United States and is also present in Canada in the provinces of southern British Columbia, Alberta and Saskatchewan.

D. variabilis (American dog tick) is a three-host tick found from the Great Plains region eastward to the Atlantic Coast of the United States and southern Canada. It has also been reported in California, southwest Oregon, southern Washington and Idaho.

Three other ticks have been incriminated in the transmission of RMSF to animals and people, but their significance is uncertain. The Lone Star tick (*Amblyomma americanum*) occurs in the United States from Texas eastward to the Atlantic coast. The brown dog tick, *Rhipicephalus sanguineus*, is found throughout the United States, southern Canada, Mexico, and South America. *Haemaphysalis leporispalustris,* the rabbit tick, resides throughout the Western Hemisphere. Although rickettsiae recovered from this tick are antigenically similar to *R. rickettsii*, they do not produce disease in laboratory animals.

Pathogenesis

R. rickettsii usually enter the body through the bite of infected ticks. Via the circulatory system, rickettsiae invade and replicate in endothelial cells of smaller blood vessels. Endothelial cell damage initiates platelet activation and activation of the coagulation system.[18,19] Results of coagulation factor analysis suggest activation of both the extrinsic and intrinsic pathways.[18] Progressive necrotizing vasculitis may be caused sequentially by complement activation, cellular chemotaxis, and subsequent vascular necrosis and extravasation of blood. Organs with endarterial circulation, such as the skin, brain, heart and kidneys, are frequently affected.

Significantly increased plasma and extracellular fluid volume have been described in experimental infections of nonhuman primates.[20] In people, accumulation of extracellular volume and electrolytes, renal water retention and edema were correlated with increased concentrations of aldosterone and antidiuretic hormone.[21] Fluid overload in the circulation and edema of the medulla oblongata in experimental animals[20] suggest that intravenous fluid therapy may be used sparingly in the management of dogs with RMSF. CNS signs and death may relate to cardiorespiratory depression through edema of medullary centers. Fulminant infection may result in peripheral vascular collapse and death in the first week of infection, before proliferative and thrombotic lesions occur. Acute renal failure, a fatal complication of RMSF in people, is not frequently seen in dogs with RMSF.

Clinical Disease

Both clinical and subclinical illnesses have been reported in dogs with naturally occurring and experimentally produced RMSF. Most dogs are presented for examination for illness during the months of March to October. Clinical signs of illness in dogs are similar to those in cases of naturally infected people and most commonly include systemic signs of fever (>37.8 C) anorexia, mental depression, lymphadenomegaly, subcutaneous edema, stiff gait, myalgia and arthralgia, petechiae of mucosae and skin, abdominal discomfort and coughing.[22–26] Funduscopic examination provide a more sensitive means of detecting these hemorrhagic lesions. Epistaxis, melena, and hematuria may be noted in severely affected animals.

Neurologic signs of generalized cerebral and spinal cord involvement have been found. Focal or localizing neurologic signs, such as vestibular disease, are common.[22,27,28]

Infected dogs may make a rapid complete recovery if they are mildly affected or with the early institution of antimicrobial therapy. Permanent organ damage may occur within 1 to 2 weeks of onset of clinical signs in severely affected dogs that survive the acute stages of illness. Necrosis of the extremities at sites of hyperemia edema may occur.[29] Dogs may die in the acute stages of illness as a result of hemorrhagic diathesis or from thrombosis of vital organs. Cardiovascular, neurologic, and renal damage are the most consistent cause of death or functional impairments. Death in some severely affected dogs has been caused by disseminated, rapidly progressing meningoencephalitis. Shock, cardiovascular collapse, icterus and oliguria become apparent only in severe terminal stages of illness.

Veterinary Public Health

The clinical manifestations in affected people closely parallel those signs seen in dogs. Therefore infection in dogs serves as both a model and sentinel for human infection. Of the more than 1000 cases of rickettsial diseases reported in people each year in the United States, approximately 90% are RMSF.[30]

Approximately 10% of reported human cases follow only known exposure to dogs or their ticks, but this should not imply an absolute association, because common exposure to the same tick population is more likely.[31] Dogs are a potential source for human infections because they carry infected ticks into closer proximity to people, who become exposed by transfer of ticks from dogs to themselves or by their contact with the engorged tick's hemolymph during tick removal or by contact with tick excreta with the person's abraded skin or conjuntivae. It is not the secretions from infected dogs but the effluents from engorged, infected ticks that pose the greater danger. Aerosol exposure from an infected dog's secretions is unlikely under natural conditions, as the organism does not survive outside host or tick cells. Aerosol exposure has only occurred in the laboratory, where inadvertent inoculation of infected tissues may also occur.

Ticks should be removed by applying constant traction with curved forceps or less desirably with tweezers, or fingers protected with facial tissue, placed as close as possible to the point of attachment.[32] Ticks should not be squeezed or crushed with bare fingers since the organism can be transmitted via tick feces or hemolymph. Hands should be washed thoroughly with soap and water after removal of the tick.

Pathology

Gross lesions, if present, consist of widespread petechial and ecchymotic hemorrhages in all tissues. Generalized hemorrhagic lymphadenopathy and splenic enlargement are usually found.

Microscopic findings consist of necrotizing vasculitis with perivascular polymorphonuclear and lymphoreticular cell infiltrations. Vascular lesions are most prominent in the skin, epididymis, testicle, GI tract, pancreas, kidneys, urinary bladder, myocardium, meninges, retina and skeletal muscle. Acute meningoencephalitis with small focal nodular gliosis is found in brain parenchyma of dogs with acute infections. Focal myocardial and hepatic necrosis and acute interstitial pneumonia are common lesions. Rickettsiae can be detected in many tissues by previously described staining and isolation procedures, but not by routine histologic methods.

Immunity

A wide variety of mammals have detectable antibodies to SFG rickettsiae. Cross-sections in dog sera develop between SFG-antigens; however, the titer is generally highest to the specific rickettsial species causing infection. There is generally minimal reaction to typhus-group or other genera of rickettsiae. Dogs on the Atlantic seaboard have between 5% to 15% seropositivity to SFG rickettsiae.[28] The prevalence of clinical illness due to RMSF is lower than seropositivity presumably because some of the positive titers to *R. rickettsii* are from exposure to nonpathogenic SFG rickettsiae.[28,33] Furthermore, subclinical or mild infections with *R. rickettsii* seem to be more common in dogs, than people, since dogs appear to be more frequently exposed and better adapted to the organism.

Dogs recovering from infection with *R. rickettsii* have been immune to reinfection when challenged 6–36 months later.[34–36] Infection with nonpathogenic rickettsiae such as *R. montana* does not seem to protect dogs from infection with the more virulent *R. rickettsii*.[34] Naturally infected dogs that recover from RMSF have never been shown to be reinfected. There are no commercial vaccines available for use in dogs or people. Experimental, inactivated, tissue culture-origin vaccines appear to offer protection against infection in experimentally inoculated people and animals.[37] Inactivated vaccine containing purified surface antigens of *R. rickettsii* produced by recombinant DNA technology was used successfully to protect mice from lethal RMSF.[38]

Diagnosis

Mild leukopenia, which may develop early in the course of illness, is followed by a moderate leukocytosis with a left shift or stress hemogram. The longer the duration of clinical signs prior to diagnosis, the more pronounced is the leukocytosis. A normocytic normochromic anemia and elevated erythrocyte sedimentation rate are nonspecific hematologic changes. Fibrinogen concentration, which increases as a result of an acute phase reaction, may be decreased in severely affected dogs developing DIC.

Thrombocytopenia has been one of the most consistent hematologic abnormalities in infected dogs. Platelet counts have ranged from 23,000 to 220,000/μl. Platelet counting is preferable to examination of blood smears because the thrombocytopenia in RMSF is often too severe and the platelet counts generally exceed 75,000/μl.

Biochemical abnormalities may include mildly increased serum glucose concentration and elevated serum alkaline phosphatase and alanine aminotransferase activities. Hypercholesterolemia and hypoalbuminemia have been more consistent findings in affected dogs. Hyponatremia, hypochloremia and metabolic acidosis are variable findings. The blood urea nitrogen concentration increases in terminal stages of the disease and corresponds with oliguria and renal failure. Proteinuria, hematuria, bilirubinuria and hyperbilirubinemia occur in some dogs. Serum creatine phosphokinase has been found to mildly to moderately increased in some dogs. CSF analysis is frequently normal; however, mildly increased protein (>25 but <100 mg/dl) and polymorphonuclear or mononuclear cells have also been found.[22,39] Analysis of synovial fluid in dogs developing polyarthritis has shown inflammatory changes, with a predominant increase in neutrophils. Results of lupus erythematosus cell, rheumatoid factor, antinuclear antibody, platelet autoantibody and Coombs' testing and of bacterial blood culture results are usually negative.

Electrocardiographic abnormalities, if present, consist of sinoatrial node dysfunction, ST segment and T wave depressions and premature ventricular contractions and second or third degree heart block. Thoracic radiography reveals diffuse increased interstitial density, especially in dogs presented for dyspnea and coughing.

Several serologic tests have been developed to detect antibodies to RMSF in humans, including Weil–Felix, complement fixation, microscopic immunofluorescence (Micro-IF), microagglutination, indirect hemagglutination, ELISA and latex agglutination (LA). The Micro-IF, ELISA and LA tests appear to be the best suited to examine canine sera.

The Micro-IF test and the ELISA have the advantages of requiring small amounts of sera and reagents, having high sensitivity, and the ability to classify antibodies to *R. rickettsii* as IgM or IgG. Measurement of IgG antibodies to *R. rickettsii* using the Micro-IF method is used by most diagnostic laboratories that test canine sera. Acute and convalescent IgG titers have been generally <1:64 in uninfected dogs or in those with ehrlichiosis, although titers will vary between laboratories. Actively infected dogs may have increased IgG titers (≥1:64) by the time clinical signs are apparent and the first sample is taken. IgG titers in experimentally infected dogs usually do not increase until 2 to 3 weeks after infection.[34,35] Since Micro-IF testing for IgG and IgM antibodies has resulted in both false-positive and false-negative results, evaluation of results of acute and convalescent samples are necessary to confirm a diagnosis of RMSF. An IgG titer increase of four-fold or greater is required to definitively document active infection. High IgG titers that develop in actively infected dogs generally decrease after 3 to 5 months, although they may remain increased (≥1:128) for at least 10 months.[22,34] Differences can be found between laboratories performing the test and within laboratories performing the same test at a later date. Therefore, it is recommended that acute and convalescent serum samples be submitted to the laboratory at the same time. When evaluating a single serum sample, simultaneous assessment of IgM and IgG titers provides more accurate information as to the time course of infection.

The IgM titers in naturally and experimentally infected dogs usually increase ($\geq$1:8) during the first week following infection and decrease after 4 weeks.[35,40] The maximum measured IgM titers are generally of 2–4 dilutions lower in magnitude than the corresponding IgG titers in the same animal.

The LA test appears to be a rapid and specific assay for recent *R. rickettsii* infection in dogs.[40] Because the sensitivity is lower than the micro-IF test, false-negative results occur, although in dogs a single increased titer ($\geq$1:32) appears indicative of active RMSF.

Direct fluorescent antibody (FA) staining of infected tissues is a valuable test for rapid clinical or postmortem diagnosis of RMSF. Direct FA procedures have been used to detect organisms in embryonated eggs or tissue culture, tissues at necropsy, ticks and skin biopsies from acutely infected people and dogs.[22,26,41] Rickettsiae can be found in approximately 75% of specimens taken from affected lesions and are rarely found in unaffected skin.[26] Formalin fixation causes some decrease in sensitivity of rickettsial detection.[41] Specimens should be obtained early in the course of infection because organisms are eliminated from the tissue within a few days, especially after antimicrobial therapy.[42] Owing to the usual absence of cutaneous petechiae in dogs, biopsy specimens can be obtained from muscosal hemorrhages or from vesicles in the buccal mucosa.

The polymerase chain reaction has been used to identify the 17 kDa antigen gene in the peripheral blood of affected humans.[43] The primers tested were specific for the SFG group. Similar primer sequences have been used to identify various *Rickettsia* spp. in infected arthropods.[44]

Bioassays involving isolation of *R. rickettsii* in susceptible species of laboratory animals such as meadow voles or guinea pigs have been a research laboratory means of diagnosing RMSF. The serum of these susceptible species may be tested for the presence of antibody to *R. rickettsii*. Tissues or blood of the affected or laboratory animal may be inoculated into embryonated chicken eggs or tissue culture to isolate and purify the agent. A staining technique using carbol basic fuchsin is widely used for the identification of SFG and typhus-group rickettsiae.[45]

Treatment

Mortality in dogs with RMSF usually relates to incorrect diagnosis and treatment or to rapidly progressive shock or severe CNS infections. Antibody titers are not always available at the time the dog is admitted, and even then, results from the first sample may not be diagnostically useful, because it may take 1 to 3 weeks for maximal

IgG response. In the clinical setting, a response to therapy is used to increase the index of suspected diagnosis. Treatment should not be delayed while awaiting laboratory results. The antibiotics used to treat RMSF are considered to be rickettsiostatic.[46] Eventual eradication from the host requires adequate immune responses; the immunodeficient patient may require prolonged therapy of up to 2 weeks duration. Tetracycline or oxytetracycline should be given at a dose of 22 mg/kg three times daily, for at least 7 days. Lipid-soluble tetracyclines, such as minocycline or doxycycline, have been shown to be as effective in treating rickettsial infections in people when they have been used for periods of less than 7 days.[47,48] Chloramphenicol is equally effective and is indicated in young (<6 month old) puppies to avoid dental staining. Enrofloxacin, a fluoroquinolone, has been shown to be effective in treatment[49] but this drug has restrictions for use in dogs less than 1.5 years. Dogs treated early in the course of illness show rapid clinical improvement, generally within 36–48 h after therapy is instituted. Delayed or incomplete recovery is associated with organ failure or with CNS damage. Antibiotics are only effective in reducing the severity of the illness if they are given prior to the development of advanced pathologic changes, such as thrombosis and tissue necrosis. Animals that develop acryl gangrene will have eventual healing of their extremities with permanent scarring or disfigurement. Supportive care must be used in dogs with shock, coagulation disorders and clinical or laboratory evidence of organ failure.

In people, use of tetracycline early in the course of illness is thought to reduce the magnitude of the serologic response that would otherwise develop, however early treatment does not appear to interfere with serodiagnosis in dogs.[34,35,49] In addition to the previously discussed drugs, josamycin, rifampin and ciprofloxacin have been found to be somewhat effective *in vitro* and experimentally against *R. rickettsii*,[50–52] but their clinical use has not been investigated.

IV fluid therapy must be used with caution because increased vascular permeability and expanded extracellular fluid volume can give rise to pulmonary and cerebral edema.

Control

The best means of prevention of RMSF in dogs is avoidance of tick-infested areas and rapid, safe removal of attached ticks. Pets should be dipped repeatedly if their housing areas are inhabited by ticks. Tick eradication in the pet's environment is impossible because of the maintenance of these vectors by rodents and other reservoir hosts. Elimination of small ground rodents is difficult, if not impossible, to achieve. Some reduction in tick numbers has been achieved locally in the eastern and southern United States by application of insecticides in the form of aqueous suspension or dust to surrounding vegetation.

References

1. McDade, J.E. and Newhouse, V.F. 1986. Natural history of *Rickettsia rickettsii*. *A. Rev. Microbiol.* **40:** 287–309.
2. Uchida, T., Tashiro, F., Funato, T. and Kitamura, Y. 1986. Isolation of a spotted fever group rickettsia from a patient with febrile exanthematous illness in Shikoku. *Jap. Microbiol. Immun.* **30:** 1323–1326.
3. Uchida, T., Uchiyama, T. and Koyama, A.H. 1988. Isolation of spotted fever group rickettsia from humans in Japan. *J. infect. Dis.* **18:** 664–665.
4. Wolach, B., Franco, S., Bogger-Goren, S., Drucker, M., Goldwasser, R.A., Sadan, N. and Bernheim, J. 1989. Clinical and laboratory findings of spotted fever in Israeli children. *Pediatr. infect. Dis. J.* **8:** 12–15.
5. Dasch, G.A., Ching, W., Kim, P.Y., Pham, H., Stover, C.K., Oaks, E.V., Dobson, M.E. and Weiss, E. 1990. A structural and immunological comparison of Rickettsial HSP60 antigens with those of other species. *Ann. N.Y. Acad. Sci.* **590:** 352–369.
6. Anderson, B.E. 1990. The 17-kilodalton protein antigens of spotted fever and typhus group rickettsiae. *Ann. N.Y. Acad. Sci.* **590:** 326–333.
7. Li, H. and Walker, D.H. 1990. Biological characterization of major polypeptides on the surface of spotted fever group rickettsiae. *Ann. N.Y. Acad. Sci.* **590:** 389–394.
8. Anacker, R.L., McDonald, G.A., List, R.H. and Mann, R.E. 1987. Neutralizing activity of monoclonal antibodies to heat-sensitive and heat resistant epitopes of *Rickettsia rickettsii* surface proteins. *Infect. Immun.* **55:** 825–827.
9. Li, H., Lenz, B. and Walker, D.H. 1988. Protective monoclonal antibodies recognize heat-labile epitopes on surface proteins of spotted fever group rickettsiae. *Infect. Immun.* **56:** 2587–2593.
10. Regnery R. 1990. Use of DNA probes for differentiation of spotted fever group and other rickettsiae. *Ann. N.Y. Acad. Sci.* **590:** 422–429.
11. Fuerst, P.A., Poetter, K.P., Pretzman, C. and Perlman, P.S. 1990. Molecular genetics of populations of intracellular bacteria: The spotted fever group rickettsiae. *Ann. N.Y. Acad. Sci.* **590:** 430–438.
12. Anderson, B.E. and Tzianabos, T. 1989. Comparative sequence analysis of a genus-common rickettsial antigen gene. *J. Bact.* **171:** 5199–5201.
13. Gilmore, R.D., Jr, Joste, N. and McDonald, G.A. 1989. Cloning expression and sequence analysis of the gene encoding the 120 kD surface-exposed protein of *Rickettsia rickettsii*. *Molec. Microbiol.* **3:** 1579–1586.
14. McDonald, G.A., Anacker, R.L. and Garjian, K. 1987. Cloned gene of *Rickettsia rickettsii* surface antigen: Candidate vaccine for Rocky Mountain spotted fever. *Science* **235:** 83–85.
15. Policastro, P.F., Anderson, B.E. and McDonald, G.A. 1990. Promoter structure and expression of the 155-kDa surface antigen gene of *Rickettsia rickettsii*. *Ann. N.Y. Acad. Sci.* **590:** 468–477.
16. Norment, B.R. and Burgdorfer, W. 1984. Susceptibility and reservoir

potential of the dog to spotted fever-group rickettsiae. *Am. J. vet. Res.* **45:** 1706–1710.

17. BISHOPP, F.C. AND TREMBLEY, H.L. 1945. Distribution of certain North American ticks. *J. Parasit.* **31:** 1–54.
18. RAO, A.K., SCHAPIRA, M., CLEMENTS, M.L., NIEWIAROWSKI, S., BUDZYNSKI, A.Z., SCHMAIER, A.H., HARPEL, P.C., BLACKWELDER, W.C., SCHERRER, J., SOBEL, E. and COLMAN, R.W. 1988. A prospective study of platelets and plasma proteolytic systems during the early stages of Rocky Mountain spotted fever. *New Engl. J. Med.* **318:** 1021–1032.
19. HERRERO-HERRERO, J.I., RUIZ-BELTRAN, R. and BATTLE-FORONDONA, J. 1988. The complement system in Mediterranean spotted fever. *J infect. Dis.* **17:** 1093–1095.
20. LIU, C.T., HILMAS, D.E., GRIFFIN, M.J., PEDERSEN. C.E., JR, HADICK, C.L., JR and BEISEL, W.R. 1978. Alterations of body fluid compartments and distribution of tissue water and electrolytes in rhesus monkeys with Rocky Mountain spotted fever. *J infect. Dis.* **138:** 42–48.
21. KAPLOWITZ, L.G. and ROBERTSON, G.L. 1983. Hyponatremia in Rocky Mountain spotted fever: role of antidiuretic hormone. *Ann. Intern. Med.* **98:** 334–335.
22. GREENE, C.E., BURGDORFER, W., CAVAGNOLO, R., PHILIP, R. and PEACOCK, M.G. 1985. Rocky Mountain spotted fever in dogs and its differentiation from canine ehrlichiosis. *Am. J. vet. Med. Ass.* **186:** 465–472.
23. HELMICK, C.G., BERNARD, K.W. and D'ANGELO, L.J. 1984. Rocky Mountain spotted fever: clinical, laboratory, and epidemiological features of 262 cases. *J. infect. Dis.* **150:** 480–488.
24. GREENE, C.E. 1987. Rocky Mountain spotted fever. *Am. J. vet. Med. Ass.* **191:** 666–671.
25. GREENE, C.E. and BREITSCHWERDT, E.B. 1990. Rocky Mountain spotted fever and Q fever. In: *Infectious Diseases of the Dog and Cat,* pp. 419–433. GREENE, C.E. (Ed.). W.B. Saunders, Philadelphia.
26. DAVIDSON, M.G., BREITSCHWERDT, E.B., WALKER, D.H., NASISSE, M.P. and SUSSMAN, W. 1989. Identification of rickettsiae in cutaneous biopsies from dogs with experimental Rocky Mountain spotted fever. *J. vet. Intern. Med.* **3:** 8–11.
27. KEENAN, K.P., BUHLES, W.C., JR, HUXSOLL, D.L., WILLIAMS, R.G. and HILDEBRANDT, P.K. 1977. Studies on the pathogenesis of *Rickettsia rickettsii* in the dog: clinical and clinicopathologic changes of experimental infection. *Am. J. vet. Res.* **38:** 851–856.
28. BREITSCHWERDT, E.B., MONCOL, D.J., CORBETT, W.T., MACCORMACK, J.N., BURGDORFER, W., FORD, R.B. and LEVY, M.G. 1987. Antibodies to spotted fever-group rickettsiae in dogs in North Carolina. *Am. J. vet. Res.* **48:** 1436–1440.
29. WEISER, I. and GREENE, C.E. 1988. Dermal necrosis associated with Rocky Mountain spotted fever in three dogs. *J. Am. vet. Med. Ass.* **195:** 1756–1758.
30. *Rocky Mountain spotted fever—United States.* 1986. M.M.W.R. **35:** 247–249.
31. GORDON, J.C., GORDON, S.W., PETERSON, E. and PHILIP, R. 1984. Rocky Mountain spotted fever in an urban canine population. *Am. J. trop. Med. Hyg.* **33:** 1026–1031.
32. NEEDHAM, G.R. 1985. Evalution of five popular methods for tick removal. *Pediatrics* **75:** 997–1002.
33. HOSKINS, J.D., BREITSCHWERDT, E.B., GAUNT, S.D., FRENCH, T.W. and BURGDORFER, W. 1988. Antibodies to *Ehrlichia canis, Ehrlichia platys* and spotted fever group rickettsiae in Louisiana dogs. *J. vet. Intern. Med.* **2:** 55–59.
34. BREITSCHWERDT, E.B., WALKER, D.H., LEVY, M.G., BURGDORFER, W.,

Corbett, W.T., Hurlbert, S.A., Stebbins, M.E., Curtis, B.C. and Allen, D.A. 1988. Clinical, hematologic, and humoral immune response in female dogs inoculated with *Rickettsia rickettsii* and *Rickettsia montana*. *Am. J. vet. Res.* **49:** 70–76.

35. Breitschwerdt, E.B., Levy, M.G., Davidson, M.G., Walker, D.H., Burgdorfer, W., Curtis, B.C. and Babineau, C.A. 1990. Kinetics of IgM and IgG responses to experimental and naturally acquired *Rickettsia rickettsii* infection in dogs. *Am. J. vet. Res.* **51:** 1312–1316.
36. Keenan, K.P., Buhles, W.C., Huxsoll, D.L., Williams, R.G., Hildebrandt, P.K., Campbell, J.M. and Stephenson, E.H. 1977. Pathogenesis of infection with *Rickettsia rickettsii* in the dog: a disease model for Rocky Mountain spotted fever. *J infect. Dis.* **135:** 911–917.
37. Ascher, M.S., Oster, C.N., Harber, P.I., Kenyon, R.H. and Pedersen, C.E., Jr. 1978. Initial clinical evaluation of a new Rocky Mountain spotted fever vaccine of tissue culture origin. *J infect. Dis.* **138:** 217–221.
38. McDonald, G.A., Anacker, R.L. and Garjian, K. 1987. Cloned gene of *Rickettsia rickettsii* surface antigen: candidate vaccine for Rocky Mountain spotted fever. *Science* **235:** 83–85.
39. Breitschwerdt, E.B., Meuten, D.J., Walker, D.H., Levy, M., Kennedy, K., King, M. and Curtis, B. 1985. Canine Rocky Mountain spotted fever: a kennel epizootic. *Am. J. vet. Res.* **46:** 2124–2128.
40. Greene, C.E., Marks, A.M., Lappin, M.R., Breitschwerdt, E.B., Burgdorfer, W. and Wolski, N. 1993. Comparison of latex agglutination, immunofluorescent antibody, and enzyme immunoassay methods in the diagnosis of Rocky Mountain spotted fever in dogs. *Am. J. vet. Res.* **54:** in press.
41. Walker, D.H., Cain, B.G. and Olmstead, P.M. 1978. Laboratory diagnosis of Rocky Mountain spotted fever by immunofluorescent demonstration of *Rickettsia rickettsii* in cutaneous lesions. *Am. J. clin. Path.* **69:** 619–623.
42. Woodward, T.E. 1984. Rocky Mountain spotted fever: epidemiological and early clinical signs are keys to treatment and reduced mortality. *J infect. Dis.* **150:** 465–468.
43. Tzianabos, T., Anderson, B.E. and McDade, J.E. 1990. Detection of *Rickettsia rickettsii* DNA in clinical specimens by enzymatic amplification using polymerase chain reaction technology. *Ann. N.Y. Acad. Sci.* **590:** 553–556.
44. Azad, A.F., Webb., L., Carl, M. and Dasch, G.A. 1990. Detection of *Rickettsiae* in arthropod vectors by DNA amplification using the polymerase chain reaction. *Ann. N.Y. Acad. Sci.* **590:** 557–563.
45. Gimenez, D.F. 1964. Staining rickettsiae in yolk sac cultures. *Stain Technol.* **39:** 135–140.
46. Wisseman, C.L. and Ordonez, S.V. 986. Actions of antibiotics on *Rickettsia rickettsii*. *J. infect. Dis.* **153:** 626–628.
47. Bella-Cueto, F., Font-Creus, B., Segura-Porta, F., Espejo-Arenas, E., Copez-Pares, P. and Munoz-Espin, T. 1987. Comparative, randomized trial of one-day doxycycline versus 10-day tetracycline therapy for Mediterranean spotted fever. *J infect. Dis.* **155:** 1056–1058.
48. Yagupsky, P., Gross, E.M., Alkan, M. and Bearman, J.E. 1987. Comparison of two dosage schedules of doxycycline in children with rickettsial spotted fever. *J infect. Dis.* **155:** 1215–1219.
49. Breitschwerdt, E.B., Davison, M.G., Aucoin, D.P., Levy, M.G., Szabados, N.S., Hegarty, B.C., Kuehne, A.L. and James, R.L. 1991. Efficacy of chloramphenicol, enrofloxacin, and tetracycline for treatment of experimental

Rocky Mountain spotted fever in dogs. *Antimicrob. Agents Chemother.* **35:** 2375–2381.

50. RAOULT, D., ROUSSELLIER, P., VESTRIS, G. and TAMALET, J. 1987. *In vitro* antibiotic sysceptibility of *Rickettsia rickettsii* and *Rickettsia conorii*: plaque assay and microplaque colorimetric assay. *J infect. Dis.* **155:** 1059–1061.
51. RAOULT, D., ROUSSELLIER, P. and TAMALET, J. 1988. *In vitro* evaluation of josamycin, spiramycin, and erythromycin against *Rickettsia rickettsii* and *R. conorii*. *Antimicrob. Agents Chemother.* **32:** 255–256.
52. MCCLAIN, J.B., JOSHI, B. and RICE, R. 1988. Chloramphenicol, gentamicin and ciprofloxacin against murine scrub typhus. *Antimicrob. Agents Chemother.* **32:** 285–286.

8

Canine Ehrlichiosis

M. RISTIC AND C. J. HOLLAND

Introduction

Following the discovery of *Ehrlichia canis,* the causative agent of canine ehrlichiosis in tick-infested dogs in Algeria in 1935, the disease was reported in dogs in many parts of Africa, the Middle East, and the Orient.[1,2] In the Western Hemisphere the disease was first identified in dogs on the island of Aruba in 1957.[3] In the United States, the first case of canine ehrlichiosis was reported in 1963 with the causative agent mistakenly identified as *Babesia canis.*[4]

The full pathogenic potential of *E. canis* for its canine host, however, was first recognized during the war in Vietnam (1968–1970) where a severe epizootic of ehrlichiosis occurred among U.S. military dogs, resulting in hundreds of cases of morbidity and mortality among these animals.[5] This severe and often fatal form of the disease is known as tropical canine pancytopenia (TCP). The disease is characterized by hemorrhage, pancytopenia and severe debilitation.[6] Since that time, numerous cases of canine ehrlichiosis have been reported in the United States and many other parts of the world. While the most common pattern of disease occurrence was that of a sporadic nature, some epizootics of canine ehrlichiosis have also been reported.[7]

An organized and intensive research effort that followed at the military and university levels resulted in the development of methods for *in vitro* cultivation of *E. canis* and serologic identification of infected dogs.[8,9] Over the past decade the use of these new means of disease detection made it possible to recognize ehrlichiosis as one of the most important canine infectious diseases in the United States, with outbreaks and isolated cases occurring in every state where the vector, the brown dog tick, *Rhipicephalus sanguineus,* exists.

The advancement in knowledge of the biological properties of *E. canis,* which followed the development of methods for *in vitro* cultivation and diagnostic serology, led to the recognition of a close antigenic and morphologic relationship between *E. canis* and *Rickettsia sennetsu*, the etiologic agent of human sennetsu fever in Western Japan.[10–12] These findings led to the inclusion of *R. sennetsu* into the genus *Ehrlichia* under the name *Ehrlichia sennetsu*.[13] The availability of the latter agent facilitated the identification and isolation of *Ehrlichia risticii*,[14] the causative agent of equine monocytic ehrlichiosis (EME; Syn., Potomac horse fever). Thus, *E. canis*, the type species of the genus *Ehrlichia*, has played a prominent role in identifying and characterizing additional members within this genus.

Causal Agent

Morphology

Ehrlichia canis and other members of the genus *Ehrlichia* are minute gram-negative cocci that stain dark blue to purple with Romanovsky stain. With the Machiavello method, they stain light red and brown-black by silver stain. Within its host cell, the blood monocyte, three developmental stages of *E. canis* may be observed microscopically. The earliest stage is represented by small elementary bodies 0.2–0.4 microns in diameter, followed by slightly larger initial bodies (0.5–4 μm diameter), and finally, even larger inclusion bodies (4–6 μm diameter). The latter growth stage, which consists of a variable number of elementary bodies, is generally referred to as a morula.[8] At the electron microscopic level, it has been shown that all three growth stages occur within a membrane-lined vacuole of host origin that separates individual organisms or a group of these from the host cell cytoplasm. Each organism is bound by its own outer and inner membrane.[15] The multiplication of the organism within the vacuole takes place by binary fission.[16] In cell cultures, certain morulae may contain more than 100 organisms and there can be 30 or more morulae within the cytoplasm of a single blood monocyte (Fig. 8.1).

Cultivation

Because *E. canis* is extremely host specific, early studies focused on the disease, its transmission, and treatment with little information on the biological properties of the organism.

In 1971, Nyindo *et al.*, at the University of Illinois, were the first to successfully culture *E. canis* in the peripheral blood monocytes obtained from experimentally infected dogs during the acute phase of

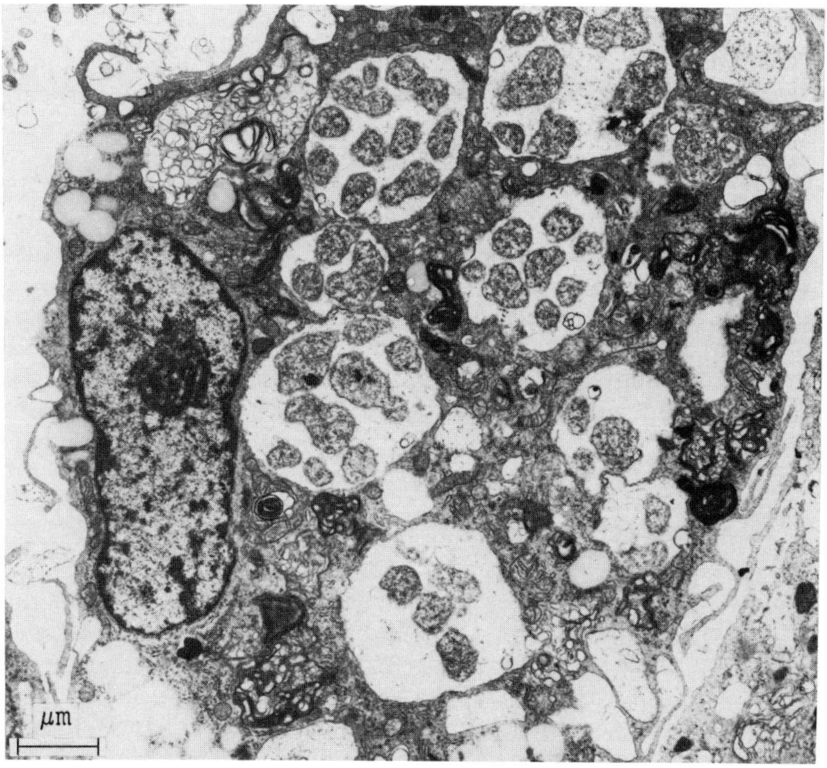

FIG. 8.1. Multiple *Ehrlichia canis* morulae in the cytoplasm of a cultured blood monocyte (× 14,800).

the disease.[8] The method of *in vitro* cultivation was later improved by transferring *E. canis*-infected monocytes to normal primary canine monocyte cell cultures obtained from noninfected dogs.[17] This method eventually resulted in the continuous *in vitro* propagation of *E. canis* in primary cultures of canine blood monocytes.

The first continuous cell line for massive propagation of *E. canis*, termed MDH, was developed by Holland and Ristic.[18,19] This *E. canis* chronically-infected cell line was developed spontaneously following cocultivation of mouse peritoneal macrophages and *E. canis*-infected canine monocytes. The mass production of *E. canis* by this method has allowed for a cost-efficient means by which large quantities of *E. canis* may be produced for various serological, antigenic and molecular genetic studies.

Other *in vitro* cultivation methods have utilized canine peritoneal macrophages,[20] human-canine hybrid cells[21] and canine macrophage cell lines.[22]

Metabolic Properties of Ehrlichiae

Metabolic studies on *E. sennetsu*, and the two isolates of *E. risticii*, provided the first biochemical evidence that rickettsia and ehrlichia carry out similar metabolic functions.[23] The *Ehrlichia* species were demonstrated to resemble rickettsiae in their apparent lack of glycolytic pathway and in their metabolism of glutamine.[24,25] In previous studies, *Rickettsia* species were demonstrated to utilize glutamate more rapidly than glutamine. However, ehrlichiae utilize glutamate to a much lesser degree than glutamine.[26,27] This may be due to the fact that ehrlichiae are enveloped by the host membrane and glutamine penetrates phagosomes better than glutamate. More recent studies showed that the incubation of *Ehrlichia* species in the presence of glutamine induces the production of low, but significant, levels of ATP.[28] The metabolic activity of ehrlichiae is greatest at pHs 7.2–8.0 and rapidly declines at a pH below 7.0.[26]

Antigenicity

Using an indirect fluorescent antibody (IFA) test, none of the specific sera against common canine bacterial and viral agents and sera against eight pathogenic rickettsial and one chlamydial agents reacted against *E. canis*, the type species of the genus *Ehrlichia*.[9] This finding supports general contention that ehrlichiae are antigenically specific, and, in that respect, unique among obligate intracellular bacteria. The lack of Weil–Felix reactivity with *E. canis* gives further support for its biologic difference from classic rickettsiae.[29]

The study of cross-antigenic reactivity among species of the genus *Ehrlichia* revealed a good degree of relationship among most agents. Only the two equine agents, *E. equi* and *E. risticii*, lack such cross-reactivity.[30] Western blot analysis showed that immune sera obtained from *E. canis*-infected dogs reacted with 160, 100, 78, 74, 64, 48, 40, 30, 24 and 21 kDa proteins of that organism.[31] The strongest common antigenicity was noted between *E. risticii* and *E. sennetsu*.[14,31] Sera of human ehrlichiosis patients in the United States reacted strongest with *E. canis*.

Epidemiology

Natural Transmission

The relationship of ticks in the transmission of *E. canis* has been closely studied. As early as 1935, the brown dog tick, *Rhipicephalus sanguineus*, was considered to be a vector of *E. canis*.[1] The importance of this tick in transmitting canine ehrlichiosis has been demonstrated in numerous cases where effective tick control prevented occurrence and spread of the disease. Subsequent studies conclusively demonstrated trans-stadial transmission of *E. canis* by *R. sanguineus* and described the development of the agent in tick tissues.[32] All three growth stages, i.e. larvae, nymphs and adults, are able to transmit the disease. In infected ticks, *E. canis* multiplies within hemocytes and cells of the salivary gland. From there, the organism eventually enters the digestive tract and infects the midgut epithelium.[33] An adult *R. sanguineus* can transmit *E. canis* for approximately 155 days after being detached from its mammalian host.[34] It is postulated that the attraction of mononuclear cells to the inflamed site of the tick bite may facilitate the infection of canine blood monocytes with *E. canis*. Two other ticks, *Amblyomma americanum* and *Octobius magnini* were more recently described as potential vectors of ehrlichiae.[35]

Experimental Infection

Experimentally, the infection with *E. canis* can be transmitted from acutely or chronically infected dogs to susceptible dogs by whole blood inoculation. Depending on the dose and virulence of the organism, experimentally infected dogs may clinically remain relatively normal and demonstrate only minor hematologic abnormalities typical of canine ehrlichiosis. With larger inoculums of the virulent organism, three phases of the disease may be identified.[18] At 10–14 days after inoculation, the first febrile phase begins. Major clinical manifestions of this phase include: intermittent fever, anorexia, weight loss, enlarged lymph nodes, frequent corneal opacity, conjunctivitis, pneumonitis, edema of legs and scrotum and occasional vomiting. Epistaxis is a pathognomonic feature primarily for German shepherd dogs but may also occur in other dog breeds. The febrile phase, which may last from a few days to 3 weeks, is followed by a subclinical phase. During the latter phase, dogs appear clinically recovered, but the total blood cell count is depressed, particularly the circulating blood platelet count. Erythrocyte sedimentation rate and total plasma proteins are elevated. Hypergammaglobulinemia, which generally develops during the febrile phase, persists during the subclinical and chronic phase of the disease.[36]

Hosts Affected and Geographical Distribution

No animal species other than the canidae are found to be susceptible to infection with *E. canis*. Accordingly, only wild and domestic canids are currently considered the natural reservoir of *E. canis*.[32] In view of the fact, however, that ticks remain infected only through trans-stadial rather than transovarial means, and because ticks most likely acquire *E. canis* during feeding on an affected animal in the acute phase of the disease, it is reasonable to suggest that other unknown reservoirs of *E. canis* may exist in nature. These could be small mammals, such as rodents, which serve as a constant source of the infection for ticks. This concept is supported by epizootics of canine ehrlichiosis, which have been occasionally observed.[37]

Canine ehrlichiosis is a worldwide disease. It has been reported from many geographic regions of the world which include: Southeast Asia, India, Ceylon, Africa, Europe, the Middle East, North America and Central America, suggesting that its distribution apparently coincides with the prevalence of the tick vector *R. sanguineus*.[38] A serologic study examining the prevalence of *E. canis* infections among United States military working dogs situated around the world showed that of 2,077 dogs examined, 233 (11%) were positive.[37] The highest antibody prevalence rate (24%) was found among a select population stationed between 40° and 45° north latitude (Japan and Okinawa).

Pathogenesis

Certain pathologic and hematologic features caused by an infection with *E. canis* are unique, and clearly different from those caused by most of the pathogenic rickettsiae.[35] Thrombosis, endothelial cell hypertrophy and vasculitis that occur with rickettsial infections are not commonly observed in ehrlichial infections. The most common finding in an acute *E. canis* infection is the extensive invasion of parenchymal organs and perivascular cuffing by plasma cells, particularly of the lungs, meninges, kidneys and spleen, suggesting an immunopathologic etiology.[39] Such an etiology was further substantiated by the finding that lymphocytes of infected dogs exert a cytotoxic effect upon autologous monocytes. This monocytotoxicity was shown to bear a temporal relationship with the disease-associated thrombocytopenia.[40]

A further contrasting characteristic between classic rickettsiae and ehrlichiae is the effect of the organism on its host cell. While rickettsiae are known to exert a cytolytic effect on an invaded tissue cell, such a phenomenon is seldom observed *in vitro* and *in vivo* with *E. canis* and other ehrlichiae.[35] Similarly, plaque formation in a monolayer of culture-infected canine monocytes is not seen. Such an effect in ehrlichiae is manifested by detachment of infected cells from the bottom of the culture flask. In common with *R. tsutsugamushi* and chlamydiae, ehrlichiae inhibit lysosomal fusion with cytoplasmic vacuoles which harbor the organism.[41]

In an infected dog, *E. canis* induces very prominent hematologic changes, while such a feature is not as pronounced in infections caused by other members of the tribe *Rickettsieae*. Leukopenia, along with a highly prominent thrombocytopenia, is a pathognomonic hematologic manifestation for canine ehrlichiosis.[42] Based on *in vitro* studies, there is a strong indication that the associated thrombocytopenia is immunologically mediated. It was first demonstrated that sera of *E. canis*-infected dogs induce inhibition of the migration of normal canine blood platelets.[40] Such an effect was shown to be maximal prior to the detection of anti-*E. canis* antibodies as demonstrated by the IFA test. Scanning electron microscopy indicated that platelet migration was interfered with by inhibiting pseudopod formation. Affected platelets became rounded and showed evidence of clumping and leakage.[40]

As a follow-up to these studies, a soluble factor, termed platelet migration inhibition factor (PMIF), was isolated from the serum of dogs with acute ehrlichiosis.[43,44] The synthesis of PMIF was found to be lymphocyte-dependent and the factor can be produced *in vitro* using lymphocytes derived from the blood of *E. canis*-infected dogs. Canine lymphocytes derived from ehrlichia-free dogs can be induced by *E. canis*-infected canine monocytes to produce significant levels of PMIF under *in vitro* conditions. The concentration of PMIF in the plasma of affected dogs is directly related to the virulence of the infecting *E. canis* isolate. The PMIF was preliminary characterized as a heat-stable glycoprotein of 160–190 kDa.[43,44]

Clinical Disease

The onset of the acute phase of the disease generally occurs within 8–20 days following the bite of an infected tick. This stage lasts 2–4 weeks and is usually characterized by fever (40°C–41.4°C), depression, anorexia, weight loss, oculonasal discharge and lymphadenopathy. Edema of the limbs and ataxia may also be present; most dogs survive the acute phase after which a subclinical phase occurs.[36] The subclinical phase is of varying duration but may persist for as long as 4–5 years. Immunocompetent dogs should be able to greatly reduce the organism load, thereby controlling the infection.[36,45]

Dogs that enter the subclinical phase may appear clinically normal; however, all blood values remain at subnormal levels when compared with values recorded prior to infection. The disease may remain at the mild chronic level with occasional episodes of fever, or develop into the severe chronic phase known as TCP. Certain breeds of dogs, such as the German shepherd dog, appear to be predisposed to acquiring the more severe manifestations of the disease.[45,46]

Characteristic features of TCP are: fever, corneal opacity, regenerative or nonregenerative anemia, and severe leukopenia and thrombocytopenia.[42] During the early phase of the disease, bone marrow hyperplasia is evident. However, as the disease progresses, cellular elements in the marrow become exhausted, producing a state of hypoplasia. Owing to the severe thrombocytopenia, epistaxis, petechiation of mucous membranes, hemorrhagic skin lesions, and peripheral edema are often observed. Death during this phase of the disease is generally due either to extensive mucosal and serosal hemorrhages or to secondary bacterial infections prompted by the dog's debilitated condition.[36]

Dogs are also susceptible to two other ehrlichiae, *Ehrlichia equi* and *Ehrlichia risticii*.[47,48] *Ehrlichia equi* organisms infect the circulating granulocytes and cause only mild, and sometimes inapparent, infections. Susceptibility of dogs to experimental infection with *E. risticii* has been reported.[48] In nature such infections have been documented by serological means, but clinically they are usually mild or not apparent.[30] There have been several recognized field cases of dogs experiencing a moderate to severe clinical disease syndrome which, based on serologic evidence, was apparently due to infection by *E. risticii*. In general, those dogs experienced moderate to severe anorexia, depression and leukopenia, along with some associated vomiting and diarrhea. In each case, dogs responded well to tetracycline therapy, resulting in full recovery from the clinical disease.[49] Infections with *E. equi* and *E. risticii* does not seem to alter the susceptibility of dogs to *E. canis*. The vector, reservoir, and mode of transmission of these two ehrlichiae are not known, although tick transmission is suspected.[45]

Hematology

The most prominent hematologic manifestations of canine ehrlichiosis are a greatly increased erythrocyte sedimentation rate, thrombocytopenia and a slight to severe pancytopenia. In recovering animals there is a gradual and spontaneous improvement in thrombocyte levels. During the chronic phase of the disease, the hematological findings are usually similar to those of the acute phase of the disease. Thrombocytopenic dogs may develop severe chronic ehrlichiosis subsequent to surgery or chemotherapy. Consequently, the severe chronic phase may be precipitated by stress or by immunosuppression after a prolonged subclinical infection.[36,45]

Prolonged bleeding times are the result of thrombocytopenia and/or platelet malfunction (see section on pathogenesis). Auto agglutination of erythrocytes and a positive Coombs' test are often present before any treatment. Hyperglobulinemia and hypoalbuminemia are characteristic findings during an early *E. canis* infection. Serum electrophoresis generally shows a polyclonal gammopathy.[45] However, only a portion of increased gammaglobulins is due to anti-*E. canis* antibodies.

According to Hoskins,[45] the initial *E. canis* infection may have occurred months earlier and persisted without being noted by the owner. Consequently, current hematologic and serum chemistry abnormalities must be considered in light of the case history and the presenting signs of illness.

Pathology

The gross lesions of acute canine ehrlichiosis are petechial and hemorrhagic lesions in the subcutaneous tissues and major organs and generalized lymphadenopathy, with mesenteric nodes being more commonly affected. Distribution, number and severity of the hemorrhages are variable, although the heart, lungs and gastrointestinal and urogenital tracts are most often affected.[39] Microscopically, the most characteristic features are altered architecture of lymphopoietic tissue, with plasmacytosis and generalized perivascular lymphoid and plasma cell accumulation. The plasma cell accumulation varies in quality and distribution, and is most prominent in meninges, kidney and lymphopoietic tissues.[39] The erythrophagocytosis and accompanying hemosiderosis in the lymph nodes accounts for the color seen grossly. The prolonged thrombocytopenia observed clinically is primarily due to depression and exhaustion of the bone marrow.

The microscopic appearance of TCP is comparable with that of immunoproliferative disease and resembles, in many respects, Aleutian mink disease,[50] equine infectious anemia[51] and lymphocytic choriomeningitis in older germfree mice.[52] Each of these diseases has a persistent infectious organism that stimulates the reticulo-endothelial (RE) system, resulting in an exaggerated RE response. The long clinical course of ehrlichiosis allows for immunoproliferative manifestations to develop. The plasma cell infiltrate of meninges, kidney and eye, however, must be considered characteristic of TCP, although by no means is this pathognomonic.[39]

Immunity

Due to its predominant intracellular location, it is reasonable to assume that the major *E. canis* effector mechanism resides in the parasite's ability to invade mononuclear phagocytes. This is in agreement with the result of a series of studies on the mechanism of protective immunity in canine ehrlichiosis, which clearly documented that the protection against clinical disease depends on infection-immunity (premunition), with cell-mediated immunity (CMI) being the functional force.[18,53]

The study of the kinetics of antibody response to *E. canis* in experimentally infected dogs revealed that the earliest antibody detectable in the IFA test appears 7 days after inoculation and resides in the immunoglobulin M (IgM) and immunoglobulin A (IgA) classes. At approximately 21 days after inoculation, the antibody resides in IgM, IgA and immunoglobulin G (IgG) classes. Thereafter, antibody concentrations of the IgG class continue to increase, while those in the other 2 immunoglobulin classes have a variable pattern.[54]

The effect of immune canine serum (ICS) and normal canine serum (NCS) on the growth of *E. canis* was studied in blood monocyte cultures derived from normal and immune dogs. It was shown that ehrlichiae treated with NCS, and then introduced into normal monocyte cultures maintained in NCS, multiplied within these cells and destroyed them.[55] On the other hand, immune serum, collected from *E. canis* carrier dogs, suppressed ehrlichial growth in normal monocytes. Also, immune macrophages, collected from *E. canis* carrier dogs maintained in NCS, were more resistant to the growth of *E. canis* than were normal macrophages maintained in NCS.[56]

Dogs infected with *E. canis* promptly produced specific antibodies regardless of the presence of clinical signs. The presence of antibody is diagnostically useful, indicating infection by the agent. However, the presence and the titer of antibody does not correlate with the presence of protective immunity. Donatien and Lestoquard were among the first investigators to demonstrate that infected dogs are refractory to disease symptoms following challenge.[57] When tetracycline compounds became available, it was demonstrated that these compounds could be effectively used to eliminate *E. canis* from infected dogs. However, elimination of the carrier state with tetracycline did not leave treated dogs fully protected against challenge infection.[42] These authors also noted that persistent antibody titers following treatment were of no protective value. A lack of protective value of anti-*E. canis* antibodies is in full agreement with our observation on chronically infected dogs which, in spite of excessively high antibody titers, may suddenly succumb and die. Moreover, a series of our immunization studies using inactivated cell culture-derived *E. canis* antigens, fortified by various adjuvants that induced good levels of antibody response, not only failed to produce evidence of protection in immunized animals, but clinical manifestations in these dogs appeared more fulminating than those in the nonimmunized control animals.[30] These findings and other related observations confirmed the lack of *in vivo* protection by anti-*E. canis* antibodies and also indicated that such antibodies may serve to augment the development of the organism in its host cell and thereby provide for more severe signs of the disease. While concrete evidence to that effect is unavailable at this time, a postulated sequence of possible events in the course of interaction between *E. canis*, its antibody, and its host cell is presented in Fig. 8.2.

There are at least two possible ways that enable the entry of *E. canis* into a macrophage, its host cell. In the first instance, the parasite uses nonspecific host cell surface sites for its entry, using the process induced primarily by phagocytosis. In the second instance, the entry takes place by way of specific receptors on the surface of macrophages. These are: Fc receptor for IgG and the C3b receptor (Fig. 8.2A). Accordingly, antibodies of the IgG class that have interacted with the organism would provide for its entry into the macrophage by way of their Fc portion (Fig. 8.2B). Similarly, a multiple interaction between several antibodies and corresponding *E. canis* antigens would trigger an activation of serum complement (C3), which in turn would provide for the entry of the organism into its host cell by way of a C3b macrophage receptor (Fig. 8.2C). When the rickettsia is in the host cell, the organism must possess a mechanism enabling it to evade destruction by lysosomal action. Also, aggregates of the organisms and corresponding antibodies may provide further support to that effect.

In accordance with the observation of other intracellular obligate parasites, cytotoxic and killer cells, as well as lymphokines produced by activated macrophages and T-cells are probably major protective elements in canine ehrlichiosis. There appears to be a similarity in the mechanism of protective immunity between cutaneous leishmaniasis and canine ehrlichiosis. As with *E. canis*, leishmania parasites exist within the macrophages of the vertebrate host in the amastigot form. Similar to canine ehrlichiosis, antibodies generated in the course of leishmaniasis also appear to be of little protective value. A series of experimental studies in the latter disease suggests that cellular immunity mediated by T-cells that produce interferon-γ (IFN-γ) and macrophage activating factor (MAF) are the functional protective force.[58]

Finally, experimental infections with *E. canis* in German shepherd dogs were shown to cause states of specific and nonspecific immunosuppression.[59] This occurrence may explain the greater clinical sensitivity of this breed of dog to infection with *E. canis* and provides a partial explanation for the difficulty in inducing adequate protection in recovered animals.

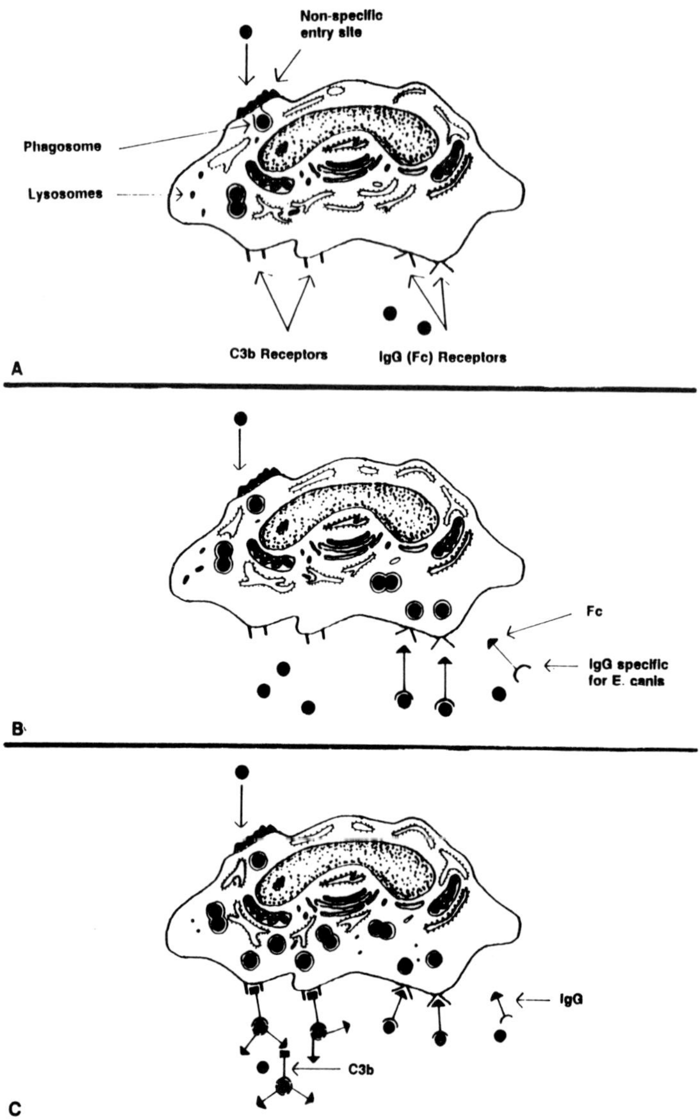

FIG. 8.2. Postulated sequence of events relevant to an interaction between *E. canis*, its antibody, and its host cell. Following its entry into blood monocyte and/or macrophage, *E. canis* multiplies by binary fission within a phagosome. The fusion of lysosomes with phagosomes is prevented through an unknown mechanism (A). The Fc portion of a specific antibody (IgG) that has interacted with the organism binds to the corresponding receptor on blood monocytes and/or macrophages. This process provides for more efficient and massive entry of the organism into the host cell (B). Two adjacent IgG molecules bound to the organism can fix many C_3b molecules, thereby enhancing the opportunity for organismal entry into the macrophage by way of the C_3b receptors (C).

Diagnosis

A diagnosis of acute ehrlichiosis by microscopic detection of the organism in Giemsa-stained blood smears or buffy coat preparations is generally difficult, if not impossible, because the percentage of infected monocytes within the peripheral blood is extremely low. An indirect fluorescent antibody (IFA) test is currently the only available specific means for detection and titration of antibodies to *E. canis*.[9] The organism generated by *in vitro* culture techniques serves as an antigen in the test.[19] The IFA test is applicable to both experimental laboratory and field diagnosis of canine ehrlichiosis. In experimentally infected dogs, the period prior to detection of antibodies at a beginning 1:10 serum dilution varies from 8 to 24 days. Analysis of the inoculation data indicates that this variation is apparently due to individual animal responses rather than to the volume of inoculum used. The serum titer in the IFA test may vary from 1:10 to 1:10,240 or greater, depending on the stage of infection, immune involvement of a given dog with the agent, and the breed of dog. In the acute stage of infection there is generally a spontaneous and rapid increase in titer, which usually reaches high levels during early convalescence. Thereafter, the titer is generally maintained at variable levels for long periods of time. Antibody titers of extremely high magnitude (i.e. 1:163,840 or greater) generally reflect a long-term chronic infection.

Persistence of IFA titers for periods longer than 6 months after appropriate treatment designed to eliminate *E. canis* infection usually indicates that the agent has not been cleared from the dog.[36] The possibility that a treated dog has been reinfected following cessation of treatment may also be a factor. Sudden decrease in IFA titers have been observed in infected dogs just prior to death. These dogs often have a severely depressed bone marrow and are hypogammaglobulinemic.

Preparation of adequate reagents, particularly cell culture-derived antigens for the IFA test, and knowledgeable test reading ability and interpretation of test results in conjunction with clinical history, carries great importance for accurate serodiagnosis of this disease. It is for this reason that some discrepancies in test results on identical serum samples have been noted between experienced and nonexperienced laboratories.

Treatment and Control

Among all therapeutics tested, tetracyclines are the most effective for treatment of *E. canis* and other ehrlichial infections of dogs. The

TABLE 8.1. *Therapeutic products available for the treatment of ehrlichial infections in dogs.**

Therapeutic Agents	Dose	Route	Frequency
First Line Antibiotics			
Tetracycline hydrochloride	22 mg/kg	Oral	Three times a day for 21 days
Oxytetracycline	25 mg/kg	Oral	Three times a day for 21 days
Doxycycline	5 mg/kg	Oral or intravenous	Two times a day for 14 days
Minocycline	20 mg/kg	Oral	Two times a day for 14 days
Second Line Antibiotics			
Chloramphenicol	50 mg/kg	Oral	Three times a day for 21 days
Imidocarb dipropionate	5 mg/kg	Intramuscular or subcutaneous	Single injection and repeat injection in 2 to 3 weeks

* From Hoskins, J.D.[45]

name of these compounds, and the dose used for treatment, are provided in Table 8.1. Following treatment with tetracycline, dogs in the early stages of the disease usually show spontaneous clinical and hematological improvement. Chronically infected dogs may respond more slowly to treatment. Some of these dogs require continuous treatment over a few months. If the treatment is effective in totally eliminating the organism from the affected dog, the IFA titer should gradually subside to a nondetectable level within 6–12 months post treatment, depending on the initial magnitude of the titer.[36] If this is not the case, the clinician may decide to repeat the treatment. For this reason periodic serological screening is recommended.

Various supportive therapies, i.e. blood transfusion, using fresh whole blood or platelet rich plasma and polyionic fluids, are frequently required, particularly for chronically infected dogs. Short-term administration of anti-inflammatory and immunosuppressive compounds may be useful for secondary immune-mediated complications. For dogs with depressed bone marrow function and pancytopenia, the use of androgenic steroids may be of some value.[45]

The only preventative therapeutic measure for canine ehrlichiosis, thus far available, is administration on a continuous basis of tetracycline at a low dosage (6.6 mg/kg/day). This may be highly effective for dogs traveling to enzootic areas. The routine use of commercially available acaricides for the control of tick infestation is strongly recommended.[36] Also, new dogs should be confirmed free of tick infestation, and their serologic status for exposure to *E. canis* determined before introducing them into an established *E. canis*-free group of dogs.[45]

References

1. DONATIEN, A. and LESTOQUARD, F. 1935. Existance en Algêrie d'une rickettsia du chien. *Bul. de la Soc. de Path. Exot.* **28:** 418–419.
2. EWING, S.A. 1969. Canine ehrlichiosis. *Adv. vet. comp. Med.* **13:** 331–353.
3. BOOL, P.H. and SUTMOLLER, P. 1957. *Ehrlichia canis* infections in dogs on Aruba (Netherlands Antilles). *J. Am. vet. Med. Ass.* **130:** 418–420.
4. EWING, S.A. 1963. Observations on leukocytic inclusion bodies from dogs infected with *Babesia canis. J. Am. vet. Med. Ass.* **143:** 503–506.
5. HUXSOLL, D.L., HILDEBRANDT, P.K., NIMS, R.M. and WALKER, J.S. 1970. Tropical canine pancytopenia. *J. Am. vet. Med. Ass.* **157:** 1627–1632.
6. WALKER, J.S., RUNDQUIST, J.D., TAYLOR, R., WILSON, B.L., ANDREWS, M.R., BARCK, J., HOGGE, A.L. JR, HUXSOLL, D.L., HILDEBRANDT, P.K. and NIMS, R.M. 1970. Clinical and clinicopathologic findings in tropical canine pancytopenia. *J. Am. vet. Med. Ass.* **157:** 43–55.
7. STEPHENSON, E.H. and RISTIC, M. 1978. Retrospective study of an *Ehrlichia canis* epizootic around Phoenix, Arizona. *J. Am. vet. Med. Ass.* **182:** 63–65.
8. NYINDO, M.B.A., RISTIC, M., HUXSOLL, D.L. and SMITH, A.R. 1971. Tropical canine pancytopenia: *in vitro* cultivation of the causative agent, *Ehrlichia canis. Am. J. vet. Res.* **32:** 1651–1658.
9. RISTIC, M. HUXSOLL, D.L., WEISIGER, R.M., HILDEBRANDT, P.K. and NYINDO, M.B.A. 1972. Serological diagnosis of tropical canine pancytopenia by indirect immunofluorescence. *Infect. Immun.* **6:** 226–231.
10. HOILIEN, C.A., RISTIC, M., HUXSOLL, D.L. and RAPMUND, G. 1982. *Rickettsia sennetsu* in human blood monocyte cultures: similarities to the growth cycle of *Ehrlichia canis. Infect. Immun.* **35:** 314–319.
11. HOLLAND, C.J., RISTIC, M., HUXSOLL, D.L., COLE, A.I. and RAPMUND, G. 1985. Adaptation of *Ehrlichia sennetsu* to canine blood monocytes: preliminary structural and serological studies with cell culture-derived *Ehrlichia sennetsu. Infect. Immun.* **48:** 366–371.
12. RISTIC, M., HUXSOLL, D.L., TACHIBANA, N. and RAPMUND, G. 1981. Evidence of a serologic relationship between *Ehrlichia canis* and *Rickettsia sennetsu. Am. J. trop. Med. Hyg.* **30:** 1324–1328.
13. RISTIC, M. and HUXSOLL, D.L. 1984. Tribe II. *Ehrlichiae.* In: *Bergey's Manual of Systematic Bacteriology,* Vol. 1, pp. 704–711. KRIEG, N.R. and HOLT, J.G. (Eds). The Williams and Wilkins Co., Baltimore.
14. HOLLAND, C.J., RISTIC, M., COLE, A.I., BAKER, J.G. and GOETZ, T.E. 1985. Isolation, experimental transmission and characterization of causative agent of Potomac horse fever. *Science* **227:** 522–524.
15. HILDEBRANDT, P.K., CONROY, J.D., MCKEE, A.E., NYINDO, B.A. and HUXSOLL, D.L. 1973. Ultrastructure of *Ehrlichia canis. Infect. Immun.* **7:** 265–271.
16. SMITH, R.D. and RISTIC, M. 1977. *Ehrlichiae.* In: *Parasitic Protozoa,* pp. 295–328. KREIER, J.P. (Ed.). Academic Press, New York.
17. HEMELT, I.E., LEWIS, G.E., JR, HUXSOLL, D.L. and STEPHENSON, E.H. 1980. Serial propagation of *Ehrlichia canis* in primary canine peripheral blood monocyte cultures. *Cornell Vet.* **70:** 37–42.

18. RISTIC, M. 1986. Pertinent characteristics of leukocytic rickettsiae of man and animals. In: *Microbiology*—1986, pp. 182–187. LEIVE, L. (Ed.). American Society for Microbiology, Washington, D.C.
19. HOLLAND, C.J. and RISTIC, M. 1990. Development of a cell line for continuous *in vitro* propagation of *Ehrlichia canis*. *Proceedings 4th International Symposium Rickettsiae and Rickettsial Diseases*. Piestany Spa, Czechoslovakia, pp. 771–775.
20. STEPHENSON, E.H. and OSTERMAN, J.V. 1977. Canine peritoneal macrophages: cultivation and infection with *Ehrlichia canis*. *Am. J. vet. Res.* **38:** 1815–1819.
21. STEPHENSON, E.H. and OSTERMAN, J.V. 1980. Somatic cell hybrids of canine peritoneal macrophages and SV-40 transformed human cells: derivation, characterization, and infection with *Ehrlichia canis*. *Am. J. vet. Res.* **41:** 234–240.
22. DAWSON, J.E., RIKIHISA, Y., EWING, S. and FISHBEIN, D.B. 1991. Serologic diagnosis of human ehrlichiosis using two *Ehrlichia canis* isolates. *J. infect. Dis.* **163:** 564–567.
23. WEISS, E. 1982. The biology of rickettsiae. *A. Rev. Microbiol.* **36:** 345–370.
24. HAHN, F.E., COHN, Z.A. and BOZEMAN, F.M. 1960. Metabolic studies of rickettsiae. Metabolism of glutamine and asparagine in *Rickettsia mooseri*. *J. Bact.* **80:** 400–405.
25. WEISS, E. 1973. Growth and physiology of rickettsiae. *Bact. Rev.* **37:** 259–283.
26. WEISS, E., DASCH, G.A., KANG, Y.H. and WESTFALL, H.N. 1988. Substrate utilization by *Ehrlichia sennetsu* and *Ehrlichia risticii* separated from host constituents by renografin gradient centrifugation. *J. Bact.* **170:** 5012.
27. WEISS, E., DASCH, G.A., WILLIAMS, J.C. and KANG, Y.H. 1990. Biological properties of the genus *Ehrlichia*: Substrate utilization and energy metabolism. In: *Ehrlichiosis: A vector-borne disease of animals and humans,* pp. 59–67. WILLIAMS, J.C. and KAKOMA, I. (Eds). Kluwer Academic Publishers, Boston.
28. WEISS, E., WILLIAMS, J.C., DASCH, G.A. and KANG, Y.H. 1989. Energy metabolism of monocytic *Ehrlichia*. *Proc. natn. Acad. Sci. U.S.A.* **86:** 1674–1678.
29. EWING, S.A. and PHILIPS, C.B. 1966. Ehrlichia-like rickettsiosis in dogs in Oklahoma and its relationship to *Neorickettsia helminthoeca*. *Am. J. vet. Res.* **27:** 67–69.
30. HOLLAND. C.J. and RISTIC, M. 1988. Unpublished data.
31. RIKIHISA, Y. 1991. Western immunoblot analysis of *Ehrlichia canis* antigens shared with other ehrlichial organisms. *Abst. ann. Mtg Am. Soc. Microbiol.* (abstr. C193), p. 374.
32. GROVES, M.G., DENNIS, G.L., AMYX, H.L. and HUXSOLL, D.L. 1975. Transmission of *Ehrlichia canis* to dogs by ticks *(Rhipicephalus sanguineus)*. *Am. J. vet. Res.* **36:** 937–940.
33. SMITH, R.D., SELLS, M., STEPHENSON, E.H., RISTIC, M. and HUXSOLL, D.L. 1976. Development of *Ehrlichia canis*, causative agent of canine ehrlichiosis, in the tick *Rhipicephalus sanguineus* and its differentiation from symbiotic rickettsia. *Am. J. vet. Res.* **37:** 119–126.
34. LEWIS, G.E., JR, RISTIC, M., SMITH, R.D., LINCOLN, T. and STEPHENSON, E.H. 1977. The brown dog tick *Rhipicephalus sanguineus* and the dog as experimental hosts of *Ehrlichia canis*. *Am. J. vet. Res.* **38:** 1953–1955.
35. RIKIHISA, Y. 1991. The tribe *Ehrlichieae* and ehrlichial diseases. *Clin. Microbiol. Rev.* **4:** 286–308.
36. RISTIC, M. and HOLLAND, C.J. 1988. Canine ehrlichiosis. In: *Manual of Small Animal Infectious Diseases,* pp. 239–243. BARLOUGH, J.E. (Ed.).
37. KEEFE, T.J., HOLLAND, C.J., SALYER, P.E. and RISTIC, M. 1982. Distribution of

Ehrlichia canis among military working dogs in the world and selected civilian dogs in the United States. *J. Am. vet. Med. Ass.* **181:** 236–238.
38. EWING, S.A. 1972. Geographic distribution and tick transmission of *Ehrlichia canis. J. med. Ent.* **9:** 597–598.
39. HILDEBRANDT, P.K., HUXSOLL, D.L., WALKER, J.S., NIMS, R.M., TAYLOR, R. and ANDREWS, M. 1973. Pathology of canine ehrlichiosis (tropical canine pancytopenia). *Am. J. vet. Res.* **34:** 1309–1320.
40. RISTIC, M., HOLLAND, C.J. and KHONDOWE, M. 1991. An overview of research on ehrlichiosis. *Eur. J. Epidemiol.* **7:** 246–252.
41. WELLS, M.Y. and RIKIHISA, Y. 1988. Lack of lysosomal fusion with phagosomes containing *Ehrlichia risticii* in $P388D_1$ cells: abrogation of inhibition with oxytetracycline. *Infect. Immun.* **56:** 3209–3215.
42. BUHLES, W.C., JR, HUXSOLL, D.L. and RISTIC, M. 1974. Tropical canine pancytopenia: Clinical, hematologic and serologic response of dogs to *Ehrlichia canis* infection, tetracycline therapy, and challenge inoculation. *J. infect. Dis.* **130:** 357–367.
43. ABEYGUNAWARDENA, I.S. 1988. Kinetics of platelet migration inhibition factor in canine ehrlichiosis: *in vivo* and *in vitro* studies. M.S. Thesis, University of Illinois, Urbana, Illinois.
44. RISTIC, M. 1990. Current strategies in research on ehrlichiosis. In: *Ehrlichiosis,* pp. 136–153. WILLIAMS, J.C. and KAKOMA, I. (Eds). Kluwer Acad. Pub., Boston.
45. HOSKINS, J.D. 1991. Ehrlichial diseases of dogs: Diagnosis and treatment. *Canine Pract.* **16:** 13–21.
46. KUEHN, N.F. and GAUNI, S.D. 1985. Clinical and hematological findings in canine ehrlichiosis. *J. Am. vet. Med. Ass.* **186:** 355–358.
47. MADEWELL, B.R., GRIBBLE, D.H. 1982. Infection in two dogs with an agent resembling *Ehrlichia canis. J. Am. vet. Med. Ass.* **180:** 512–514.
48. RISTIC, M., DAWSON, J.E., HOLLAND, C.J. and JENNY, A.L. 1988. Susceptibility of dogs to infection with *Ehrlichia risticii,* causative agent to Potomac horse fever. *Am. J. vet. Res.* **49:** 1497–1500.
49. HOLLAND, C.J. 1992. Unpublished data.
50. HELMBOLDT, C.F. and JUNGHERR, E.L. 1957. The pathology of Aleutian disease of mink. *Am. J. vet. Res.* **19:** 212–222.
51. SQUIRE, R.A., MONTALI, R.J. and BUSH. M. 1989. Pathogenetic aspects of equine infectious anemia. *J. Am. vet. Med. Ass.* **155:** 355–358.
52. POLLARD, M. and SHARON, N. 1969. Immunoproliferative choriomeningitis virus in germ-free mice. *Proc. Soc. exp. biol. Med.* **132:** 242–246.
53. LEEFLANG, P. 1972. Relation between carrier-state oxytetracycline administration and immunity in *Ehrlichia canis* infections. *Vet. Rec.* **90:** 703–704.
54. WEISIGER, R.M., RISTIC, M. and HUXSOLL, D.L. 1975. Kinetics of antibody response to *Ehrlichia canis* assayed by the indirect fluorescent antibody method. *Am. J. vet. Res.* **36:** 689–694.
55. LEWIS, G.E., HILL, S.L. and RISTIC, M. 1978. Effect of canine immune serum on the growth of *Ehrlichia canis* within nonimmune canine macrophages. *Am. J. vet. Res.* **39:** 71–76.
56. LEWIS. G.E. 1977. The effect of serum and macrophages derived from *Ehrlichia canis*-immune dogs on the *in vitro* growth and development of *Ehrlichia canis.* Ph.D. Thesis. University of Illinois, Urbana, Illinois.
57. DONATIEN, A. and LESTOQUARD, F. 1936. Existence de la premunition dans la rickettsiose naturelle ou experimentale du chien. *Bull. Soc. Path. Exot.* **29:** 378–383.

58. LIEW, F.Y. 1986. Cell-mediated immunity in experimental cutaneous leishmaniasis. *Parasit. Today* **2:** 264–270.
59. NYINDO, M., HUXSOLL, D.L., RISTIC, M., KAKOMA, I., BROWN, J.L., CARSON, C.A. and STEPHENSON, E.H. 1980. Cell-mediated and humoral immune responses of German shepherd dogs and beagles to experimental infection with *Ehrlichia canis*. *Am. J. vet. Res.* **41:** 250–254.

9

Human Ehrlichiosis

M. RISTIC AND C. J. HOLLAND

Introduction

Before the report of the first case of human ehrlichiosis in the United States (U.S.) in 1988, *Ehrlichia sennetsu*, the causative agent of sennetsu fever in Southeast Asia, was the only species of *Ehrlichia* that was known to be infectious for human beings. The description of the first human case of ehrlichiosis in the U.S. has been determined to be caused by an *Ehrlichia canis*-like agent as documented by clinical, serological and microscopic evidence. During the last few years more than 150 cases of human ehrlichiosis have been reported and at least three mortalities have been indirectly related to the disease. Thus far, the disease has been recognized in 16 states of the U.S. with a greater prevalence in the southeastern region of the country. In a majority of cases, the infection has been related to tick bites. There has been no evidence that the infection was acquired by contact with *E. canis*-infected dogs. Because of clinical similarities between Rocky Mountain spotted fever (RMSF) and ehrlichiosis, a great number of cases of human ehrlichiosis have been presumptively diagnosed as RMSF but subsequently confirmed as ehrlichiosis following serological examination.

The putative causative agent of human ehrlichiosis has recently been identified. All evidence indicates that the organism is a unique species of ehrlichia that is antigenically closely related to *E. canis*.

Sennetsu Fever

The causative agent of sennetsu fever was originally isolated in the 1950s from a 25 year old Japanese male in Fukuoka, Japan.[1] The symptoms of this patient became progressively worse with signs of a severe headache, lumbago, anorexia, sleeplessness, profuse sweating and constipation. Homogenates of the bone marrow, blood and lymph nodes were inoculated into mice. Eight to ten days postinoculation, the mice developed anorexia, lymphadenopathy, lymphopenia and prostration, followed by death. Human volunteers were inoculated with emulsified lymph nodes from diseased mice. These volunteers developed clinical signs typical of infectious mononucleosis, with atypical lymphocytes in the peripheral blood.

Preliminary studies of the causative agent indicated that it was a new species of rickettsiae and the organism was named *Rickettsia sennetsu*.[2] Subsequent series of studies by Ristic and his associates,[3–5] which included *in vitro* propagation, morphologic characterization at microscopic and electron microscopic levels, and cross-antigenic reactivity, showed that the organism is closely related to the members of the genus *Ehrlichia*. Consequently, *R. sennetsu* was reclassified as *Ehrlichia sennetsu* and included as a new member of the genus *Ehrlichia* in 1984.[6] The disease is presumed to be transmitted by ticks, however, no conclusive evidence to that effect has been provided.

For many years the consensus of opinion was that the existence of *E. sennetsu* and sennetsu fever in man were geographically limited to regions in Western Japan. The development of methods for more efficient *in vitro* propagation of *E. sennetsu* provided sufficient quantities of antigen for a large-scale seroepidemiologic study.[7,8] Between 1980 and 1983, more than 3000 sera from regions of Southeast Asia, other than Japan, were examined by the indirect immunofluorescent antibody (IFA) test for anti-*E. sennetsu* antibodies. Approximately one-third of the sera, the majority originating from Malaysian patients with febrile illness of undetermined etiology, contained *E. sennetsu*-specific antibodies. At least three *E. sennetsu*-like agents have been isolated from the blood of some of the above affected individuals. Isolation was accomplished following inoculation of blood from these patients into mice, and subsequent cultivation of the organism in primary canine blood monocytes and a continuous murine macrophage cell line ($P388D_1$).[9] These studies concluded that either *E. sennetsu*, or an agent which shares a dominant antigenic epitope with *E. sennetsu*, is present in Malaysia and possibly other regions of Southeastern Asia.

A more recent study in the U.S. on sera from 98 patients who experienced symptoms of infectious mononucleosis, but were negative in the "monospot" test, revealed that 30 sera (31%) were positive for anti-*E. sennetsu* antibodies.[10]

Human Ehrlichiosis in the U.S.A.

Early Inconclusive Studies

Several reports in the literature suggest a role for *E. canis* in human disease. *Ehrlichia canis*-like organisms were detected in blood monocytes of a splenectomized male with pancytopenia[11] and from several patients with acquired immune deficiency syndrome (AIDS).[12] In another study, two children with Kawasaki disease were found to have low titers of antibody to *E. canis*.[13] However, neither an etiologic relationship to the disease process, nor absolute identity of the microorganism were established in these cases.

First Human Ehrlichiosis Case

In April 1986, a 51 year old male was admitted to a Detroit Hospital for an acute illness characterized by fever, headache, myalgia, pancytopenia, confusion, abnormal liver function tests and renal failure, but no rash. Ten days before the onset of symptoms, the patient had been bitten by ticks while in Arkansas.[14]

Laboratory examination revealed a white blood cell count of 4600/mm^3, marked thrombocytopenia, elevated creatinine, decreasing hemoglobin levels and evidence of disseminated intravascular coagulation. The differential diagnosis included RMSF, leptospirosis and tularemia. The initial therapy administered was chloramphenicol. However, no clinical improvement was observed. Therapy was then changed to doxycycline. The patient gradually recovered and was released from the hospital 12 weeks later.

Serological tests were negative for *Rickettsia rickettsii*, as well as *Rickettsia typhi*, *Coxiella burnetii*, *Leptospira interrogans*, *Francisella tularensis*, hepatitis A virus and hepatitis B virus. The etiological relationship of the causative agent to *E. canis* was established by Ristic and his research team on the basis of serologic examination of the patient's sera.[14] Examination of the sera collected during the acute and early convalescence phases of the disease in the IFA test revealed titers at 1:640 for *E. canis*. Thereafter, the titer gradually declined to a level of 1:40 at six months after the onset of the disease. A week after the onset of the illness, microscopic examination of the patient's peripheral blood samples revealed the presence of inclusions in the leukocytes. The rickettsial nature of these inclusions was established by electron microscopic examination (Fig. 9.1A).

Other Retrospective and Prospective Studies

Prompted by the discovery of the first human ehrlichiosis case, scientists at the Center for Disease Control (CDC) and those at the University of Illinois initiated retroactive serological studies of patients that were hospitalized during October 1, 1985 and September 30, 1986, for RMSF-like illness but were serologically

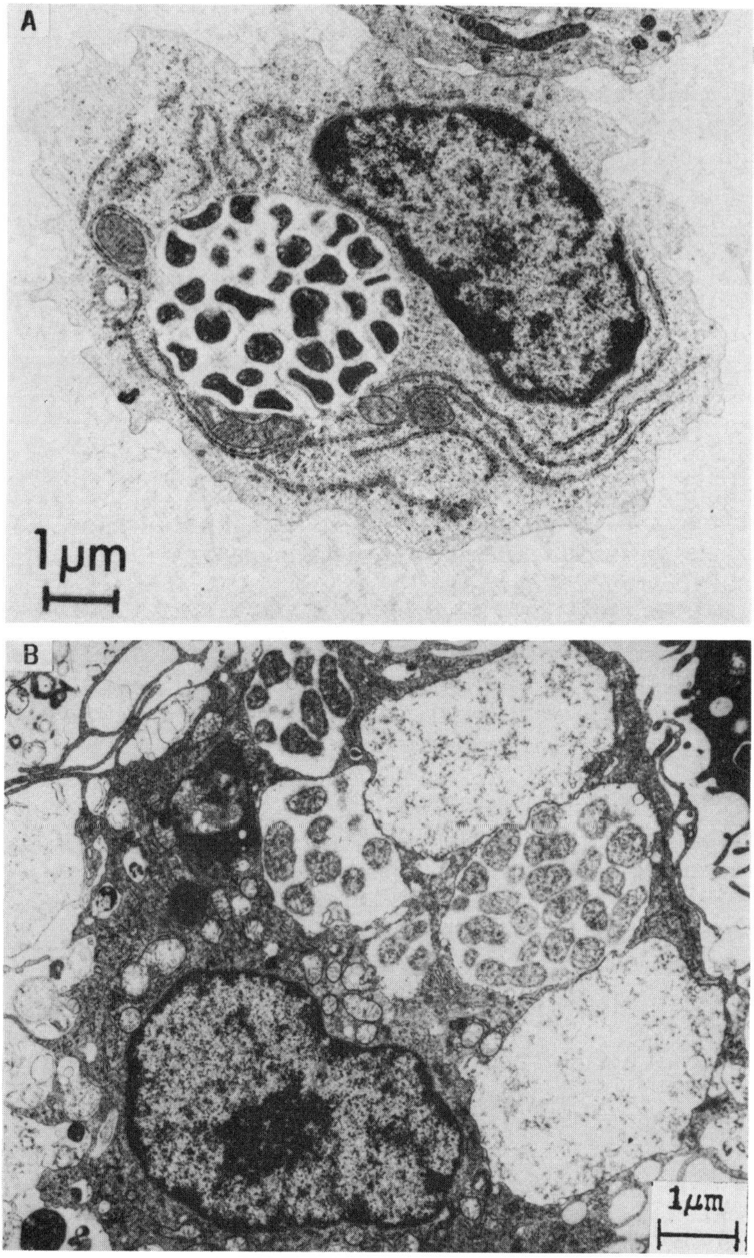

FIG. 9.1. Electron micrographs demonstrating (A) An *Ehrlichia canis*-like inclusion body observed within the cytoplasm of a lymphocyte derived from the blood of a patient affected with ehrlichiosis (× 10,300) and; (B) Cultured human monocyte infected with *E. canis* derived from an acutely infected dog (× 10,300). (Fig. 9.1A—reprinted by permission of the senior author (Ref. 14) and the New Engl. J. Med.)

negative for *R. rickettsii*, as well as for *R. typhi*, *C. burnetii*, *B. burgdorferi* and *F. tularensis*. A four-fold rise or fall in serum antibody titers to *E. canis* in some of these patients provided confirmatory evidence of ehrlichiosis.[14,15] In these and subsequent studies between CDC and several departments of health with the Oklahoma State Department of Health being the most prominent, more than 150 cases of human ehrlichiosis have been identified.[16,17] The majority of these cases occurred in 16 states of the southeastern region of the country. The disease has been seasonally reported, with the majority of clinical cases being recognized from late spring through to early fall.[16]

The median incubation period in patients with a history of a tick bite was 12 days. The most common signs and symptoms in these patients were: fever, anorexia, headache, myalgia, chills, nausea, weight loss and, occasionally, vomiting and confusion. While these signs are similar to those of RMSF, only 20% of the ehrlichiosis patients had a rash, compared with 88% of those affected by RMSF. Among the prominent hematologic abnormalities were leukopenia and thrombocytopenia.[18]

The therapy of choice for treatment of human ehrlichiosis is tetracycline.[19] Signs of recovery and a subsiding fever are usually noted within 24 to 48 h after the start of the treatment.

The specific tick involved in human transmission has not been identified. The vector of canine ehrlichiosis, the brown dog tick (*Rhipicephalus sanguineus*), does not appear to be the vector, as this tick very rarely feeds on people in the U.S.[20] Also, epidemiologic studies showed that the disease is not transmitted to humans by contact with *E. canis*-infected dogs.[21,22] It is more likely that wildlife, including some types of rodents, should be considered as possible reservoirs of the causative *Ehrlichia* species.

Etiologic Agent of Human Ehrlichiosis

Serologic evidence, the history of tick bites, hematologic abnormalities, i.e. thrombocytopenia and leukopenia, in the majority of patients and microscopic evidence of ehrlichia-like inclusion bodies in blood leukocytes of the first human ehrlichiosis case, strongly suggests that the etiologic agent is a species of *Ehrlichia*. This organism appears to be antigenically closely related to the causative agent of canine ehrlichiosis, *E. canis*. In contrast, the only known human ehrlichia species to date, *E. sennetsu*, is antigenically the most closely related to *Ehrlichia risticii*, the causative agent of equine monocytic ehrlichiosis (Syn., Potomac horse fever), rather than *E. canis*.[7,9]

The prototype strain of *Ehrlichia canis* has been considered to be extremely host specific. Previous attempts to infect other animal species, or to propagate the organism in cell cultures other than those of canine origin, have failed. Recently, however, virulent *E. canis*, isolated in primary canine monocyte cultures from the blood of a dog during the acute stage of ehrlichiosis, was successfully adapted to growth in primary human monocyte cell cultures.[23] Initially, the infection rate of human monocytes was slow, with atypical, loosely-packed morula formation being observed using light microscopy. As time in culture progressed, the percentage of infected cells increased significantly with *E. canis* morulae becoming more typical of those observed in cultured canine monocytes (Fig. 9.1b). The significance of this study with respect to the natural susceptibility of humans to the classical strain of *E. canis* is yet to be determined, particularly since no human infections have been recognized following contact with *E. canis*-infected dogs.

Recently, an *E. canis*-like agent was isolated from the blood of a patient with human ehrlichiosis and successfully propagated *in vitro* using DH82 cell cultures.[24] It is still not clear as to whether this is a variant strain of *E. canis* or a unique ehrlichia that is responsible for human ehrlichiosis. Studies on this human isolate, using 16S rDNA gene sequencing, indicate that this agent is a unique *Ehrlichia spp.* and has been named *Ehrlichia chaffeensis*.[25] This putative causative agent of human ehrlichiosis appears to be very closely related to *E. canis*, having a 98.2% 16S rDNA homology, and less related to *E. equi*, *E. phagocytophila*, *E. sennetsu* and *E. risticii*, respectively. Because of the extreme host-specificity of *E. canis*, the pathogenicity of the newly isolated agent should be tested in subhuman primates in order to further elucidate its potential as a human pathogen.

Conclusion

The pathogenic potential of members of the genus *Ehrlichia* has been clearly recognized only during the last 30 years of this century, and some species. i.e. *E. risticii* and *E. platys*, have been discovered more recently. Lately, biological properties of ehrlichiae and their importance to human and animal health have been the subject of considerable scientific studies and reports in human and veterinary medicine. It is unfortunate that the purported etiological agent of human ehrlichiosis has not yet been identified in and isolated from more patients. This may be in part due to the fact that affected individuals were promptly treated with tetracycline compounds which adversely affected the opportunity for successful isolation. Nevertheless, future efforts towards the isolation of the putative ehrlichia from additional suspected human patients must continue. It is apparent that a tick is the principal vector of human ehrlichiosis, although the identity of the tick species has not been confirmed; *Dermacentor spp.* and, possibly, *Amblyomma spp.* seem to be the most likely candidates. The transmission cycle of the causative ehrlichia, including the role of wildlife and rodents as reservoirs of this agent, needs to be studied. It is obvious that the emergence of Lyme disease and ehrlichiosis has greatly contributed to an increase in scientific interest in tick-borne zoonoses in the U.S. and elsewhere. The first case of human ehrlichiosis contracted outside of the U.S., in Mali, was recently reported.[26] It is strongly suspected that the disease is established in other countries as well. Consequently, one can expect that, in time, more research data will be generated to allow for a better understanding of human ehrlichiosis.

References

1. MISAO, T. and KOBAYASHI, Y. 1954. Studies on infectious mononucleosis I. Isolation of etiologic agent from blood, bone marrow and lymph node of a patient with infectious mononucleosis by using mice. *Tokyo Iji Shinshi.* **71:** 683–686.
2. MISAO, T., KOBAYASHI, Y., KATSUTA, K., KUWASHIMA, K., ASO, M., NOMASA, M., SHIRAKAWA, M., KATSURA, S., IKEDA, O., OSHIMA, M., YANO, T., KAGEYAMA, T., FUJIMOTO, T. and TARAKA, M. 1956. Study on infectious mononucleosis II. In special relation to the characteristics of the pathogenic agent and its nomenclature. *Tokyo Iji Shinshi.* **73:** 191–198.
3. RISTIC, M., HUXOLL, D. L., TACHIBANA, N. and RAPMUND, G. 1981. Evidence of a serologic relationship between *Ehrlichia canis* and *Rickettsia sennetsu. Am J. trop. Med. Hyg.* **30:** 1324–1328.
4. HOLLAND, C.J., RISTIC, M., HUXSOLL, D.L., COLE, A. I. and RAPMUND, G. 1985. Adaptation of *Ehrlichia sennetsu* to canine blood monocytes: Preliminary structural and serological studies with cell culture-derived *Ehrlichia sennetsu. Infect. Immun.* **48:** 366–371.
5. HOILIEN, G.A., RISTIC, M., HUXSOLL, D.L. and RAPMUND, G. 1982. *Rickettsia sennetsu* in human blood monocyte cultures; similarities to the growth cycle of *Ehrlichia canis. Infect. Immun.* **35:** 314–319.
6. RISTIC, M. and HUXSOLL, D.L. 1984. Ehrlichieae. In: *Bergey's Manual of Systematic Bacteriology,* pp. 704–709. KRIEG, N.R. and HOLT, J.G. (Eds). Williams and Wilkins, Baltimore.
7. RISTIC, M. 1986. Pertinent characteristics of leukocytic rickettsiae of human and animals. In: *Microbiology*—1986, pp. 182–187. LEIVE, L. (Ed.). American Society for Microbiology, Washington D.C.
8. COLE, A.I., RISTIC, M., LEWIS, G.E., JR and RAPMUND, G. 1985. Continuous propagation of *Ehrlichia sennetsu* in murine macrophage cell culture. *Am. J. trop. Med. Hyg.* **34:** 774–780.
9. RISTIC, M. 1990. Current strategies in research on ehrlichiosis. In: *Ehrlichiosis,* pp. 136–153. WILLIAMS, J.C. and KAKOMA, I. (Eds). Kluwer Academic Publishers, Dordrecht.
10. SEGRETI, J., KESSLER, H., COLE, A.I., HOLLAND, C., RISTIC, M. and LEVIN, S.

1986. Seroprevalence of antibodies to *Ehrlichia sennetsu* in patients with symptoms of mononucleosis. *Clin. Res.* **34:** 533a.

11. KALLICK, C.A., LEVIN, S. and REDDI, K.T. 1973. Association of a rickettsia-like agent identified in human bone marrow failure with *Ehrlichia canis* and tropical canine pancytopenia (Abstract 1). In: *Program and Abstracts of the 13th Interscience Conference on Antimicrobial Agents and Chemotherapy*. American Society for Microbiology, Washington, D.C.
12. KALLICK, C.A., THADHANI, K., RISTIC, M., KESSLER, H. and LEVIN, S. 1983. Association of acquired immunodeficiency syndrome (AIDS) with ehrlichia-like organisms (Abstract 223). In: *Program and Abstracts of the 23rd Interscience Conference on Antimicrobial Agents and Chemotherapy*. American Society for Microbiology, Washington, D.C.
13. EDLINGER, E.A., BENICHOU, J.J. and LABRUNE, B. 1980. Positive *Ehrlichia canis* serology in Kawasaki disease. *Lancet.* **1:** 1146–1147.
14. MAEDA, K., MARKOWITZ, N., HAWLEY, R.C., RISTIC, M., COX, D. and MCDADE, J. 1987. Human infection with *Ehrlichia canis*, a leukocytic rickettsia. *New Eng. J. Med.* **316:** 853–856.
15. RISTIC, M., HOLLAND, C.J. and KHONDOWE, M. 1991. An overview of research on ehrlichiosis. *Eur. J. Epidemiol.* **7:** 246–252.
16. MCDADE, J.E. 1990. Ehrlichiosis—A disease of animals and humans. *J. infect. Dis.* **161:** 609–617.
17. ENG, T.R., HARKESS, J.R., FISHBEIN, D.B., DAWSON, J.E., GREEN, C.N., REDUS, M.A. and SATALOWICH, F.T. 1990. Epidemiologic, clinical and laboratory findings of human ehrlichiosis in the United States, 1988. *J. Am. vet. Med. Ass.* **264:** 2251–2258.
18. ENG. T.R. and GILES, R. 1989. Zoonosis Update: Ehrlichiosis. *J. Am. vet. Med. Ass.* **194:** 497–500.
19. Human ehrlichiosis—United States, 1988. *M.M.W.R.* **37:** 275–277.
20. NELSON, V.A. 1969. Human parasitism by the brown dog tick. *J. Econ. Ent.* **62:** 710–712.
21. FISHBEIN, D.B., SAWYER, L.A., HOLLAND, C.J., HAYES, E.B., OKOROANYANWU, W., WILLIAMS, D., SIKES, R.K., RISTIC, M. and MCDADE, J.E. 1987. Unexplained febrile illness after exposure to ticks. *J. Am. vet. Med. Ass.* **257:** 3100–3104.
22. HARKESS, J.R., EWING, S.A., CRUTCHER, J.M., KUDLAC, J., MCKEE, G. and ISTRE, G.R. 1989. Human ehrlichiosis in Oklahoma. *J. infect. Dis.* **159:** 576–579.
23. HOLLAND, C.J., KAKOMA, I. and RISTIC, M. 1988. Adaptation of *Ehrlichia canis* to growth in primary human monocyte cultures (Abstract 208). In: *Program and Abstracts of the 37th Annual Meeting of the American Society of Tropical Medicine and Hygiene*. Washington, D.C.
24. DAWSON, J.E., ANDERSON, B., FISHBEIN, D.B., SANCHEZ, J., GOLDSMITH, C., WILLSON, K. and DUOTHY, C. 1991. Isolation and characterization of an *Ehrlichia sp.* from a patient diagnosed with human ehrlichiosis. *J. clin. Microbiol.* **29:** 2741–2745.
25. ANDERSON, B.T., DAWSON, J.E., JONES, D.C. and WILSON, K.H. 1991. *Ehrlichia chaffeensis*, a new species associated with human ehrlichiosis. *J. clin. Microbiol.* **29:** 2838–2842.
26. UHAA, I.J., MACLEAN, J.D., GREENE, C.R. and FISHBEIN, D.B. 1992. A case of human ehrlichiosis acquired in Mali: Clinical and laboratory findings. *Am. J. trop. Med. Hyg.* **46:** 161–164.

10

Canine Infectious Cyclic Thrombocytopenia (Ehrlichia Platys Infection in Dogs)

T. W. FRENCH AND J. W. HARVEY

Introduction

Ehrlichia platys was first reported in 1978 following the observation of intrathrombocytic inclusions on a blood film from a thrombocytopenic dog in Florida. The designation "infectious cyclic thrombocytopenia" was coined to denote the nature of the cause and the most notable laboratory feature of the clinically mild, self-limiting, experimental infections.[1] Subsequent studies of experimental infections, using isolates from the U.S., also reported mild or no clinical signs despite transient episodes of severe thrombocytopenia.[2–4] Recently, however, experimental infections using a Greek strain of *E. platys* have been reported to cause fever, anorexia and petechial hemorrhage in addition to thrombocytopenia.[5] Natural infections often occur in combination with other rickettsial and protozoal agents, thus questioning the role of *Ehrlichia platys* in the clinical syndrome in such cases.[2,5–7] Published[8] and unpublished reports from the southern U.S. indicate that some natural cases of *E. platys* infection alone can manifest a symptomatic course. In addition, some naturally occurring infections with *E. platys* of Greek origin appear to cause fever, anorexia and petechial hemorrhage[5] in the absence of other concomitant infections. Hence, *E. platys* infection is relevant in that it may cause or contribute to clinical disease, and it should be considered in the differential diagnosis of thrombocytopenia in the dog.

The Causative Agent

Light Microscopic Morphology

The organism can be seen by light microscopic examination of infected platelets on blood films stained with Romanowsky-type

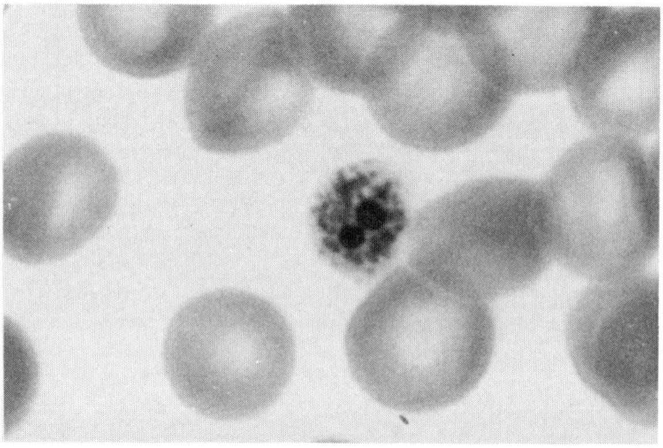

FIG. 10.1. Light microscopic appearance of *Ehrlichia platys* within a platelet. Two densely-stained morulae are present, although the constituent organisms cannot be discerned. Wright–Giemsa stain, ×2400. (From HARVEY, J.W., SIMPSON, C.F. and GASKIN, J.M. 1978. Cyclic thrombocytopenia induced by a *Rickettsia*-like agent in dogs. *J. infect. Dis.* **137:** 182–188. Reprinted with permission.)

hematology stains (Fig. 10.1). Individual organisms appear as round to oval basophilic inclusions of about 1 μm in diameter. Morulae are larger, 2–3 μm in diameter, although the constituent organisms can be difficult to discern due to the compact nature of the cluster. Platelets may contain multiple individual organisms or, less commonly, multiple morulae. Staining of unfixed air-dried blood films with 0.5% new methylene blue in physiologic saline is useful in demonstrating the organism, permitting better visualization of the individual organisms within morulae (Fig. 10.2).[1]

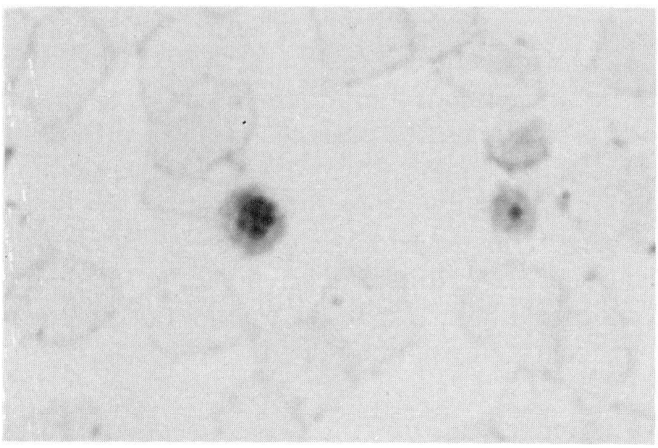

FIG. 10.2. Light microscopic appearance of *Ehrlichia platys* within platelets stained with new methylene blue. Individual organisms within a morula are apparent in the larger platelet. A single organism is present within the second platelet. NMB stain, ×2400.

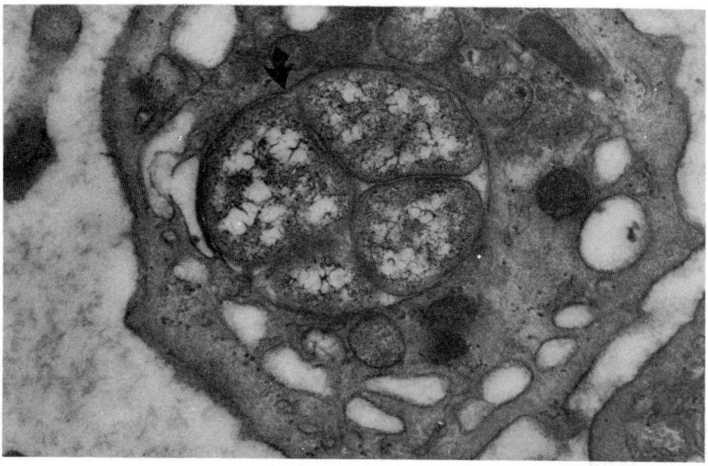

FIG. 10.3. Ultrastructure of *Ehrlichia platys* organisms within a platelet. Division of an organism is shown (arrow) by infolding of the membrane surrounding the organism. × 15,000. (From HARVEY, J.W., SIMPSON, C.F. and GASKIN, J.M. 1978. Cyclic thrombocytopenia induced by a *Rickettsia*-like agent in dogs. *J. infect. Dis.* **137**: 182–188. Reprinted with permission.)

Ultrastructural Morphology

When examined by electron microscopy,[1,4] the individual organisms are oval to bean shaped, and range from 350–1,250 nm in diameter (Fig. 10.3). Morulae in platelets contain 1–8 organisms, and as many as three morulae may be present in a single platelet. Each organism is surrounded by a double membrane. Morulae consist of multiple organisms surrounded by a membrane which roughly conforms to the external surfaces of the individual organisms. Deep infoldings occur in the membranes of some organisms (Fig. 10.3), suggesting replication by binary fission within platelets. Internal components of the organisms consist of fibrillar material and small electron-dense granules. Such granules appear to be nucleoprotein composed of both RNA and DNA. The ultrastructure of the organism is similar to that of *E. canis*.

Cultural Characteristics

Successful *in vitro* culture of the organism has not been reported. A common impetus for efforts to establish conditions for culture is lacking, due to the relative ease with which large amounts of *E. platys* antigen can be obtained from the platelets of acutely infected dogs.[2] Antigen harvested in this way has been sufficient for producing slides for serologic testing, production of antisera in rabbits, and preparation of inoculums for long-term storage.

The infectivity of the agent can be retained for long periods of time (at least five years) in a frozen state. One successful method uses a mixture of whole blood with equal volumes of 15% glycerol in phosphate-buffered 0.9% NaCl solution at pH 7.2. This mixture is then placed in sealed ampules and stepped down to freeze in liquid nitrogen.[1] Freezing of heparinized blood with 15% DMSO at −80°C also has been successfully used to preserve the organism.[8]

Antigenic Characteristics

The rapid and vigorous development of serum antibodies in dogs with acute experimental infections indicates that *E. platys* presents a potent antigenic stimulus. As determined by indirect fluorescent antibody testing (IFAT), cross reaction between *E. platys* and *E. canis* appears to be minimal. High titer sera from dogs with experimental acute *E. platys* infection did not react with *E. canis* antigen. Conversely, in a group of 23 clinical cases with high titers (>1:160) to *E. canis*, 35% of the sera failed to react with *E. platys* antigen. Hence, serum samples with high titers to both of these agents may result from dual infections, rather than cross-reactivity of antibodies.[2]

E. platys has not been extensively tested for cross-reaction with other rickettsial agents, but serum samples from 10 horses with Potomac horse fever were negative for antibodies to *E. platys* antigen by IFAT using a proven anti-horse IgG conjugate (T. W. French, unpublished results). Further testing of the antigenic relatedness of *E. platys* to other ehrlichial agents is needed, using newer, more sensitive techniques such as protein immunoblotting.[9]

Epidemiology

Natural Transmission

Transmission of *E. platys* in nature generally has been presumed to occur via ticks. Circumstantial evidence for this theory includes the common occurrence of coinfection with other hematoparasites known to be transmissible by ticks, especially *E. canis*. Clinically, ticks are commonly observed on animals with naturally occurring *E. platys* infection.[1,5] Furthermore, the rate of seropositivity among dogs from heavily tick-infested areas is very high.[6]

Experimental confirmation of this possibility is lacking. Only one study has attempted to prove a tick vector. Using *Rhipicephalus sanguineus* under experimental conditions similar to those which have supported transmission of *E. canis*, no transmission of *E. platys* was established.[10] Nevertheless, the possibility that this or other ticks can act as biological vectors cannot be excluded. Given the magnitude of the initial parasitemias seen in experimental infections, mechanical transmission by mosquitoes and/or fleas is also plausible.

Experimental Infections

Infection can be reliably established in dogs by intravenous injection of citrated or heparinized fresh whole blood or frozen preserved blood from infected dogs.[1,8] The age of the animal appears to have no significant effect on the course of the infection; clinical and hematologic findings in a group of three weanling puppies were similar to that in mature dogs (J.W. Harvey, unpublished results). The infection in splenectomized dogs is clinically similar to intact dogs, although the henatologic pattern is slightly more dramatic (see hematology section).

Hosts Affected

Fully confirmed natural or experimental infection has been reported only in dogs. Attempts to infect cats by intravenous injection of blood from an acutely infected dog were unsuccessful.[11] Although infection in humans has not been fully documented, some human sera from a prospective study of *E. canis* infection in coastal Georgia were reactive to *E. platys* antigen using an IFA test; these sera also reacted to *E. canis* antigen in a similar test (T. W. French, unpublished).

Geographic Distribution

E. platys infection in the U.S. appears to have a distribution similar to that of *E. canis* and other tick-borne infections.[2,6] It is endemic in the southern U.S., especially in the lower eastern seaboard and Gulf coast states. The agent also appears to be endemic in Arizona and California (T. W. French, unpublished). Sporadic cases have been documented in dogs from many other areas of the U.S., but the exposure may have occurred during the course of travels to endemic areas in many of these cases. A very high frequency was established in one survey of dogs in Louisiana, in which 41% of clinically ill dogs with thrombocytopenia and 54% of clinically normal kennel dogs had significant titers (>1:100) to *E. platys* by the IFA test.[6] The healthy kennel dogs were mostly hunting dogs from heavily tick-infested areas. Many of these dogs also had serum antibodies to *E. canis* and to *Rickettsia rickettsii*, the causative agent of Rocky Mountain spotted fever.

The infection also occurs in Greece[5] and southern Italy.[7]

Pathogenesis

The mode of entry, though not proven, is most likely via the bite of a tick or possibly other arthropods. It appears likely that the organisms subsequently gain access to platelets by endocytosis, and that the vacuole containing organisms is lined by membrane derived from the platelet surface.[11] Electron micrographs suggest that the agent is capable of replication by binary fission within platelets.[1] Aside from the blood platelets, no tissue or organ has been clearly shown to harbor intact, viable organisms. *E. platys* antigen was demonstrated in macrophages of liver, spleen, bone marrow and lymph nodes from experimentally infected dogs at 14 days postinoculation by immunofluorescent staining of frozen tissues using a dog anti-*E. platys* antiserum.[3] This may represent the fate of infected platelets, however, rather than a site of multiplication. Immunocytochemical staining of tissues from acutely infected dogs using an avidin–biotin immunoperoxidase complex failed to identify *E. platys* antigens in any tissue, although the same procedure readily demonstrated reactive antigen in blood platelets.[12] No antigen was detected in megakaryocytes from acutely infected dogs using an indirect immunofluorescent technique,[13] and organisms have not been observed in megakaryocytes using Wright's stained smears.

The pathogenesis of the thrombocytopenia has not been fully established. Results of coagulation screening tests performed on blood from acutely infected puppies remained within the normal range (J. W. Harvey, unpublished observations). Hence, the thrombocytopenia does not appear to be caused by a consumptive coagulopathy such as disseminated intravascular coagulation. The percentage of platelets seen to be infected decreases dramatically in successive parasitemias, but the associated thrombocytopenic episodes remain severe. This finding has prompted speculation that the initial parasitemia triggers immunologic mechanisms which are the cause of subsequent thrombocytopenias. Plasma samples from acutely infected dogs were shown to be positive for anti-platelet antibody using the platelet factor-3 release test and an indirect ELISA method, but megakaryocytes were negative for surface immunoglobulin by direct immunofluorescence.[13] These findings suggest that an antibody against antigens present on normal platelets may play a role in the development of thrombocytopenia.

The *in vitro* aggregation response of platelets from acutely infected dogs has been studied.[4] Platelet rich plasma aggregation responses to collagen were unchanged, but were decreased when tested using a low dose of ADP (0.1 mM). This finding is compatible with prior reversible activation of platelets occurring as a feature of the infection.

Megakaryocytes in marrow increase during the acute phase of infection, consistent with a response to thrombocytopenia caused by shortened platelet survival,[3,4] although direct measurement of platelet lifespan has not been reported. The spleen does not appear to play a pivotal role in the pathogenesis, since infection of splenectomized dogs results in episodes of thrombocytopenia similar to those seen in intact dogs.[1]

Little evidence is available with regard to the occurrence of a carrier state following acute infection. Infection was transmitted in one instance using blood from a clinically normal, nonparasitemic, seropositive dog.[2]

Clinical Disease

Prepatent Period

The prepatent period, here defined as the time elapsed between the introduction of infective agent into the host and the first appearance of infected platelets in the blood, has not been established for naturally-occurring infections. Evidence from experimental infections suggests that the prepatent period depends on the dose of viable infective organisms injected. Prepatent periods ranging from 3 days to 3 weeks have been observed, following injection of organism-rich fresh whole blood and a five year old frozen inoculum, respectively (T. W. French, unpublished observations). In most published studies, prepatent periods of 7–14 days have been reported.[1,2,5,8]

Clinical Signs in Natural Infections

Clinical signs directly attributable to *E. platys* infection in naturally-occurring cases often are difficult to establish due to the frequent coinfection with other hematoparasites. The dog from which *E. platys* was originally isolated was clinically normal at the time of examination.[1] However, fever, anorexia, lethargy, and loss of condition have been reported in some dogs from Greece with *E. platys* infection, in the absence of other recognizable concomitant diseases.[5]

Bilateral uveitis, fever, and mucosal pallor were reported in a well-documented case of natural *E. platys* infection.[8] Anemia, thrombocytopenia, intrathrombocytic inclusions, and a high serum antibody titer to *E. platys* (1 : 100 by IFAT) were present, consistent with the acute stages of infection. Serum antibodies to *E. canis* were not detected, and no evidence of other diseases was found. The dog recovered fully following a two week course of oral tetracycline and topical application of ophthalmic antibiotics, dexamethasone and atropine. The hematologic findings appeared compatible with an uncomplicated *E. platys* infection. Although other causes of uveitis could not be entirely excluded, this case may well represent an ocular manifestation of acute *E. platys* infection. Uveitis has also been recognized in association with *E. canis* infections.[11]

Clinical Signs in Experimental Infections

Reports of clinical signs in experimentally infected dogs vary in detail, but generally are relatively mild. Death due to *E. platys* infection has not been reported in published studies.

In the initial report describing this agent, clinical signs of illness in four experimentally infected dogs were virtually absent.[1] Two of the four had slight fever (39.4–40.2°C) at the time of the first parasitemia. There was no evidence of spontaneous hemorrhage, although the bleeding time, as measured by wounding the muscosa of the oral labia, was greatly prolonged (>30 min) during episodes of severe thrombocytopenia.

Experimental infections using a Greek strain of *E. platys* produced a more severe clinical syndrome.[5] Fever and mucosal pallor were observed coincident with the first parasitemia, and petechia of the oral mucosa and skin (abdomen, inner thighs) developed a few days later when the platelet count was low. Decreased appetite and loss of condition were also reported.

Hematology

The hematologic hallmarks of infection with *E. platys* are thrombocytopenia and the presence of the characteristic intrathrombocytic inclusions. Parasitemia in experimental infections is cyclic, with a periodicity of 7–14 days.[1] Platelet concentration decreases rapidly concomitant with each parasitemia, and may remain at very low levels (<15,000/μl) for 2–3 days (Fig. 10.4). Organisms usually are not identifiable in blood during the period of severe thrombocytopenia. The platelet count rebounds sharply to preinoculation levels (or greater) between parasitemic episodes. The first parasitemia is of the greatest magnitude. The percentage of platelets with inclusions

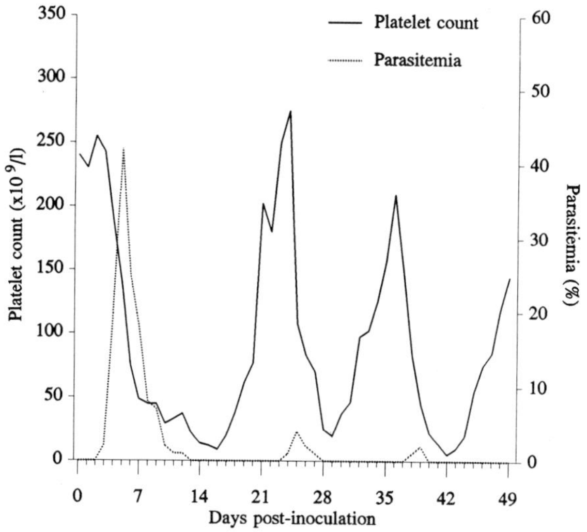

FIG. 10.4. Platelet counts and parasitemias from a dog with acute experimental *Ehrlichia platys* infection. Successive parasitemias are of decreasing magnitude, but the associated episodes of thrombocytopenia remain severe.

builds over 3–4 days before reaching a maximum of 31–63%. Subsequent parasitemias are of progressively decreasing amplitude, but the associated episodes of thrombocytopenia typically remain severe through at least the first 6–8 cycles. Such periodicity has not been documented in naturally acquired infections. The degree of the thrombocytopenia diminishes with time, and the platelet count gradually returns to normal. Visible organisms are absent or very rare during this period.

Infections in splenectomized dogs are similar, although the magnitude of parasitemias tends to be greater[1] (T. W. French, unpublished observations). The high preinoculation platelet counts, common in recently splenectomized dogs, result in an even more dramatic oscillations in platelet counts through the period of recurring parasitemias. This combination of the high starting platelet count and high grade parasitemia is advantageous in the research setting, in that large numbers of infected platelets are circulating. Platelet-rich plasma prepared from such blood is a rich source of antigen.[1]

Anemia has been reported in both natural and experimental infections. Moderate, nonregenerative, tetracycline-responsive anemia (PCV=21%) accompanied thrombocytopenia in a report of naturally-occurring infection in a Louisiana dog.[8] Mild anemia was noted in a study of experimental acute infection. On day 14 postinfection, hematocrits reached a mean low level of 35%; concomitant decreases in serum iron concentration and total iron binding capacity in the face of plentiful stainable iron in marrow were considered compatible with the anemia of inflammation.[14] Anemia was more severe (PCV = 23–25%) in experimental infections using a Greek strain; lowest levels were reached during the period when the petechial hemorrhages occurred.[5]

Decreased leukocyte counts may accompany the first few parasitemic episodes, although this is less consistent than thrombocytopenia.[1,5,14] The decrease is attributable to lowered numbers of neutrophils, lymphocytes and eosinophils.[1,14] The leukopenia tends to be transient, relatively mild and unaccompanied by complicating secondary bacterial infections. Margination of leukocytes in small vessels in histologic sections of tissues from acutely infected dogs has been reported,[1] and may account for decreased cell counts in the circulating pool. Granulopoiesis in marrow remains morphologically normal.[14]

Changes in serum protein concentrations may occur in association with *E. platys* infection. In a study of acute infection using a Louisiana isolate, significant elevations in alpha and gamma globulins were demonstrated, consistent with increased acute phase proteins and immunoglobulins, respectively. These changes were counterbalanced by decreased albumin ("negative" acute phase reaction) and beta-1 globulins, however, such that total protein levels were not changed.[14] In a study using a Greek strain of *E. platys*, total plasma protein increased from 6.5 to 9.0 g/dl and remained elevated through 21 months postinoculation. Serum protein electrophoresis was not included in this study, but increased immunoglobulin and/or acute phase protein concentrations are most likely to account for the increase.[5]

Pathology

Gross lesions of acute *E. platys* infections may be absent,[1] or consist of generalized lymphadenopathy. Microscopic lesions are generally similar to, but milder than, those of acute *E. canis* infection and consist of hyperplasia of lymphoid tissue and tissue macrophages. A significant difference between the two is the lack of apparent vasculitis or endothelial cell injury in acute *E. platys* infection.[3]

Lymph node follicles were hyperplastic; increased numbers of plasma cells and erythrophagocytic macrophages were present in the medullary cords and sinuses. Spleens from acutely infected dogs also had follicular hyperplasia and increased numbers of sinusoidal plasma cells and erythrophagocytic macrophages. Slight necrosis of follicular lymphocytes with karyorrhectic debris was evident in the lymph nodes and spleen. Additional splenic lesions included increased prominence of periarteriolar macrophage sheaths, hyperplasia of periarteriolar lymphoid sheaths, extramedullary hematopoiesis and crescent shaped areas of hemorrhage at the periphery of periarteriolar lymphoid sheaths.[3]

Hepatic lesions consist of multifocal Kupffer cell hyperplasia. Lymphocyte and plasma cell infiltrates occurred in the renal cortical interstitium around glomeruli and subcapsular veins. Overall bone marrow cellularity was consistently increased; megakaryocyte numbers were normal to increased.[3,4] Mild interstitial pneumonia was identified in one study of acute *E. platys* infection,[1] but no pulmonary lesions were noted in another.[3]

Immunity

No studies have been performed to assess the question of protective immunity in *E. platys* infection. It is not known if antibodies detectable by IFAT confer effective immunity to reinfection. It is possible that the presence of circulating antibodies indicates persistent infection, rather than protection against infection.

Diagnosis

In acutely infected dogs, organisms can be detected by microscopic examination of blood films stained with new methylene blue or Romanowsky type stains. Preparation of buffy coat smears increases sensitivity in detecting low grade parasitemias by allowing examination of a larger number of platelets. The appearance of the organism in such preparations is quite characteristic. In Romanowsky stained preparations, *E. platys* stains a deep blue. Putative remnants of megakaryocyte nuclei and aggregated/large platelet granules occasionally can mimic the organism, but tend to stain more purple and reddish, respectively. Identification of organisms in varying stages of development (i.e. single, paired and morula forms) also helps to increase confidence of diagnosis.

An immunocytochemical staining procedure using an avidin–biotin immunoperoxidase complex has been described which can specifically identify *E. platys* antigen in blood platelets. This method can distinguish *E. platys* organisms from large platelet granules and/or remnants of megakaryocyte nuclei.[12]

An indirect fluorescent antibody test for detection of serum antibodies to *E. platys* was described, and appeared to be relatively specific and sensitive.[2] Platelets isolated from the blood of acutely infected splenectomized dogs with high grade parasitemias were utilized as a source of antigen. Experimentally infected dogs first developed detectable serum antibodies 7–19 days postinoculation, shortly after, or coincident with, the peak of the first parasitemia.[2,3] The antibody titer rose quickly during the next 7–14 days. The kinetics of antibody response were similar in dogs experimentally infected with a Greek strain of *E. platys*.[5]

Serum antibodies detectable by IFA persisted at high levels (1:1000) up to 6 months after experimental infection.[5] In one naturally occurring infection, serum antibodies were detected (1:160) more than 5 years after initial diagnosis, although the possibility of repeated exposures during that period cannot be excluded.[2]

Coinfection with other rickettsial and protozoal parasites appears to be common. In a report of clinical cases in Greece, serologic and/or morphologic evidence of concomitant infection with *E. canis*, a granulocytic ehrlichial agent, *Rickettsia conorii, Babesia canis* and *Hepatozoon canis,* in varying combinations, were seen in some dogs.[5]

Treatment and Control

As with other rickettsial agents, the tetracycline group of antibiotics appear to be clinically effective treatment for *E. platys* infections.[5,7,8] Tetracycline hydrochloride or oxytetracycline (22 mg/kg T.I.D., P.O.), and doxycycline (10 mg/kg O.I.D., P.O. or I.V.) are most commonly employed.[15] Therapy probably should be continued for a minimum of 3–4 weeks. Chloramphenicol may also be effective against the organism, but generally is less desirable due to the potential marrow suppressive effects.

Oral tetracycline was used to treat one experimentally infected dog during the acute stage of the disease and appeared to be very effective (T. W. French, unpublished observations). This dog was allowed to progress through two episodes of parasitemia and thrombocytopenia. Oral tetracycline therapy was initiated when organisms reappeared at the start of the fourth parasitemia (Fig. 10.5). Although tetracycline abolished the cycles of parasitemia and thrombocytopenia in this acutely infected dog, it is not known if such treatment totally clears the organism from the body.

As no vaccine is available, preventing exposure is the only means of controlling infection. Although not proven, ticks seem to be the most likely vector for transmitting the organism.

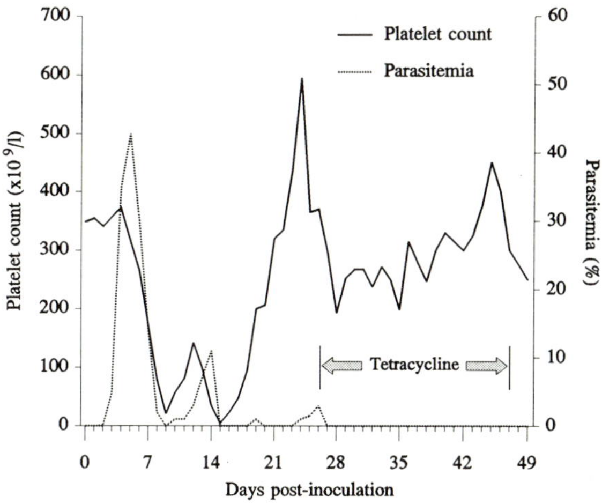

FIG. 10.5. Platelet counts and parasitemias from a dog with acute experimental *Ehrlichia platys* infection. Tetracycline (22 mg/kg T.I.D., P.O.) was given during the period indicated by the arrow, and was effective in halting the cycles of parasitemia and associated thrombocytopenia.

References

1. HARVEY, J.W., SIMPSON, C.F. and GASKIN, J.M. 1978. Cyclic thrombocytopenia induced by a *Rickettsia*-like agent in dogs. *J. infect. Dis.* **137:** 182–188.
2. FRENCH, T.W. and HARVEY, J.W. 1983. Serologic diagnosis of infectious cyclic thrombocytopenia in dogs using an indirect fluorescent antibody test. *Am. J. vet. Res.* **44:** 2407–2411.
3. BAKER, D.C., SIMPSON, M., GAUNT, S.D. and CORSTVET, R.E. 1987. Acute *Ehrlichia platys* infection in the dog. *Vet. Path.* **24:** 449–453.
4. GAUNT, S.D., BAKER, D.C. and BABIN, S.S. 1990. Platelet aggregation studies in dogs with acute *Ehrlichia platys* infection. *Am. J. vet. Res.* **51:** 290–293.
5. KONTOS, V.I., PAPADOPOULOS, O. and FRENCH, T.W. 1991. Natural and experimental canine infections with a Greek strain of *Ehrlichia platys. Vet. clin. Path.* **20:** 101–105.
6. HOSKINS, J.D., BREITSCHWERDT, E.B., GAUNT, S.D., FRENCH, T.W. and BURGDORFER, W. 1988. Antibodies to *Ehrlichia canis, Ehrlichia platys,* and spotted fever group Rickettsia in Louisiana dogs. *J. vet. Intern. Med.* **2:** 55–59.
7. PENNISI, M.G., FRENCH, T.W. and CATARSINI, O. 1989. Infectious cyclic thrombocytopenia *(Ehrlichia platys)* of dogs in Italy. *Atti della Societa Italiana delle Scienze Veterinarie* **XLIII:** 1341–1344.
8. GLAZE, M.B. and GAUNT, S.D. 1986. Uveitis associated with *Ehrlichia platys* infection in a dog. *J. Am. vet. Med. Ass.* **188:** 916–917.
9. NYINDO, M., KAKOMA, I. and HANSEN, R. 1991. Antigenic analysis of four species of the genus *Ehrlichia* by use of protein immunoblot. *Am. J. vet. Res.* **52:** 1225–1230.
10. SIMPSON, R.M., GAUNT, S.D., HAIR, J.A., KOCAN, K.M., HENK, W.G. and CASEY, H.W. 1991. Evaluation of *Rhipicephalus sanguineus* as a potential biologic vector of *Ehrlichia platys. Am. J. vet. Res.* **52:** 1537–1541.

11. GREENE, C.E. and HARVEY, J.W. 1984. Canine Ehrlichiosis. In: *Clinical Microbiology and Infectious Diseases of the Dog and Cat*, pp. 545–561. GREENE, C.E. (Ed.). W.B. Saunders Co., Philadelphia.
12. SIMPSON, R.M. and GAUNT, S.D. 1991. Immunocytochemical detection of *Ehrlichia platys* antigens in canine blood platelets. *J. vet. diagn. Invest.* **3:** 228–231.
13. FRENCH, T.W., SHELLY, S.M. and HARVEY, J.W. 1987. Investigation of the mechanism of thrombocytopenia in dogs with acute *Ehrlichia platys* infection (abstract). In: *Proceedings 38th Annual Meeting Am. Coll. Vet. Path.* p. 25.
14. BAKER, D.C., GAUNT, S.D. and BABIN, S.S. 1988. Anemia of inflammation in dogs infected with *Ehrlichia platys. Am. J. vet. Res.* **49:** 1014–1016.
15. WOODY, B.J. and HOSKINS, J.D. 1991. Ehrlichial diseases of dogs. *Vet. clin. North Am. Small Anim. Pract.* **21:** 75–98.

11

Equine Ehrlichiosis

J. E. MADIGAN

Introduction

Equine ehrlichiosis, caused by *Ehrlichia equi*, is a seasonal disease of horses first reported by Gribble in horses in northern California in 1969.[1,2] While initially thought to be of low incidence, the disease is now commonly recognized in this region.[3,4] Clinical signs in horses include high fever, depression, partial anorexia, limb edema, petechiation, icterus, ataxia and reluctance to move. Hematological changes include leukopenia, thrombocytopenia, anemia and the presence of *E. equi* inclusion bodies found principally in neutrophils and occasionally eosinophils. Diagnosis is made by clinical signs and observing characteristic morulae in the neutrophils of stained blood smears. Mortality is low unless secondary infection develops or injury occurs due to incoordination. Treatment with tetracycline results in defervescence of fever and gradual improvement of other clinical signs. Chronic infections with *E. equi* do not occur. The disease may be confused with other conditions including encephalitis, liver disease, purpura, and equine infectious anemia.

The Causative Agent

The causative agent, *Ehrlichia equi*, is observable in the cytoplasm of neutrophils or eosinophils on blood smears stained with Giemsa or new methylene blue stains. Inclusion bodies consist of one or more coccoid or cocci-bacillary organisms approximately 0.2 μm in diameter to large granular structures (morulae) approximately 0.5 μm in diameter.[1] Inclusion bodies are often pleomorphic and more than one inclusion body may be found in an individual cell (Fig. 11.1). Organisms are readily visible under high, dry or oil emersion with light microscopy and stain a deep blue to pale blue gray with

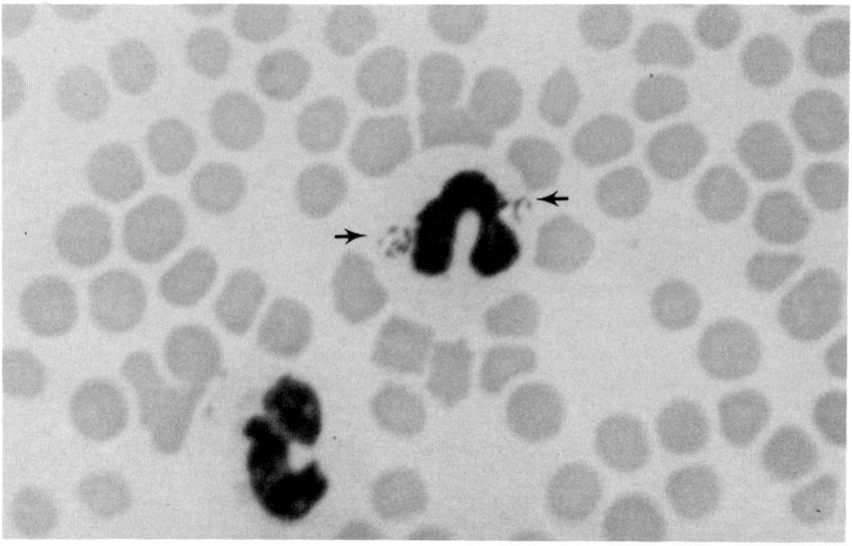

FIG. 11.1. Peripheral blood smear demonstrating intracytoplasmic inclusions of *Ehrlichia equi* within the neutrophils of a horse during the acute phase of equine ehrlichiosis (arrows). Giemsa, ×1500 (Courtesy of C. J. Holland.

Giemsa or Wright–Leishman stains.[1] They are gram- and PAS-negative and are fluorescent with acridine orange.[1]

Electron microscopy reveals the organisms to be contained within membrane-lined cytoplasmic vacuoles of neutrophils with ovoid, round and rod-shaped appearances.[5] Individual organisms are surrounded by a cell wall and plasma membrane.[5] A variable number of organisms (1–33) may be observed in individual cytoplasmic vacuoles.

The organism has not been propagated in cell culture. The organism is maintained by passage in susceptible horses with fresh or frozen blood obtained from experimental or naturally occurring cases of *E. equi*. Approximately 20 ml of fresh heparinized blood from a horse with fever and parasitemia will produce infection in susceptible horses when inoculated intravenously. The organism remains viable for up to 2 years when infected blood is stored at −70°C.

Recently, the application of SDS-Page and Western blot methods have provided information on the antigenicity of *E. equi*.[6] *Ehrlichia equi* has been found, based on homologous reactions, to have 5 immunodominant polypeptides (13, 16, 23, 25 and 45 kDa). Antiserum to *E. equi* does not recognize antigens of *E. risticii* and vice versa.[6,7] Antiserum to *E. equi* recognized 15 polypeptides of *E. sennetsu*, and anti *E. sennetsu* serum reacted with 8 *E. equi* polypeptides, suggesting a closer relationship between these species than previously believed.

Epidemiology

The natural host of *E. equi* is the equine species, including donkeys. Horses of any age are susceptible, but the clinical manifestations are less severe in horses under 3 years of age.[1,4] The majority of cases are seen in the late fall, winter and spring in northern California.[3] The disease has been reported in horses in Florida,[8] Colorado,[9] New Jersey,[10] Washington,[11] Switzerland[12] and Sweden.[13] The mode of transmission, vectors and reservoir of infection are unknown.

A number of animal species can become infected with *E. equi* experimentally, but do not show significant clinical signs unlike the horse. This includes monkeys, baboons, sheep, goats, cats and dogs.[14] Two dogs undergoing immunosuppression chemotherapy became naturally infected with *E. equi* following a visit to an endemic area of northern California.[15]

Pathogenesis

Because of the presence of ticks on a large percentage of infected horses and the seasonality of clinical disease, tick transmission is suspected but unproven. The organism has been found only in circulating neutrophils and eosinophils. The disease manifestations are due to a vasculitis. The thrombocytopenia, which occurs during the acute clinical phase, does not appear to be due to a consumption of platelets associated with the vasculitis. The author has experimentally blocked vasculitis manifestations in horses with concurrent administration of corticosteroids, and the horses still developed a thrombocytopenia. This suggests a direct bone marrow suppression of platelet release or maturation. The carrier state of the causative agent does not appear to exist.[16]

Clinical Disease

The prepatent period following experimental inoculation of infectious blood into susceptible horses is 3–10 days. Blood that has been frozen generally has a longer incubation period. With naturally acquired infections, the incubation period is believed to be less than 14 days based on two clinical cases whereby the affected horses had visited an endemic area for a single trail ride and then returned to a nonendemic area and, subsequently, developed the disease within that time period.

Clinical signs evolve over several days. Initially there is fever (38.4–41.6°C; 101–107°F) and mild depression. The disease progresses with continued fever, which fluctuates from 38.4–41.6°C (101–107°F), along with partial anorexia, ataxia, limb edema, reluctance to move and icterus. Younger horses (<1 year) may experience only a short period of fever without any other signs. In general, the disease is less severe in horses under 3 years of age. The clinical signs last for 7–14 days followed by gradual improvement. Mortality is low, but deaths have occurred due to secondary infection and injury resulting from severe incoordination.

A recently identified symptom in some clinical cases is the development of cardiac arrhythmias. A ventricular tachycardia and premature ventricular contractions have been observed in association with the usually recognized clinical signs. Treatment with antiarrhythmia medication, as well as therapy for the ehrlichia infection, has produced resolution of the cardiac manifestations. Experimentally, horses have been shown to develop a myocardial vasculitis[17] and presumably this may account for the manifestation of transient cardiac arrythmia.

Pathology

The characteristic gross lesions observed by Gribble[1] consisted of hemorrhages, petechiae, ecchymoses and edema. Edema is worse in the limbs, and hemorrhages were most common in the subcutaneous tissues, fascia, and epimysium of the distal limbs.[1] Histologically, there is inflammation of the small arteries and veins. Vasculitis lesions may be necrotizing with perivascular accumulation of monocytes, lymphocytes and some neutrophils.[1] Mild inflammatory lesions develop in the brain, heart and kidneys.[1]

Immunity

Inoculation studies performed by Gribble[1] demonstrated that horses are refractory to challenge after a 20 month period. There is a substantial cell-mediated immune response as well as humoral immunity following infection and natural recovery.[16] Serum antibodies persisted for at least 300 days and cell mediated immunity for 200 days postexperimental infection.[16] Treatment of recovered horses with tetracycline and rechallenge failed to produce a second infection, suggesting that a chronic active or latent basis of infection is not responsible for the long-lasting immunity associated with *Ehrlichia equi* infection.[16]

Based on the indirect immunofluorescence assay, horses residing in endemic areas of the foothills of California have a higher prevalence of seropositivity (10.4%) to *E. equi* than horses from nonendemic areas of the central valley of California (3.1%).[4] The seroprevalence rate on two farms, where only single cases of *E. equi* infection have been diagnosed yearly, was nearly 50%, indicating that many horses are exposed but develop subclinical infection.[4]

Diagnosis

Diagnosis is based on an awareness of the geographic regions where *E. equi* may be found, typical clinical signs, abnormal laboratory findings, and the finding of characteristic ehrlichia morulae in the cytoplasm of neutrophils or eosinophils. More than one inclusion body (morulae) should be observed when making a definitive diagnosis, in order to rule out the possibility of artifact error. During the first 24–48 h of infection, inclusion bodies are rarely observed. By 3–5 days of infection, they are readily apparent on slides stained by the Giemsa method. Because horses are leukopenic, a greater percentage of neutrophils can be examined by use of the buffy coat smear and subsequent staining. An indirect fluorescent antibody (IFA) test is available[4] and paired serum testing can be performed to confirm recent infection. Since inclusion bodies are always visible during the mid stages of the febrile period, IFA testing is not required at this time to make a definitive diagnosis. However, the test, using paired titers, is highly reliable in confirming equine ehrlichiosis during the late acute/early convalescent phase of the disease when the percentage of infected neutrophils in the peripheral blood is markedly decreased.

Treatment and Control

Treatment with intravenous administration of oxytetracycline at a rate of 7 mg/kg once daily has been highly effective. A prompt reduction in fever occurs in all cases within 12–24 h. Indeed, a failure of defervescence with treatment during this time period would suggest re-evaluation of the diagnosis of equine ehrlichiosis. Penicillin, chloramphenicol and streptomycin are of no therapeutic value.[17] Treatment with oxytetracycline should continue for 7 days when infection is detected in the early stages of the disease. Several cases have reoccurred within 3–4 weeks following shorter durations of treatment. The prognosis should be considered excellent in uncomplicated cases. Since concurrent infections may become exacerbated during the time of leukopenia, a thorough physical examination should be performed.

No vaccination against *E. equi* is presently available. Control measures are limited because the vector is unknown. However, it seems prudent to suggest arthropod vector control wherever possible, particularly tick control.

References

1. Gribble, D.H. 1969. Equine ehrlichiosis. *J. Am. vet. Med. Ass.* **155:** 462–469.
2. Stannard, A.A., Gribble, D.H. and Smith, R.S. 1969. Equine ehrlichiosis: A disease with similarities to tick-borne fever and bovine petechial fever. *Vet. Rec.* **84:** 149–150.
3. Madigan, J.E. and Gribble, D.H. 1987. Equine ehrlichiosis in northern California: 49 cases (1968–1981). *J. Am. vet. Med. Ass.* **190:** 445–448.
4. Madigan, J.E., Heitala, S., Chalmers, S. and DeRock, E. 1990. Seroepidemiologic survey of antibodies to *Ehrlichia equi* in horses in northern California. *J. Am. vet. Med. Ass.* **196:** 1962–1964.
5. Sells, D.M., Hildebrandt, P.K., Lewis, G.E., Nyindo, M.B.A. and Ristic, M. 1976. Ultrastructural observation on *Ehrlichia equi* organisms in equine granulocytes. *Infect. Immun.* **13:** 273–280.
6. Nyindo, M., Kakoma, I. and Hansen, R. 1991. Antigenic analysis of four species of the genus *Ehrlichia* by use of protein immunoblot. *Am. J. vet. Res.* **52:** 1225–1230.
7. Holland, C.J., Ristic, M., Cole, A.I., Johnson, P., Baker, G. and Goetz, T. 1985. Isolation, experimental transmission, and characterization of causative agent of Potomac horse fever. *Science* **227:** 522–524.
8. Brewer, B.D., Harvey, T.W. and Mayhew, I.G. 1984. Ehrlichiosis in a Florida horse. *J. Am. vet. Med. Ass.* **185:** 446–447.
9. Rich, L.J. 1974. *The Morphology of Canine and Feline Blood Cells, Including Equine References,* p. 31. Ralston Purina Co., St. Louis.
10. Ziemer, E.L., Keenan, D.P. and Madigan, J.E. 1987. *Ehrlichia equi* infection in a New Jersey foal. *J. Am. vet. Med. Ass.* **190:** 199–200.
11. Gribble, D.H. 1986. Personal communication.
12. Hermann, M., Baumann, D., Lutz, H. and Wild, P. 1985. Erster diagnostizierter Fall von equiner Ehrlichiose in der Schweiz. *Pferdeheilkunde* **1:** 247–250.
13. Bjoersdorff, A., Johnson, A., Sjostrom, A.C. and Madigan, J.E. 1990. *Ehrlichia equi*-infektion diagnostiserat hos hast. *Svensk Veterinar Tidning* **42:** 357–360.
14. Lewis, G.E., Huxsoll, D.L., Ristic, M. and Johnson, A.J. 1975. Experimentally induced infection in dogs, cats and nonhuman primates with *Ehrlichia equi,* etiologic agent of equine ehrlichiosis. *Am. J. vet. Res.* **36:** 85–88.
15. Madewell, B.R. and Gribble, D.H. 1982. Infection in two dogs with an agent resembling *Ehrlichia equi. J. Am. vet. Med. Ass.* **180:** 512–514.
16. Nyindo, M.B.A., Ristic, M., Lewis, G.E., Huxsoll, D.L. and Stephenson, E.H. 1978. Immune response of ponies to experimental infection with *Ehrlichia equi. Am. J. vet. Res.* **39:** 15–18.
17. Gribble, D.H. 1970. Equine ehrlichiosis. Ph.D. thesis. University of California, Davis, California.

12

Equine Monocytic Ehrlichiosis (Syn., Potomac Horse Fever)

C. J. HOLLAND AND M. RISTIC

Introduction

Equine monocytic ehrlichiosis (EME; Syn., Potomac horse fever) was first recognized in 1979 as a unique clinical disease entity affecting horses in Montgomery County, Maryland.[1] A new awareness of the disease syndrome was followed by the recognition of clinical cases in Virginia, Pennsylvania and New Jersey.[1,2] Initially, the disease was characterized by fever, anorexia, depression and diarrhea.[1] The mortality rate of affected horses was reported to be 30%.[2] Early studies on EME revealed that the disease was not contagious but, rather, transmissible only through the inoculation of whole blood derived from acutely infected to susceptible horses.[2,3] Despite early intensive efforts to determine the cause of this devastating disease, the etiologic agent remained evasive. A corona-like virus[4] and several common bacteria and toxins,[5] isolated from naturally infected horses, were each suspected as the causative agent. However, these agents failed to induce the disease when inoculated into horses. Additional serologic studies with antigens of known equine pathogens also proved unsuccessful in identifying the etiologic agent of the disease.

In 1984, the search for the etiologic agent resulted in a major breakthrough when convalescent sera obtained from both naturally and experimentally infected horses were examined against major antigens of the genus *Ehrlichia* and found to react strongly with *E. sennetsu*.[2,6,7] Isolation and identification of the etiologic agent from the blood of an acutely infected horse soon followed.[6] The isolated agent was found to be a unique member of the genus *Ehrlichia* and named *Ehrlichia risticii*.[8] Confirmation of *E. risticii* as the etiologic agent of EME was subsequently documented by other investigators who independently isolated a bacterium morphologically and antigenically indistinguishable from the original isolate.[9,10]

The development of methods for the continuous *in vitro* propagation of *E. risticii*[6,7,8,9] facilitated the establishment of serologic methods for the confirmatory diagnosis of EME and for use in various seroepidemiologic studies.[11,12,13]

Currently, EME is well established throughout the United States (U.S.) as well as some regions of Canada.[11,14,15,16,17] There is also evidence that *E. risticii* and, consequently, EME, is also present in various countries abroad.[18,19]

Causal Agent

The etiologic agent of EME was originally isolated in cultured equine monocytes derived from the blood of a horse experimentally inoculated with whole blood obtained from a clinically affected horse.[6,7] Subsequently, two independent research groups isolated in cell culture an identical agent from the blood monocytes of acutely infected horses.[9,10] Various laboratory studies, and the fulfillment of Koch's postulates, confirmed the agent to be a unique new species of the genus *Ehrlichia* and named *Ehrlichia risticii* in honor of Miodrag Ristic's pioneering contributions to the study of leukocytic and erythrocytic rickettsiae.[8]

Morphology

Because of the apparently low percentage of infected circulating monocytes within the peripheral blood of affected horses, morphological characterization of *E. risticii* at the light microscopic level has been confined to cell culture-derived organisms. Similar to other ehrlichiae, *E. risticii* is an obligate intracellular parasite that appears singly, in clusters or as inclusions (morulae) within the cytoplasm of host cells (Fig. 12.1).[6–8,11,20]. The organism is gram-negative and stains bluish purple using Wright–Giemsa stain. At the electron microscopic level, organisms were shown to be contained either singly or as inclusions within cytoplasmic phagosomal vacuoles.[6–9,20–22] The organisms display a high degree of pleomorphism appearing as round, oval or elongated in shape and surrounded by a double plasma membrane and a highly rippled cell wall (Fig. 12.2).[7,20] The size of individual organisms varies considerably, with the smaller, more electron-dense cells ranging from 0.2 to 0.4 μm in diameter and larger electron-dense or electron-lucent cells ranging from 0.6 to 1.5 μm in diameter.[8,20] Individual organisms have been shown to replicate by binary fission.[8,20] In general, inclusion bodies

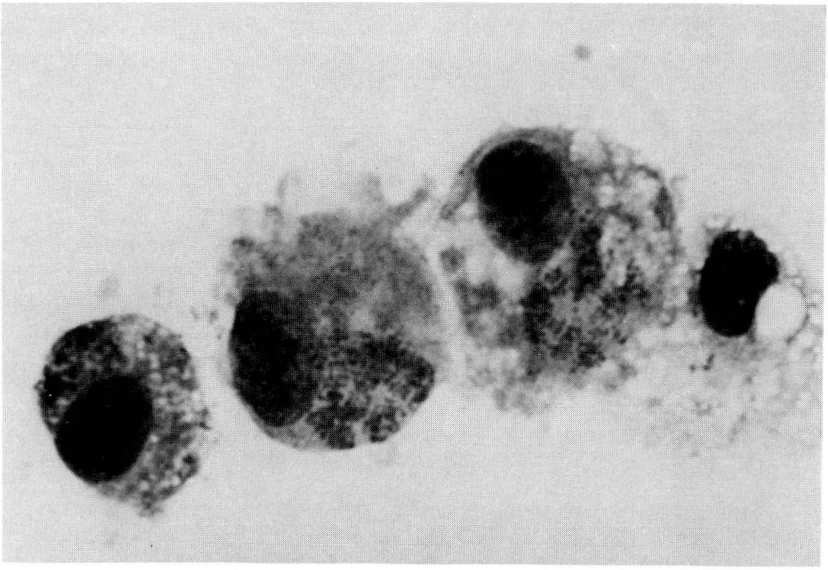

FIG. 12.1. *Ehrlichia risticii* in cultured equine monocytes derived from the blood of a horse during the acute phase of EME. The organisms may appear either singly or as small inclusions within the cytoplasm of host cells (Wright–Giemsa, × 1,500).

(morulae) are generally smaller, containing 5–20 organisms per phagosomal vacuole,[20] as compared to *E. canis*, in which inclusion bodies may contain up to 200 organisms per vacuole.[23] The more electron-lucent organisms are usually located on the periphery of the phagosome, and appear to have an affinity for attachment to the vacuolar membrane.[20] This intimate relationship may also be observed at the light microscope level, whereby organisms freed by host-cell disintegration or disruption maintain a firm attachment to cytoplasmic remnants,[11] making it more difficult to obtain organisms totally separated from host-cell components.[8,24]

Cultural Properties

Ehrlichia risticii is an obligate intracellular parasite that is readily propagated *in vitro* using cell cultures belonging to the monocyte/macrophage series.[6–9,21] The organism has been successfully propagated in primary equine and canine cell cultures[6–8] and several established cell lines including P388D1,[6–8] MDH[8] and the human histiocyte cell line U937.[9] Routine culture medium consists of Medium 199 or RPMI 1640 supplemented with 1% L-glutamine and

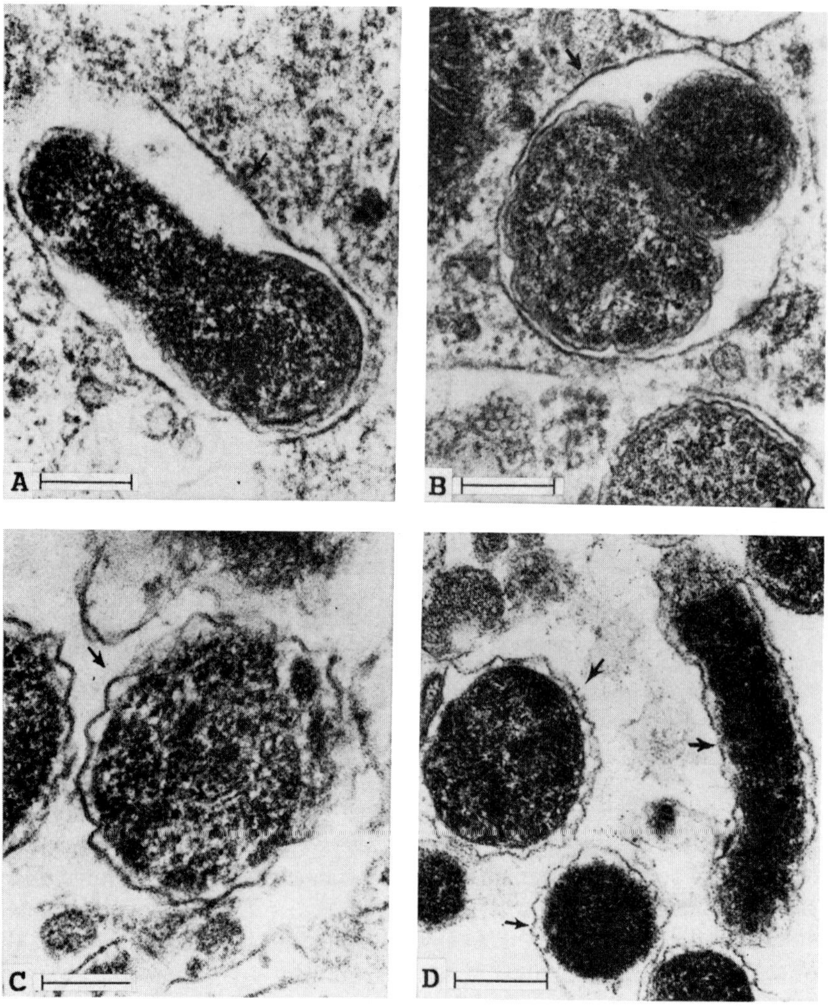

FIG. 12.2. Electron micrograph of *Ehrlichia risticii* in $P388D_1$ cell cultures. Single microorganisms and inclusions are surrounded by a distinct cytoplasmic vacuolar membrane (A and B, arrows). Note the highly rippled outer membrane (C, D) and high degree of pleomorphism (D) of the microorganism (× 34,000). Scale bar, 0.1 μm.

10% fetal bovine serum (heat-inactivated), adjusted to a pH of 7.2–7.4 using sodium bicarbonate, 5% w/v.[8] Optimal growth is achieved at 37–38°C under normal atmospheric conditions or in the presence of 5% CO_2, depending on the requirements of the host cell.[8,24]

Similar to other ehrlichiae, *E. risticii* preferentially metabolizes L-glutamine *in vitro*[24–26] and an acid pH inhibits the metabolism of exogenously supplied substrates.[26] The growth of *E. risticii* is greatly impaired by the incorporation into the medium of low concentrations of antibiotics such as penicillin, streptomycin, gentamycin, rifampin, tetracycline and oxytetracycline, with the latter proven to be the most deleterious.[27] Wells and Rikihisa showed that, by an undetermined mechanism, *E. risticii* is able to inhibit phagosome–lyosome fusion, thereby allowing for survival of the organism within the phagosome of the macrophage.[28] However, when oxytetracycline is added to the medium at a relatively low concentration (10 μg/ml), there is a rapid abrogation of inhibition of lysosomal fusion, thereby allowing for lysosomal destruction of the organism.[28] A more recent study conducted by Rikihisa and Park[29] showed that certain macrophage-activating and Ca^{2+} mobilizing agents are able to destroy *E. risticii* in mouse peritoneal macrophages propagated *in vitro*. The calcium ionophore A23187 at ≥ 0.75 μM, concanavalin A at ≥ 1 μg/ml and recombinant murine interferon gamma (rMu IFN-γ) at ≥ 25 U/ml, when incorporated at 3 h postinfection (p.i.), were able to almost totally eliminate *E. risticii* infection by 4–5 days postinfection. A23187 at 1μM and rMu IFN-γ at 100 U/ml were also able to effectively inhibit growth when incorporated at 1 day preinfection or 3 days postinfection. The method of ehrlichia-cidal activity by these two agents remains to be investigated.

Antigenic and Molecular Aspects

Serologic cross-reactivity using monospecific sera to 12 major rickettsiae by the indirect fluorescent antibody test (IFAT) revealed a lack of antigenic relatedness between *E. risticii* and members of the genus *Rickettsia*.[6–8] At the molecular level, however, the 58 to 65 kDa antigens of *E. risticii*, as well as *E. sennetsu*, were found to react with a monoclonal antibody against *Rochalimaea quintana* 60 kDa antigen, which is an evolutionally conserved heat-shock protein similar to that found in several species of the tribe *Rickettsieae*.[30]

Antigenic studies using the IFAT and serologic cross-adsorption revealed that *E. risticii* is antigenically most closely related to, but unique from, *E. sennetsu*, the causative agent of human sennetsu fever in Southeast Asia.[6,7,8] *Ehrlichia risticii* shows a lesser degree of antigenic relatedness to *E. canis* and *Neorickettsia helminthoeca*, and no antigenic cross-reactivity with *E. equi* or *E. phagocytophila*.[31]

Using Western immunoblot analysis, nine major proteins of *E. risticii* have been detected: 100, 86, 70, 55, 51, 49, 44, 33 and 28 kDa.[31,32] Of these, the 51, 33 and 28 kDa antigens seem to be the most immunogenetic in horses.[32,33] Although a number of antigens are shared between *E. risticii* and *E. sennetsu*, the 44 kDa antigen appears to have the strongest degree of cross-reactivity.[30] This antigen also appears to have the greatest degree of reactivity with sera of horses following recovery from clinical EME.[33]

Molecular cloning and analysis of 3 major recombinant antigens of *E. risticii* revealed the 70, 55 and 44 kDa peptides to be unique and measuring 3.5, 3.5 and 4.8 kb in size, respectively.[32] Mice, which were immunized with an affinity-purified 55 kDa recombinant antigen, produced a high titer of antibody that gave a monospecific reaction by Western immunoblot analysis but showed a low degree of protection from clinical infection following challenge exposure to *E. risticii*.[32] In contrast, ponies infected with virulent *E. sennetsu* showed clinical protection following challenge exposure to *E. risticii*.[33] Thus, based on this data and Western immunoblot analysis, it appears that the 44 kDa peptide is most likely a surface protein that plays a major role in protective immunity.[34]

Epidemiology

When EME was first recognized as a unique clinical disease of horses in 1979, it was believed to be limited to a narrow zone adjacent to the Potomac River in Montgomery County, Maryland.[1] However, clinical signs characteristic of EME were subsequently recognized in a number of horses throughout Maryland as well as in Virginia and Pennsylvania.[1–3] The origin of EME is not known but is now believed to have existed for years prior to its recognition as a disease entity but was misdiagnosed, e.g. salmonellosis and colitis x. While earlier reports between 1979 and 1984 were limited to the eastern seaboard, a retrospective serologic study of sera obtained from horses in the state of Washington between 1979–1981 indicates that EME was already established in the northwest region of the U.S.[35] The disease has now been confirmed in at least 41 states of the U.S., including Alaska, as well as Canada and France.[11,17,18] The disease is also suspected in several other countries and serologic evidence indicates that *E. risticii* is present in Australia.[19] It is the author's belief that *E. risticii* and, consequently, EME is established in a number of countries other than the U.S. but continues to be misdiagnosed.

Field observations have revealed that horses of all ages, breeds, purposes (e.g. pleasure, racing, show) and both sexes are at risk of contracting EME.[2,36] There appears to be no difference in the degree of susceptibility with respect to horses that are stabled or reside on pasture. Horses less than one year of age appear to be less affected by *E. risticii*.[36] Although the vector in nature remains elusive, the disease is believed to be arthropod-borne based on its seasonability and the fact that *E. risticii* can only be experimentally transmitted by blood inoculation.[2,3] The seasonal prevalence of EME in the more temperate regions of the U.S. occurs April–October.[2,11] However, the disease may be prevalent year-round in warmer regions of the country that are less temperate, e.g. Florida, Arizona, Texas and California.[15,36] Seroepidemiologic studies have determined that clinical cases represent only the "tip of the iceberg" with respect to field exposure. Studies conducted in Illinois, Ohio, Maryland, Arizona, California and South Dakota indicate that 17–25% of healthy horses examined have been exposed to *E. risticii*.[14,15,36,37]

A number of studies have been conducted to determine the natural biological and/or mechanical vector of *E. risticii*. Although the distribution of EME closely correlates with that of the American dog tick, *Dermacentor variabilis*, all attempts to infect and transmit the disease by this arthropod have failed.[11,38] Studies involving the transmission of *E. risticii* by other arthropod vectors, e.g. black flies (*Simulium* spp.), fleas, flies (*Tabinus* spp., *Hybomitra* spp., *Stomoxys* spp., *Haematobia* spp.) and mosquitos (*Aedes* spp., *Anopholus* spp., *Culex* spp. and *Psorophora* spp.) have all, thus far, proven negative.[39–41] It is hoped that work will continue in order to determine the arthropod vector(s) involved in the natural transmission of *E. risticii*.

A number of other studies aimed at determining the susceptibility of additional animal species have been conducted. Mice, dogs, cats and Rhesus monkeys (*Macacca mullata*) have been shown to be experimentally susceptible to infection by *E. risticii*, with mice showing the most severe clinical signs.[6,42–44] Serological evidence indicates that cats, dogs, foxes and wild rabbits are susceptible to natural field exposure.[11] More recent evidence indicates that dogs may be susceptible to clinical disease following natural exposure to *E. risticii*.[45] Clinical signs are variable but may include fever, depression, anorexia, vomiting, diarrhea and leukopenia. Antibody titers are greater to *E. risticii* than to *E. canis* and the dogs respond readily to tetracycline therapy.

Pathogenesis

It is believed that horses become exposed to *E. risticii* following the bite of an infected arthropod vector. The organism is then taken up by cells of the monocyte/macrophage series. Based on experimental studies, ehrlichemia is most prominent during the prepatent and early patent phase of infection. Although clinical signs of disease do not become apparent until day 12–18 p.i., the organism is most readily cultured from peripheral blood monocytes between days 7–14 p.i., with the infective titer of organisms decreasing through day 20 p.i. Unlike other members of the genus *Ehrlichia*, which appear to have a tissue tropism for the microvasculature and major organs (e.g. lung, meninges and spleen),[46] *E. risticii* tends to migrate towards reticuloendothelial cells situated within the wall of the colon, in particular the large colon, of affected horses,[26,31] which is apparently the cause of diarrhea in 40–45% of horses affected by EME.[31,46] Aside from the blood and various lymphoid tissues, *E. risticii* has been detected in macrophages, crypt endothelial cells and mast cells in the wall of the large colon, small colon, cecum and small intestine and has been isolated in cell culture from mesenteric and colonic lymph nodes.[26,31,47] While little or no gross pathologic alterations are observable upon necropsy of affected animals,[2,3,31] it appears that the associated diarrhea may either be the result of endotoxemia caused by microscopic perforations in the intestinal wall or as a result of an electrolyte imbalance created during localized infection of cells within the gastrointestinal tract. According to a study conducted by Rikihisa *et al.*,[22,31] microscopic examination of sections of the large colon of infected horses revealed focal degeneration and/or dedifferentiation and hyperplasia of glandular epithelial cells, depletion of goblet and Paneth cells and monocytic infiltration. This resulted in a net lack of Na^+ and Cl^- movement within the colon.

Since the recognition of the disease, veterinarians have noticed an increasing incidence of abortions in mares following recovery from clinical EME.[47] Necropsy results of aborted fetuses, along with routine uterine cultures and biopsies and various blood assays from affected mares in order to determine the etiology, have been inconclusive. One case concerned a thoroughbred broodmare in Kentucky.[48] This mare developed EME at 2 months of gestation and aborted a nearly full-term fetus at $10\frac{3}{4}$ months of gestation. Gross pathologic examination of the fetus revealed partially aerated lungs, tracheal froth, and hemorrhage in the shoulder joint. The amnion showed infarcts and calcified plaques. No significant histopathologic changes or adventitious bacteria were observed or cultured by standard bacteriological techniques. A serum sample collected from the fetus was negative for equine rhinopneumonitis virus and various leptospira species, but positive against *E. risticii* at a titer of 1:320. At the time of abortion, the dam was serologically positive at a titer of 1:2560 against *E. risticii*. Thus, transplacental infections of the fetus may occur when mares are exposed to *E. risticii* during gestation. This is supported by the finding of precolostral *E. risticii*-specific antibodies that have been detected in some foals born to mares with a history of naturally acquired EME at some point during gestation.[48] Experimental studies have provided stronger evidence to support transplacental infection by *E. risticii*. In a limited study, *E. risticii* was isolated from the bone marrow, spleen, mesenteric and colonic lymph nodes of a 7 month old fetus whose dam was experimentally infected at 3 months gestation.[47,48] The organism was not isolated from the corresponding tissues of the dam. In a larger more recent study designed to further examine fetal infectivity by *E. risticii* in pregnant mares, six mares were infected intravenously with virulent cell culture-derived *E. risticii* at 120 days of gestation.[36,49] Two mares served as noninfected controls. All six infected mares developed clinical signs of EME. The organism was isolated in cell cultures from the blood of each infected mare and all responded serologically by the IFAT. Although all infected mares recovered from the disease, four of the six mares aborted between days 75 and 100 postinfection. Each aborted fetus was subjected to necropsy. Tissue samples from the bone marrow, liver, spleen and mesenteric lymph nodes were processed and inoculated into primary canine monocyte cell cultures. *Ehrlichia risticii* was isolated *in vitro* from three of the four aborted fetuses. All four aborted fetuses demonstrated similar pathological findings, including lymphoid hyperplasia of the mesenteric lymph nodes and spleen, enterocolitis and periportal hepatitis.[36] The remaining two infected mares delivered normal, healthy foals, with one foal seropositive for *E. risticii* using precolostral serum while the remaining foal was seronegative. The two control mares remained healthy and seronegative throughout the study. This study has overwhelmingly confirmed that *E. risticii* is able to cross the equine placenta and infect the fetus *in utero* and provides further supportive evidence that *E. risticii* may induce abortions in affected mares.

Clinical Disease

The disease, in its most recognizable form, is generally characterized by an acute onset of depression, anorexia and fever (38.9–41.7°C).[2,10,36,50] The fever is usually biphasic, whereby an initial increase in rectal temperature of limited duration (12–18 h) may occur several days prior to the onset of depression and anorexia. Based on experimental studies, clinical manifestations are generally evident by day 12–18 postinoculation (p.i).[2,10] The clinical course of disease then progresses to include any or all of the following: subcutaneous edema of the lower limbs and ventral abdomen, colic, mild to profuse diarrhea and laminitis.[2,10,36,50]

Colic of variable severity, ranging from mild abdominal discomfort to a severe intense pain resembling "surgical" colic, may precede the onset of diarrhea in approximately 25% of the cases.[2]

Prior to the diarrheic phase, which develops in approximately 50–60% of recognized cases, moderate abdominal distention may be noticed. Mucous membranes become muddy and a prominent "toxic ring", represented by a blue ring surrounding the teeth, may be present.[36,51] Horses may also exhibit a mild to moderate tachypnea and tachycardia. Auscultation of the intestinal tract generally reveals a significant decrease in borborygmus. Occasionally, loud gaseous sounds may also be noted. Auscultation and percussion of the abdomen often reveals hyperresonance, or a "cecal ping", in the right paralumbar fossa.[51]

The diarrhea, which develops in some affected horses, usually begins between 3 and 6 days following the initial febrile phase and may vary from a soft "cowpie" to a profuse, brown, watery "pipestream" in character, with a duration of 24 h to 10 days.[2,36,51] The severity of shock in some affected horses with diarrhea has been shown to be directly proportional to the rapidity and extent of fluid loss in the liquid stool.

Mild to severe laminitis may develop following the onset of diarrhea.[36,51] As a result, there is rotation of the third phalynx, with sloughing of all four hooves occurring in some cases. Horses that develop laminitis are often euthanized for humane reasons. Experimental studies indicate that ponies are less susceptible to EME-induced laminitis than are horses.[36,52]

Clinical EME has been shown to vary greatly, ranging from transient mild fever and depression to severe diarrhea followed by hypovolemic shock and death, regardless of treatment.[36,51] The disease course has been observed to be as short as 2 or 3 days and as long as 2–3 weeks.

Based on serologic studies, it is apparent that the majority of exposed horses do not experience clinical disease. Prior to recognition of *E. risticii* as the etiologic agent and, consequently, the implementation of a more effective therapeutic regimen, the mortality rate in affected horses was about 30%.[2] Over the past several years, there has been a significant reduction in mortality, now estimated to be about 7%, which is attributed to an earlier recognition and diagnosis of EME, leading to a more rapid initiation of the appropriate treatment.[36]

Pathology

Necropsy examination of horses that succumb to EME reveals very few, if any, gross pathologic changes. The only observed lesions, which are by no means pathognomonic for the disease, include small ulcerative lesions within the small and large colon[2,3] and patchy hyperemia along the wall of the large intestine.[31] Unlike that observed with acute salmonellosis, there is a lack of foul odor, gross bowel destruction and evidence of significant infiltration by inflammatory cells.[2,3,31] Histopathologic examination of the colon reveals marked depletion of goblet cell mucous, reduced height and increased basophilia of mucosal epithelial cells, dilation of intestinal glands, and entrapment of cell debris in gland lumens.[31] Mesenteric lymph nodes were shown to contain prominent sheets of histiocytes, macrophages and some giant cells, and were severely depleted of lymphoid cells.[22,31] Using electron microscopy, *E. risticii*-infected macrophages, mast cells and crypt endothelial cells within the lamina propria and submucosa of the colon, small colon, cecum and small intestine have been observed.

There are very limited hematologic changes that may occur during clinical EME. Leukopenia may develop early in the course of infection, followed by leukocytosis during the late phase of illness.[2,36,53] A mild thrombocytopenia, which occurs in some cases, usually becomes more marked in horses that succumb to the infection.[53] The only changes that may occur in hematocrit and erythrocyte counts occur in horses that experience severe diarrhea, leading to a significant level of hemoconcentration. These horses usually require massive amounts of fluid therapy to prevent shock and death. Generally, there is a variable increase in plasma fibrinogen levels in horses affected with EME.[51,53] Horses that experience severe clinical disease show a significant increase in plasma fibrinogen levels, plasma factor VIII: coagulant values, activated partial thromboplastin times and a lower concentration of factor V, just prior to death.[53]

Immunity

Horses that become infected with *E. risticii* generally develop detectable antibody responses of the IgG class, as measured by the IFA and enzyme-linked immunosorbent assay (ELISA) test methods, by the time clinical signs become evident.[11–13] Occasionally, a horse may be seronegative at this point, but a serum sample collected 2–3 days later will show a significant seroconversion to a positive status.[11,13] Experimentally, the IgG class of antibody is first detectable at 11–14 days p.i.[11] This is preceded by an IgM antibody response that may be detectable by the ELISA method as early as 5 days p.i. and peaking at 12–18 days p.i.[12,13] Thereafter, IgM titers usually decline over an approximate 2 month period, at which time IgM antibody is no longer detectable. In contrast, IgG antibody titers usually reach peak levels during the early convalescent phase of disease and continue to persist, albeit at lower levels, for more than a year following infection.[11,12,13]

Immunity to *E. risticii* appears to depend primarily on both the cell-mediated immune response (CMI) and humoral immunity.[46,50] In various studies on protective immunity to *E. risticii*, it was shown that recovery from infection results in resistance to clinical disease after homologous challenge.[46,50,54,55] Furthermore, similar to the immunity induced by infection with *E. equi*,[56] protective immunity to *E. risticii* appears to be of the sterile type since all attempts to recover the microorganism from the blood and solid tissues (e.g. spleen, liver, bone marrow and colonic/mesenteric lymph nodes) following recovery have failed.[47,50,54,55] A recently conducted study revealed that mice, which received purified anti-*E. risticii* IgG by passive transfer, were protected from clinical disease upon challenge with virulent *E. risticii* at Day −3 or Day 0 of antibody inoculation.[57] Studies have yet to be conducted to determine whether a similar degree of protection may be induced in horses using this method.

Diagnosis

Based on the fact that clinical signs of EME may vary greatly in affected horses and that many of the associated manifestations are not clearly distinguishable from a number of other febrile and diarrheal diseases of horses, diagnosis made solely on clinical presentation is difficult.[2,11,36] Some of the differential diagnoses taken into consideration include acute salmonellosis, colitis x, colic or upper respiratory tract infection.[36] Examination of peripheral blood smears is of no value as *E. risticii*-infected monocytes are present in such small concentrations in the blood and are very difficult to detect. Isolation in cell cultures of *E. risticii* derived from the blood of horses during the acute phase of infection is the best method for confirming clinical diagnosis of EME.[11,36] However, this method is costly, laborious, time-consuming (requiring 7–14 days) and requires specialized equipment and highly trained personnel. Thus, at present, the best method for confirmatory diagnosis of EME is based on serology.[11–13] Two tests that have been developed for this purpose are the IFAT[11] and the ELISA,[12,13] although the IFAT is used most often for this purpose. A monoclonal antibody-mediated competitive enzyme-linked immunosorbent assay (CELISA) for serodiagnosis of EME has also been developed.[58] This test appears to have a greater degree of sensitivity than that of the IFAT or ELISA. Paired serum samples, collected at a minimum of 3 days apart, are optimal for providing a confirmatory serodiagnosis of EME since a single positive sample may only be indicative of previous exposure. Since

IgG antibody titers generally peak rapidly, it is important to obtain the first sample as early in the course of disease as possible, since the ideal 4-fold change in titer may not be reflected with samples collected late in the disease and during convalescence.[11,36] Nevertheless, a single serum sample having a titer of 1:640 or greater, in conjunction with compatible clinical signs, strongly suggests a diagnosis of EME. Since its development in 1984, the IFAT has proven highly valuable for the confirmatory serodiagnosis of EME[6,11] as well as for use in various seroepidemiologic studies.[14–16,37]

A number of laboratories have been trying to develop suitable test methods for the detection of *E. risticii* in the blood of acutely infected horses. Detection by way of immunoperoxidase staining is one such method being explored.[59] Thacker *et al.*[60] have been successful in developing a DNA gene probe that may be used to detect as little as 0.5 pg of *E. risticii* within the peripheral blood monocytes of experimentally infected horses beginning at day 7 p.i. and peaking during the height of clinical illness at days 14–17 p.i. This test should prove to be of great value if successful in detecting *E. risticii* antigen in the blood of naturally infected horses.

Treatment and Control

The recommended treatment for EME consists of supportive treatment as well as specific antimicrobial chemotherapy.[36,51,61] Following recognition of the etiologic agent as an ehrlichia, various studies determined that oxytetracycline, administered intravenously at a dosage of 6.6 mg/kg s.i.d. for 7–10 days, is highly effective in the treatment of EME.[51,61] In case salmonellosis is also suspected, other antibiotics such as Gentocin (Schering–Plough Animal Health; Kenilworth, New Jersey), amikacin, chloramphenicol and potentiated sulfas may also be administered, particularly if septicemia may be evident.[36] Supportive therapy may consist of fluids, electrolytes and antidiarrheics, such as Pepto-Bismol. Suspected endotoxemia may be treated with Banamine or Endoserum (IMMVAC Inc.; Columbia, Missouri).[36,51,61] DMSO, given intravenously, may aid in the prevention of laminitis.[36] Other prophylactic treatments for laminitis may consist of frog support, heparin and acepromazine.

A killed adjuvant-fortified vaccine (PHF-VAX; Schering–Plough Animal Health; Kenilworth, New Jersey) was commercially developed and received USDA approval in 1988. Experimental studies have determined the vaccine to be 80% effective in completely preventing clinical disease following experimental intravenous challenge of vaccinated horses.[54] With over 1.5 million horses thus far vaccinated, PHF-VAX has shown a high degree of safety and efficacy under field conditions.[36] The vaccine is initially administered, prior to the onset of the EME season, in 2 doses given 3 weeks apart. Horses are then given an annual booster dose to provide for continued protection. In regions where the climate is less seasonal, in which the potential vector may be active year-round, booster doses given at 4 to 6 month intervals have been recommended.[36,54] A second vaccine against EME, Potomovac™ (Pitman–Moore; Mundelein, Illinois), has more recently become available. However, there is no experimental or field data available with respect to its efficacy.

Although the vector is not yet known, all researchers agree that some biting arthropod(s) is involved.[11,14,38–41] Thus, routines should be established to eliminate or decrease various factors that attract biting arthropods, such as stagnant water, certain types of lights, manure piles, etc. In addition, horses should be checked for ectoparasites and sprayed on a regular basis with repellents during the insect season. Since dogs and cats residing near horses might also serve as a host for the vector, they should also be monitored and dipped with acarasides on a routine basis.

References

1. Knowles, R.C., Anderson, D.W., Shipley, W.D., Whitlock, R.H., Perry, B.D. and Davidson, J.P. 1983. Acute equine diarrhea syndrome (AEDS): A preliminary report. *Proc. Am. Ass. Equine Pract.* **29:** 353–357.
2. Whitlock, R.H., Palmer, J.E., Benson, C.E., Acland, H.M., Jenny, A.L. and Ristic, M. 1984. Potomac horse fever: Clinical characteristics and diagnostic features. *Am. Ass. vet. Lab. Diag. 27th Annu. Proc.* 103–124.
3. Jenny, A.L. 1984. Potomac horse fever—National Veterinary Services Laboratories (USDA) report. *Am. Ass. Equine Practnr. Newslett.* **2:** 64–66.
4. Huang, J.C.M., Wright, S.L. and Shipley, W.D. 1983, Isolation of a corona virus-like agent from horses suffering from acute equine diarrhea. *Vet. Rec.* **113:** 262–263.
5. Ehrich, M., Perry, B.D., Troutt, H.F., Dellers, R.W. and Magnusson, R.A. 1984. Acute diarrhea in horses of the Potomac River area: Examination for clostridial toxins. *J. Am. vet. Med. Ass.* **185:** 433–435.
6. Holland, C.J. 1986. The etiology of Potomac horse fever. Ph.D. Thesis. University of Illinois; Urbana, Illinois.
7. Holland, C.J., Ristic, M., Cole, A.I., Johnson, P., Baker, G. and Goetz, T. 1985. Isolation, experimental transmission, and characterization of causative agent of Potomac horse fever. *Science* **227:** 522–524.
8. Holland, C.J., Weiss, E., Burgdorfer, W., Cole, A.I. and Kakoma, I. 1985b. *Ehrlichia risticii* sp. nov.: Etiologic agent of equine monocytic ehrlichiosis (syn., Potomac horse fever). *Int. J. Syst. Bact.* **35:** 524–526.
9. Rikihisa, Y. and Perry, B.D. 1985. Causative ehrlichial organisms in Potomac horse fever. *Infect. Immun.* **49:** 513–517.
10. Dutta, S.K., Myrup, A.C., Rice, R.M., Robl, M.G. and Hammond, R.C. 1985. Experimental reproduction of Potomac horse fever in horses with a newly isolated *Ehrlichia* organism. *J. clin. Microbiol.* **22:** 265–269.

11. RISTIC, M., HOLLAND, C.J., DAWSON, J.E., SESSIONS, J. and PALMER, J.E. 1986. Diagnosis of equine monocytic ehrlichiosis (syn., Potomac horse fever) by indirect immunofluorescence. *J. Am. vet. Med. Ass.* **189:** 39–46.
12. PRETZMAN, C.I., RIKIHISA, Y., RALPH, D., GORDON, J.C. and BECH-NIELSEN, S. 1987. Enzyme-linked immunosorbent assay for Potomac horse fever disease. *J. clin. Microbiol.* **25:** 31–36.
13. DUTTA, S.K., RICE, R.M., HUGHES, T.D., SAVAGE, P.K. and MYRUP, A.C. 1987. Detection of serum antibodies against *Ehrlichia risticii* in Potomac horse fever by enzyme-linked immunosorbent assay. *Vet. Immun. Immunopath.* **14:** 85–92.
14. RIKIHISA, Y., REED, S.M., SAMS, R.A., GORDON, J.C. and PRETZMAN, C.I. 1990. Serosurvey of horses with evidence of equine monocytic ehrlichiosis (Potomac horse fever). *J. Am. vet. Med. Ass.* **197:** 1327–1332.
15. MADIGAN, J.E., DEROCK, E. and LAVAN, R.P. 1989. Clinical significance of a recent serologic survey of the incidence of Potomac horse fever in California. *Proc. Ann. Con. AAEP* **34:** 571–576.
16. OLCHOWY, T.W.J., AMES, T.R. and MOLITOR, T.W. 1990. Serodiagnosis of equine monocytic ehrlichiosis in selected groups of horses in Minnesota. *J. Am. vet. Med. Ass.* **196:** 1967–1970.
17. JONES, W.W. 1990. Ventral edema in horses testing positive for Potomac horse fever. *Can. vet. J.* **31:** 531.
18. VIDOR, E., BISSUEL, G., MOREAU, Y., MADEC, J.L. and CADORE, J.L. 1988. Positive serologic reaction for *Ehrlichia risticii* in a mare showing clinical signs of equine ehrlichiosis. *Prat. vet. Equine* **20:** 5–10.
19. BOND, M. 1990. Potomac horse fever detected in WA titers. *Aust. Vet. J.* **67:** N261.
20. RIKIHISA, Y. 1990. Ultrastructural of rickettsiae with special emphasis on ehrlichia. In: *Ehrlichiosis: A Vector-Borne Disease of Animals and Humans,* pp. 22–31. WILLIAMS, J.C. and KAKOMA, I. (Eds). Kluwer Academic Publishers, Boston.
21. RIKIHISA, Y. 1990. Growth of *Ehrlichia risticii* in human colonic epithelial cells. In: *Rickettsiology: Current Issues and Perspectives,* pp. 104–110. HECHEMY, K., PARETSKY, D., WALKER, D.H. and MALLAVIA, L.P. (Eds). New York Academy of Science, New York.
22. RIKIHISA, Y., PERRY, B.D. and CORDES, D.O. 1985. Ultrastructural study of rickettsial organisms in the large colon of ponies experimentally infected with Potomac horse fever. *Infect. Immun.* **49:** 505–512.
23. NYINDO, M.B.A., RISTIC, M., HUXSOLL, D.L. and SMITH, A.R. 1971. Tropical canine pancytopenia: *In vitro* cultivation of the causative agent—*Ehrlichia canis. Am. J. vet. Res.* **32:** 1651–1658.
24. WEISS, E., DASCH, G.A., KANG, Y.-H. and WESTFALL, H.N. 1988. Substrate utilization by *Ehrlichia sennetsu* and *Ehrlichia risticii* separated from host constituents by renografin gradient centrifugation. *J. Bact.* **170:** 5012–5017.
25. WEIS, E., WILLIAMS, J.C., DASCH, G.A. and KANG, Y.-H. 1989. Energy metabolism of monocytic *Ehrlichia. Proc. natn. Acad. Sci. U.S.A.* **86:** 1674–1678.
26. WEISS, E., DASCH, G.A., WILLIAMS, J.C. and KANG, Y.-H. 1990. Biological properties of the genus *Ehrlichia*: Substrate utilization and energy metabolism. In: *Ehrlichiosis: A Vector-Borne Disease of Animals and Humans,* pp. 59–67. WILLIAMS, J.C. and KAKOMA, I. (Eds). Kluwer Academic Publishers, Boston.
27. RIKIHISA, Y. and JIANG, B.M. 1988. *In vitro* susceptibility of *Ehrlichia risticii* to eight antibiotics. *Antimicrob. Agents Chemother.* **32:** 986–991.
28. WELLS, M.Y. and RIKIHISA, Y. 1988. Lack of lysosomal fusion with phagosomes

containing *Ehrlichia risticii* in P388D1 cells: Abrogation of inhibition with oxytetracycline. *Infect. Immun.* **56:** 3209–3215.

29. RIKIHISA, Y. and PARK, M. 1991. Ehrlichiacidal mechanism by macrophage Ca^{2+} mobilization. In: *Rickettsiae and Rickettsial Diseases,* pp. 758–761. KAZAR, J. and RAOULT, D. (Eds). Proceedings of the IVth International Symposium. Slovak Academy of Sciences, Bratislava.
30. DASCH, G.A., WEISS, E. and WILLIAMS, J.C. 1990. Antigenic properties of the ehrlichiae and other rickettsiaceae. In:. *Ehrlichiosis: A Vector-Borne Disease of Animals and Humans,* pp. 32–58. WILLIAMS, J.C. and KAKOMA, I. (Eds). Kluwer Academic Publishers, Boston.
31. RIKIHISA, Y. 1991. The tribe Ehrlichieae and ehrlichial diseases. *Clin. Microbiol. Rev.* **4:** 286–308.
32. DUTTA, S.K., SHANKARAPPA, B. and MATTINGLY-NAPIER, B.L. 1991. Molecular cloning and analysis of recombinant major antigens of *Ehrlichia risticii. Infect. Immun.* **59:** 1162–1169.
33. RIKIHISA, Y., PRETZMAN, C.I., JOHNSON, C., REED, S.M., YAMAMOTO, S. and ANDREWS, F. 1988. Clinical and immunological responses of ponies to *Ehrlichia sennetsu* and subsequent *Ehrlichia risticii* challenge. *Infect. Immun.* **56:** 2960–2966.
34. SHANKARAPPA, B., DUTTA, S.K. and MATTINGLY-NAPIER, B.L. 1992. Identification of the protective 44-kilodalton recombinant antigen of *Ehrlichia risticii. Infect. Immun.* **60:** 612–617.
35. MYHRE, B., DILBECK, P., EVERMANN, J., BAYLY, W. and HOLLAND, C. 1987. Occurrence of horses positive for *Ehrlichia risticii* antibody in Washington State. Abst. Fifth Int. Conf. Equine Infect. Dis., Lexington, Kentucky, October 7–10, 1987.
36. GOETZ, T.E., HEANEY, K., HOLLAND, C.J., PETERSON, D., REED, S.M., STUBER, R.M. and WYCHARA, S. 1992. Potomac horse fever—proceedings of a round table, October 22, 1991. pp. 1–31. Schering–Plough Animal Health, Kenilworth, New Jersey.
37. GOETZ, T.E., HOLLAND, C.J., DAWSON, J.E., RISTIC, M., SKIBBE, K., KEEGAN, K., JOHNSON, P., SCHAEFFER, D. and BAKER, G. 1989. Monthly prevalence (in 1986) of antibody titers against equine monocytic ehrlichiosis in apparently healthy horses in Illinois. *Am. J. vet. Res.* **50:** 1936–1939.
38. SCHMIDTMANN, E.T., ROBL, M.G. and CARROLL, J.F. 1986. Attempted transmission of *Ehrlichia risticii* by field-captured *Dermacentor variabilis* (Acari: Ixodidae). *Am. J. vet. Res.* **47:** 2393–2395.
39. SCHMIDTMANN, E.T., RICE, R.M., ROBLE, M.G. and AZAD, A.F. 1988. Search for an arthropod vector of *Ehrlichia risticii.* In: *Proceedings from a Symposium on Potomac Horse Fever,* May 29, 1987, pp. 9–16, Louisville, Kentucky. Veterinary Learning Systems, Lawrenceville, New Jersey.
40. BURG, J.G., POWELL, D.G., KNAPP, F.W. and MCCOMB, W.C. 1988. Potential vectors of Potomac horse fever and future entomological research. In: *Proceedings from a Symposium on Potomac Horse Fever,* May 29, 1987, pp. 17–20, Louisville, Kentucky. Veterinary Learning Systems, Lawrenceville, New Jersey.
41. GORDON, J.C., BECH-NIELSON, S., FARRAR, W., FOSTER, W., PARSONS, M. and KOHN, K. 1988. Epidemiologic investigation of affected farms. In: *Proceedings from a Symposium on Potomac Horse Fever,* May 29, 1987, pp. 21–26, Louisville, Kentucky. Veterinary Learning Systems, Lawrenceville, New Jersey.
42. JENKINS, S.J., JONES, N.K. and JENNY, A.L. 1985. Potomac horse fever agent in mice. *Vet. Rec.* **117:** 556–557.

43. Ristic, M., Dawson, J.E., Holland, C.J. and Jenny, A.L. 1988. Susceptibility of dogs to infection with *Ehrlichia risticii*, causative agent of Potomac horse fever. *Am. J. vet. Res.* **49:** 1497–1500.
44. Dawson, J.E., Abeygunawardena, I., Holland, C.J., Buese, M. and Ristic, M. 1988. Susceptibility of cats to infection with *Ehrlichia risticii*, causative agent of equine monocytic ehrlichiosis. *Am. J. vet. Res.* **49:** 2096–2100.
45. Holland, C.J. 1992. Unpublished data.
46. Ristic, M. 1990. Current strategies in research on ehrlichiosis. In: *Ehrlichiosis: A Vector-Borne Disease of Animals and Humans,* pp. 136–153. Williams, J.C. and Kakoma, I. (Eds). Kluwer Academic Publishers, Boston.
47. Dawson, J.E., Ristic, M., Holland, C.J., Whitlock, R.H. and Sessions, J. 1987. Isolation of *Ehrlichia risticii*, the causative agent of Potomac horse fever from the fetus of an experimentally infected mare. *Vet. Rec.* **121:** 232.
48. Dawson, J.E., Ristic, M., Holland, C.J., Whitlock, R.H. and Sessions, J.E. 1988. Isolation of *Ehrlichia risticii* from the fetus of a mare with Potomac horse fever. In: *Proceedings of the Fifth International Conference on Equine Infectious Diseases,* Lexington, Kentucky, October 7–10, 1987, pp. 214–216. University of Kentucky Press.
49. Long, M.T., Goetz, T.E., Kakoma, I., Whiteley, H.E., Lock, T.S., Holland, C.J., Ewert, K.M., Baker, G.J. and Foreman, J.H. 1991. Preliminary investigation of the fetal infectivity of *Ehrlichia risticii* in brood mares. *Abstr. Conf. of Res. Workers in Anim. Dis.* **72:** 5.
50. Holland, C.J. 1990. Biologic and pathogenic properties of *Ehrlichia risticii*: The etiologic agent of equine monocytic ehrlichiosis. In: *Ehrlichiosis: A Vector-Borne Disease of Animals and Humans,* pp. 68–77. Williams, J.C. and Kakoma, I. (Eds). Kluwer Academic Publishers, Boston.
51. Palmer, J.E., Whitlock, R.H. and Benson, C.E. 1988. Clinical signs and treatment of equine ehrlichial colitis. In: *Proceedings from a Symposium on Potomac Horse Fever*; May 29, 1987, pp. 49–54, Louisville, Kentucky. Veterinary Learning Systems, Lawrenceville, New Jersey.
52. Goetz, T.E. and Holland, C.J. 1988. Unpublished Data.
53. Morris, D.D., Messick, J., Whitlock, R.H., Palmer, J., Ward, M.V. and Feldman, B.F. 1988. Effect of equine ehrlichial colitis on the hemostatic system in ponies. *Am. J. vet. Res.* **49:** 1030–1036.
54. Ristic, M., Holland, C.J. and Goetz, T.E. 1988. Evaluation of a vaccine for equine monocytic ehrlichiosis (Potomac horse fever). In: *Proceedings of the Fifth International Conference on Equine Infectious Diseases,* Lexington, Kentucky, October 7–10, 1987, pp. 206–213. University of Kentucky Press.
55. Palmer, J.E., Benson, C.E. and Whitlock, R.H. 1990. Resistance to development of equine ehrlichial colitis in experimentally inoculated horses and ponies. *Am. J. vet. Res.* **51:** 763–765.
56. Nyindo, M.B.A., Ristic, M., Lewis, G.E., Jr, Huxsoll, D.L. and Stephenson, E.H. 1978. Immune responses of ponies to experimental infection with *Ehrlichia equi. Am. J. vet. Med. Res.* **39:** 15–18.
57. Kaylor, P.S., Crawford, T.B., McElwain, T.F. and Palmer, G.H. 1991. Passive transfer of antibody to *Ehrlichia risticii* protects mice from ehrlichiosis. *Infect. Immun.* **59:** 2058–2062.
58. Shankarappa, B., Dutta, S.K., Sanusi, J. and Mattingly, B.L. 1989. Monoclonal antibody-mediated, immunodiagnostic competitive enzyme-linked immunosorbent assay for equine monocytic ehrlichiosis. *J. clin. Microbiol.* **27:** 24–28.
59. Gaunt, S. 1991. Personal communication.

60. Thacker, S.R., Dutta, S.K., Adhya, S.L. and Mattingly-Napier, B.L. 1990. Molecular cloning of *Ehrlichia risticii* and development of gene probe for the diagnosis of Potomac horse fever. *J. clin. Microbiol.* **28:** 1963–1967.
61. Palmer, J.E., Benson, C.E. and Whitlock, R.H. 1986. Treatment and control of equine monocytic ehrlichiosis (syn., Potomac horse fever). In: *Microbiology—1986*, pp. 203–204. Leive, L. (Ed.). Am. Soc. Micro., Washington, D.C.

13

Tick-Borne (Pasture) Fever

Z. WOLDEHIWET AND G. R. SCOTT

Introduction

Tick-borne fever (TBF) is a febrile disease of domestic and wild ruminants in the temperate regions of Europe. By itself, TBF is regarded as benign but because of its immunosuppressive effects it predisposes to other conditions such as tick pyemia, abortions and respiratory infections. The disease was fortuitously discovered in 1932.[1] In an experiment initally designed to investigate the transmission of louping ill by ticks, it was shown that the tick, *Ixodes ricinus* was apparently harboring an agent different from that which caused louping ill.[1] After reproducing the disease in sheep by subinoculating blood from infected sheep and establishing that the agent was distinct from that which caused louping ill, Gordon and his coworkers[2] gave the disease a provisional name "tick-borne fever". Further studies at the Moredun Institute, Edinburgh, established that the causative agent was found in the cytoplasm of the granular leucocytes and monocytes of infected sheep.[3]

Pasture fever is a seasonal syndrome limited to lactating heifers and cows. It was first described in 1950 by Hudson.[4] He had spent most of his career in East Africa and when he returned to the U.K. to head a research unit he instituted procedures that were routine in Africa where haemoparasites were a major disease problem. Within weeks Hudson had discovered parasitized neutrophils and had identified them as *Cytocetes (Ehrlichia) phagocytophila*. Tuomi's seminal studies in the 1960s showed that a well-known disease of cattle called "pasture fever" in Finland was also bovine tick-borne fever.[5] He characterized the disease as an annual minor epidemic syndrome that occurred when dairy heifers and cows were turned out of their indoor winter quarters in the spring and early summer onto pastures full of newly questing ixodid ticks. Within days milk yield plummeted, appetites were cut, coughing occurred, depression set and ears drooped. Clinical signs were more obvious and lasted longer in newly purchased animals than home-bred animals first infected as calves. The pasture fever syndrome has since been recognized elsewhere in Europe where in-wintered cattle spent summers on tick-infested pastures, e.g. in Austria,[6] Spain[7] and Switzerland.[8]

Causal Agent

Classification

When the causative agent of TBF was first recognized[2] it was thought that it belonged to the Rickettsia in general and in 1951[9] the organism was classified as *Rickettsia phagocytophila*. However, because of its striking morphology and preference to infect polymorphnuclear cells it was later proposed that it be included in the genus *Cytoecetes* in the tribe *Erhlichieae* as *C. phagocytophila* to distinguish it from the members of the genus *Erhlichia* of the same tribe; the latter being reserved for those animal rickettsiae which infected mononuclear cells.[10] This was in recognition of the morphological similarities of the causative agent of TBF with *C. microti* which infects the granulocytes of voles.[11] After subsequent electron-microscopic studies, Finnish workers[12] proposed that the organism should be given an intermediate place between the Rickettsia and the Chlamydiae. They argued that although the organism is similar to the rickettsiae on the basis of its transmission by an arthropod and its morphology, its location within cytoplasmic vacuoles and its susceptibility to sulfonamides make it similar to the chlamydiae. In the latest edition of *Bergey's Manual of Systematic Bacteriology*, it has been included in the genus *Erhlichia* as *E. phagocytophila*.[13] However, the two generic names *Erhlichia* and *Cytoecetes* have been used by several workers either alone or with the other one in parenthesis. Recent phylogenetic studies have shown that at least one member of the tribe *Erhlichieae, Ehrlichia risticii* is closely related to *Rickettsia prowazekii*.[14] Recently, Anderdson *et al.*[15] compared the 16S rRNA gene sequences of two strains of *E. phagocytophila* with those of *E. canis, E. risticii, E. sennetsu* and the newly recognized cause of human ehrlichiosis, *E. chaffeensis*.

Their results suggest that while a genetic relationship exists between all members of the tribe *Erhlichieae*, the five known *Erhlichia* species and the new human isolate fall into three genetically recognizable groups. *E. chaffeensis* and *E. canis*, and *E. risticii* and *E. sennetsu* constitute two distinct and closely related groups. *E. phagocytophila* and *E. equi* formed a distinct third group. *E. phagocytophila* is closely related to the *E. canis* and *E. chaffeensis* group, with a sequence divergence of 7.3% for *E. chaffeensis* and 7.6–7.7% for *E. canis*. It is distantly related with the *E. risticii* and *E. sennetsu* group, with a sequence divergence of 15.0% for *E. sennetsu* and 15.1% for *E. risticii*. Most significantly, there was no genetic difference between the two strains of *E. phagocytophila* examined and between *E. phagocytophilà* and *E. equi*. These findings indicate that *E. phagocytophila* and *E. equi* may be strain variants of the same species and it has been suggested that they be recognized as one species.[15]

Morphology

Cytoplasmic inclusions in white cells were first reported in 1940[3] and detailed descriptions of the organisms were subsequently published.[9,16,17] Foggie[9] carried out detailed studies to establish whether or not the varied morphological types in the cytoplasmic inclusions represented stages of development similar to that of the chlamydiae. Although evidence was presented as to transformation of the "elementary" bodies into large homogenous initial bodies which in turn developed into "morulae",[17] these various forms do not indicate a clear developmental cycle similar to the chlamydia.[18] Typical forms of the organisms under the light microscope are shown in Fig. 13.1.

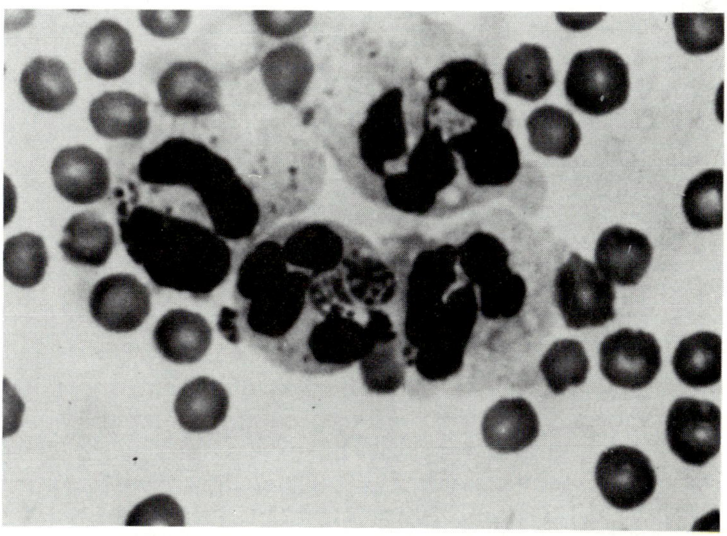

FIG. 13.1. Ovine granulocytes with intracytoplasmic inclusions 5 days after experimental infection with *C. phagocytophila* ($\times$ 1600).

Ultrastructure

There are very few published reports on the ultrastructure of the organism. Studies using ultrathin sections of infected leucocytes demonstrated that what were appearing as irregularly shaped masses under the light microscope were aggregates of particles closely packed together inside cytoplasmic vacuoles.[12,18] These vacuoles were clearly separated from the host cell cytoplasm. It is possible to find one cell with more than one vacuole containing rickettsiae of different sizes (Fig. 13.2). The organisms inside the vacuole are

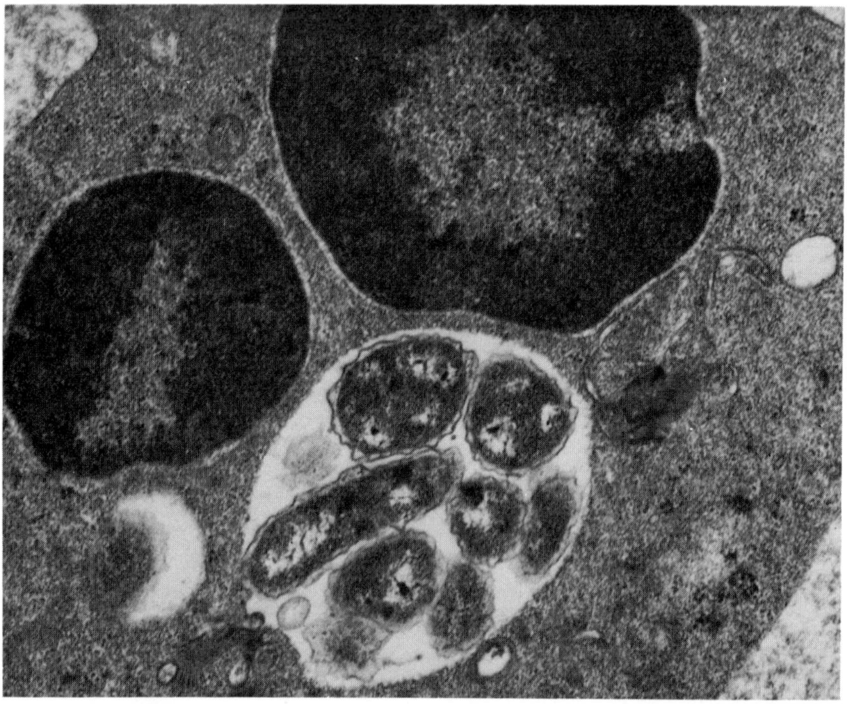

FIG. 13.2. An electron micrograph of an ovine granulocyte obtained 4 days after experimental infection with *C. phagocytophila*, showing rickettsiae of variable sizes within a clearly defined vacuole (×24,000).

surrounded by a rippled double-membrane and their arrangements inside the vacuoles are variable; thus providing an explanation for the different forms seen under the light microscope. Using ultrastructural and microscopic studies of infected leucocytes cultured for 24–48 h, Woldehiwet and Scott[18] postulated that the organism has simple developmental stages in which small organisms are taken up by phagocytic cells and divide by binary fission within clearly defined cytoplasmic vacuoles. Although it had been reported that the plasma was infectious,[9] the morphology of the organism outside the host cell has only recently been investigated. Preparations from the plasma of sheep experimentally infected with TBF contain typical rickettsial structures with an outer membrane and a cell wall.[19]

Cultural Characteristics

The organism is an obligate parasite of the polymorphonuclear cells and monocytes. Early attempts to cultivate the organism in bacteriological media were unsuccessful.[2] It has not been cultivated in embryonated hen eggs or cell culture systems.[4,20–22] However, the organism continues to multiply in granulocytes obtained from infected blood using a whole blood cell culture system[23] or peripheral blood leucocytes separated from other blood components[24] (Woldehiwet, unpublished).

Strain Differences

The presence of various strains of *C. phagocytophila* was first recognized when Hudson[4] reported TBF in cattle. He noticed that the strains isolated from cattle caused less severe disease than strains isolated from sheep. Foggie[9] reported that he could not reproduce TBF in cattle after experimental inoculation with ovine strains and Foggie and Allison[25] could not reproduce TBF in sheep experimentally inoculated with bovine strains. Tuomi[26] reported that most bovine strains were, in general, less virulent to sheep while a few were as virulent to sheep as they were to cattle. Even among ovine strains or among bovine strains there is a great deal of variation in virulence as measured by percentage of infected granulocytes, the degree and duration of parasitemia and the length of incubation period.[2,9]

Antigenicity

The antigenic composition of *C. phagocytophila* is not known. This is largely due to the fact that methods for obtaining pure organisms have not been developed recently.[19] Nevertheless, sheep and cattle infected with the organism develop antibodies which could be detected by the complement fixation test,[27,29] by the indirect immunofluorescent antibody assay[29] and by the counter-current immunoelectrophoresis test.[30] There is so far no serological test that can differentiate the organism into serotypes but cross-protection tests and complement fixation tests using homologous and heterologous antigens have been used to separate them into different groups.[31,32] The antigenic heterogeneity of strains of *C. phagocytophila* was highlighted by Tuomi's[31] observations that "it was rather exceptional for infection by any single strain to result in protection against heterologous strain". Despite this heterogeneity, it has been shown that all strains of the organism share common antigens as demonstrated by the complement fixation test and by the immunofluorescent test.[32,33] Although animals immune to one strain react with fever and parasitemia upon challenge with a heterologous strain, the magnitudes and durations of fever and parasitemia are minimal.[28]

Physico-chemical Properties

The organism can remain infective in citrated blood up to 10 days at room temperature and up to 14 days at 4°C.[4,9] When small volumes of infected blood were kept at −79°C, the organism remained infective for at least 18 months in the presence of glycerol or dimethyl sulphoxide (DMSO) as cryoprotectants.[34] The behavior of the organism outside the host cell has not been studied sufficiently. The early observations that both the plasma and serum of experimentally infected sheep were infective to susceptible sheep,[9] have been reinforced by the recent demonstration that cell-free infective organisms could be obtained from the plasma by density gradient centrifugation.[19] Furthermore, *C. phagocytophila* which was released from infected leucocytes by ultrasonic vibration and purified by density gradient centrifugation remained infective for at least six months when maintained at −114°C in sucrose phosphate glutamate (SPG) buffer,[35] with 10% DMSO as a cryopreservative.[19]

Sensitivity to Drugs

Sulphamethazine suppresses the organism in the blood stream but infection is not always eradicated.[9,36] The organism is sensitive to oxytetracycline but resistant to penicillin.[25,36–38] Tuomi[36] found the organisms were less sensitive to chloramphenicol than to oxytetracyclines or sulphamethazine. Neither streptomycin nor ampicillin are effective but the organism is reported to be relatively sensitive to tylosin.[37,38,39] It has also been reported that long-acting tetracyclines are effective in preventing the onset of clinical disease when given 1–5 days before experimental infection.[40]

Epidemiology

Geographical Distribution

The disease appears to be limited to the temperate climates of Europe although similar organisms have been described without further confirmation in India and from the Natal region of South Africa.[41,42] The disease was first recognized in Scotland but was later reported from other parts of the United Kingdom.[4,43,44] The diseases known as tick-borne fever in sheep[45] and as pasture fever in cattle[5,6,7,8] are also widespread in Europe. Pasture fever and TBF are particularly endemic in Finland, Norway and the Netherlands.[24,45,46]

Host Range

The disease naturally affects domestic and wild ruminants.[2,4,9,47–49] The main domestic ruminants affected are sheep and cattle but isolated outbreaks have been reported in goats.[47] In wild ruminants, the organism has been isolated from feral goats and from red, fallow and roe deer.[48,49] Experimentally, TBF can be readily transmitted to sheep, cattle and goats[9,20,46] but attempts to transmit the disease into laboratory animals have largely been unsuccessful.[4,9,20] The only partially successful transmission was that reported by Foggie and Hood[50] in splenectomized mice and guinea pigs. However, it has subsequently been reported that when mice and guinea pigs were splenectomized, organisms similar to *C. phagocytophila* may be present even in those which were not experimentally infected.[51] These observations have not been confirmed by other workers.

Transmission

The disease is transmitted by the temperate tick *Ixodes ricinus*.[52] The organism can be transmitted trans-stadially but not transovarially.[52,53] Thus adult ticks infected as larvae or nymphs can transmit the disease as can nymphs infected as larvae but infections do not appear to pass from the adult female to the larva via the egg.[9]

The agent can survive in infected ticks for long periods[53] and because *I. ricinus* can survive unfed for over one year awaiting a new host, ticks infected in their previous instar can still be infective after long periods of hibernation.

The ready transmission of infection by injecting infected blood suggests that the organism could be transmitted mechanically by biting insects but the role of ticks other than *I. ricinus* and other arthropods is not well-established. However, after the discovery of the disease in areas of England where *I. ricinus* is not known to be present, it has been suggested that other vectors such as *Haemophysalis punctata* may be involved.[54] If the organisms reported in India by Raghavachari and Reddy[41] and in Southern Africa by Neitz[42] are indeed *C. phagocytophila*, it is most likely that ticks other than *I. ricinus* are involved.

Animal Reservoirs

The ecological survival of the organisms seems to be guaranteed not only by the fact that infected ticks passed it on to the following stages but also by the fact that animals which had recovered from clinical disease may harbor the organisms for long periods. Foggie[9] reported that sheep which have recovered from clinical disease harbored the organism in their blood for as long as two years. In contrast, cattle appear to be poor carriers.[4,20] The presence of the organism in wild ruminants suggests that they may serve as natural reservoirs of infection[48,49] but the epidemiology of the organism in wild ruminants has not been sufficiently studied.

Pathogenesis

After a blood meal by an infected tick or experimental inoculation of infected blood, the organism may not be recovered for at least 24 h.[51] The initial sites of rickettsial multiplication are not known but the results of one study suggest that the organisms appeared in the lung before they were present in the peripheral blood.[51] Three to seven days after experimental infection or infestation with infected ticks, cytoplasmic inclusions appear in the eosinophils, neutrophils and monocytes, in that order.[22] However, blood is infective to susceptible sheep at least 24 h before cytoplasmic inclusions could be detected.[9] Cytoplasmic inclusions could be detected at least 24 h earlier by culturing infected blood.[23] Cytoplasmic inclusions can be detected in neutrophils for 2–3 weeks. It is not known whether the organism multiplies in cells other than peripheral blood leucocytes but the organisms have been demonstrated in Kupffer cells and in the alveolar macrophages alveolar epithelial cells.[55] It appears that the polymorphonuclear cells do not acquire the organisms before entering the peripheral blood. After treating sheep infected with TBF with betamethasone, the number of polymorphonuclear cells in peripheral blood is dramatically increased but the percentage of polymorphonuclear cells bearing cytoplasmic inclusions is significantly reduced, suggesting that the PMN acquire infections after entering the circulatory system.[56] It is not yet clear how the fever is generated. In general the febrile reactions in bacterial infections are believed to be mediated by endogenous pyrogens but an attempt to demonstrate the presence of endogenous pyrogens in goats experimentally infected with TBF was unsuccessful.[46]

During and after the period of parasitemia the disease is characterized by severe hematological changes. The hematological picture is characterized by severe leucopenia, due to early lymphocytopenia and prolonged neutropenia, and thrombocytopenia.[57,58] The lymphocytopenia which accompanies TBF is due to a significant reduction in the number of cells bearing surface immunoglobulins and T lymphocytes.[59] The B cells and all but the CD4–CD8- (gamma/delta) T lymphocytes are reduced in numbers during the period of parasitemia.[60]

The severe hematological changes which accompany the disease are regarded as the main predisposing causes for secondary infections.[61] The febrile period of TBF is often followed by a sequel of other diseases such as tick-pyemia,[57] louping ill,[53] listeriosis[62] and pasteurellosis.[63]

However, there have been very limited attempts to explain the phenomenon of immunosuppression in TBF. The limited published information on the subject suggests that the reduction in the number of circulating PMN and lymphocytes and the down-regulation of their functions may be responsible for the apparent susceptibility to infection and poor immune responses to viral and bacterial antigens.[61,64–67]

For example, leucocytes obtained from TBF-infected sheep are less efficient at phagocytosing and killing *Staphylococci aureus* and their lymphocytes are less responsive to mitogens *in vitro*.[67,68] After observing that PMN infected with *C. phagocytophila* showed less diapedesis *in vivo*, Foster and Cameron[69] concluded that infection with TBF impairs their functional integrity. Infected PMN are also significantly less likely to adhere to glass or plastic surfaces.[67] The fact that sheep infected with TBF develop a more severe pneumonia after exposure to *P. haemolytica* is probably due to an increased susceptibility of infected polymorphonuclear cells to the cytotoxin of *P. haemolytica* (Woldehiwet, unpublished observations).

Clinical Disease

In natural infections the incubation period may vary from 4 to 8 days.[2] Sheep experimentally exposed to infected ticks develop clinical signs within 4–14 days[53] but after intravenous incubation with infected blood the incubation period is shortened to 3–4 days.[2,9] The incubation period may be lengthened and the febrile period reduced if the animals had been previously infected by a homologous or heterologous strain.[10,20,28] The incubation period is reported to be longer in cattle than in sheep.[20]

The clinical disease is characterized by an abrupt rise in rectal temperature.[52] The duration and magnitude of fever may vary according to the strain of *C. phagocytophila*, and the type and immunological status of the host.[20,28,70] The highest point of thermal reaction is usually attained on the second day of parasitemia.[67] The thermal response is usually monophasic but secondary thermal reactions may occur.[4,9,20] The duration and magnitude of febrile response is influenced by the strain of *C. phagocytophila* and by the type and immunological status of the host.[24,28,31]

In sheep other signs are either absent or mild but the animals generally appear as dull and may loose weight.[2,3] The respiratory and the pulse rates of affected animals are usually raised and often animals may be coughing.[1,4,20]

In dairy cattle affected by TBF milk yields may be significantly reduced.[4,20,25,43] Although febrile responses do occur in cattle, often veterinary advice is sought after an abrupt fall in milk yield. The reductions in milk yield could be in excess of 50%.[20]

Despite the relative mildness of the clinical disease, TBF is often followed by other major complications including tick pyemia, abortions and respiratory infections.

Tick Pyemia

The most common complication of lambs infected with TBF is tick pyemia.[57,64,71] Tick pyemia is a disease of lambs characterized by crippling lameness and paralysis during periods of tick activity. Before TBF was recognized as a disease entity some workers had already associated pyemia of lambs with tick activity. MacLeod[53] for example, concluded that earlier description of pyemic conditions of lambs in North Wales[72] were probably due to prior infection wih TBF. Gordon[71] observed that lambs infected with TBF suffered from loss of body condition and in many instances they had pyogenic infections. Stewart and Ponsford[73] reported that nearly 50% of lambs dying from louping-ill had abscesses and in the majority of cases the latter was responsible for death. McEwen[11] observed lameness and abscess formation in a lamb 7 days after infection with TBF. In some instances, the staphylococcal infections become septicemic.[74] Experimental studies later showed that experimentally infected lambs were more susceptible to experimental infection with *S. aureus* during the period of neutropenia, and that 13 of 40 TBF-infected lambs developed staphylococcal infections.[64,75]

During this period too the capacity of peripheral blood leucocytes to phagocytose and kill *Staphylococcus aureus*, the common cause of tick-pyemia, is significantly reduced.[65,67] In addition, the capacity of neutrophils to migrate *in vivo* and *in vitro* was reduced, thereby possibly affecting their inflammatory responses.[69,76]

Abortions

Tick-borne fever was suspected as a cause of abortion in sheep after it was noticed that outbreaks of abortions occurred when pregnant ewes were moved from tick-free to tick infested areas.[77,78] The incidence of abortions was a high as 30%.[78,79] Subsequent field observations confirmed that indeed abortion is a common sequel to TBF, particularly in animals which were new to tick-infested pastures.[79,80] High percentages of ewes could abort and some of them may die. For example, Jamieson[79] reported that 41 of 80 gimmers aborted 3 months after introduction to a tick-infested farm. Sixteen of those which aborted died and TBF was confirmed in 18 animals. Similar high death rates following infection with TBF and abortions were also reported by Littlejohn.[80] It is not known whether the abortions and subsequent deaths were due to TBF *per se* or were due to bacterial complications.

Experimental studies have subsequently substantiated the field observations.[79,81] For example, Stamp and Watt[81] found that 5 of 10 susceptible pregnant ewes aborted after experimental infection with TBF compared to only one abortion in 9 pregnant ewes which were born and reared in tick-infested pasture prior to experimental infection with TBF. Jamieson[79] experimentally infected with TBF one group of 10 gimmers from tick-free farm and another group of ten 5–6 year old ewes from a tick-infested farm during late gestation. All the gimmers obtained from the tick-free farm gave birth to dead or very weak premature lambs compared to normal full-term deliveries in the ewes from the tick-infested farms, suggesting the latter group were apparently immune to TBF as a result of previous exposure.

Outbreaks of abortions and stillbirths have been reported to occur when pregnant nonimmune cattle were moved from tick-free to tick-infested areas.[44,82] In one outbreak, 28 of 120 cows aborted or gave birth to dead fetuses within 2 months of arriving in a tick-infested farm.[82] These abortions were associated with TBF after *C. phagocytophila* was demonstrated in the blood of 5 heifers which aborted and by reproducing TBF in sheep inoculated with blood from 10 of 11 aborting heifers. There is also some evidence which suggests that bulls and rams infected with TBF may suffer from reduced fertility. In one study,[83] it was reported that four of 17 rams became infertile shortly after introduction to tick-infested pastures and that pooled infected blood inoculated into susceptible rams produced semen abnormalities. Abnormal spermatozoal counts were also reported in experimentally infected bulls.[84]

Respiratory Infections

When TBF was first described in cattle,[4] the main reason why veterinary attention was sought was that there was a sudden loss of milk yield and some of the animals were coughing. Several outbreaks of pneumonia in sheep have been associated with TBF. Foggie[9] reported that 41% of sheep infected with TBF developed pneumonia due to *Pasteurella* spp. or other bacteria and Foster and Cameron[70] reported pericarditis due *P. haemolytica* in a lamb infected with TBF. It was also noted that resistance of lambs to infections with *Pasteurella* spp. may be lowered as a result of infection with TBF.[85]

Three groups of workers have produced pneumonia by experimental infection of sheep with TBF followed with bacterial or viral agents. In one study, lambs infected simultaneously with *C. phagocytophila* and PI-3 virus had higher magnitudes of fever and showed respiratory distress compared to lambs infected with *C. phagocytophila* or PI-3 virus alone.[61] When lambs were infected with PI-3 virus at the onset of TBF parasitemia, 20% of lambs died. In another study,[86] 7 four week old specific pathogen-free lambs were infected with *C. phagocytophila* and seven days later they were exposed to aerosols of *Pasteurella hemolytica*. It was shown that lambs infected with both agents had significantly more severe disease and gross lesions than groups of lambs infected with one agent alone. A third group of workers[55] found that dual infection of lambs wih TBF and *Chlamydia psittaci* results in significantly more severe pathological lesions and respiratory signs compared to infection with one agent alone.

Other Complications

Natural and experimental infections with TBF may aggravate other infections. Early workers had observed that infections due to louping ill might be aggravated by the simultaneous presence of TBF.[10,16,87] Recent experimental studies support these early observations. Reid and his coworkers[88] experimentally infected ten sheep with louping-ill virus five days after infection with *C. phagocytophila*. Other groups of sheep were infected with *C. phagocytophila* or louping-ill virus alone. Their findings indicated that infection with *C. phagocytophila* enhanced the pathogenicity of louping-ill virus and that, operating together, the two pathogens facilitated fungal invasion of the central nervous system.

A hemorrhagic syndrome was reported to occur following experimental infection with TBF[89] and some workers[90] associated a necrotic mycosis in the ileum of a lamb which died nine days after experimental infection with *C. phagocytophila* to the neutropenia of TBF. Tick-borne fever has also been implicated as a major complicating factor in Johne's disease, enterotoxemia, braxy, septicema due to latent infections wih *Listeria monocytogenes* and mucosal disease.[9,62,91,92]

Pathology

Hematology and Clinical Pathology

TBF is accompanied with significant hematological changes.[57] It was shown early in the study of TBF that the disease was characterized by leucopenia.[4,9,20] The leucopenia started with the onset of febrile reaction and returned to normal levels very gradually.[20] The leucopenia was initially due to lymphocytopenia during the first 4 days of illness. Then neutropenia develops progressively, becoming very marked at about ten days postinoculation.[9] The number of circulating eosinophils are also depressed for up to two weeks.[20,51,67] After the febrile period has subsided, the number of monocytes starts to increase.[67,93] The cells which are infected with the organism are eosinophils, neutrophils and monocytes, in that order.[21,67,93] The monocytes are predominantly infected during the later stages of parasitemia while the granulocytes were infected throughout the period of parasitemia.[67]

Recent studies with monoclonal antibodies which recognize surface markers for lymphocyte subsets have revealed that both T and B lymphocytes are reduced.[60] Only the subpopulation of T lymphocytes which had neither helper nor suppressor/cytotoxic function (gamma/delta T cells) were increased transiently.[60] The number of circulating thrombocytes is also reported to be depressed during the febrile period.[58,94] The occasional hemorrhagic syndromes associated with TBF[89] are probably related to the reduction in circulating thrombocytes but Unruh[94] found the depressed levels of circulating platelets did not significantly affect the coagulation and bleeding times. Unruh[94] found that fibrinogen levels were increased and Van Miert and coworkers[46] found that the serum alkaline phosphatase activity and the levels of zinc and iron in blood were significantly reduced in goats experimentally infected with TBF, probably due to the increased production of leucocyte endogenous mediator (LEM) which is usually responsible for the reduction in circulating zinc and iron during fever.[95] However, they could not demonstrate LEM in the plasma of the TBF-infected goats.

Ultrastructural studies of infected leucocytes revealed that the organisms are present in cytoplasmic inclusions without apparent structural damage to host cells.[12,18]

Gross Pathology and Histopathology

There is very little published information on the gross-pathological effects of TBF in naturally or experimentally infected animals. Splenic enlargement was reported by three groups of workers.[2,4,5] The enlarged spleens had no histopathological abnormalities[2] but the results of one study indicated that there was a depletion of lymphocytes from lymphoid organs in general.[4] Limited pulmonary lesions, characterized by diffuse cellular infiltration on the alveolar walls, have also been reported within 24 h of experimental infection of lambs.[55] In some areas there was increased septal thickness and considerable narrowing of the lumina of the alveoli due to mononuclear cell infiltration. They detected only a few heavily infected alveolar macrophages or epithelial cells. The organism has also been detected in Kupffer cells of the spleen and liver.[96] Hemorrhages of the colon and serosal surfaces and petechiations of the intestinal mucosa and the thymus may be occasionally present.[16] There has been one reported case of fatal pericarditis in a lamb infected with TBF.[16]

Immunity to TBF

Innate Resistance

There is some degree of innate resistance related to age and breed. Tuomi[5] reported that TBF was more common in some breeds of Finnish cattle than others. Although the severity of TBF is reported to be influenced by age, the organism readily invades the leucocytes of adults as well as neonates.[5,16,20]

Acquired Immunity

Animals exposed to TBF develop a degree of protective immunity[27] but the degree of protection would vary according to the strain of the organism, the type and age of the host and the time and frequency of challenge.[5,27,30] It has been suggested[5] that immunity to TBF is probably dependent on repeated exposure and that removal for a period of six months to tick-free pastures results in a marked lowering of immunity.[5] Although some workers[4] had reported that resistance to reinfection develops five weeks after primary infection, all the available evidence indicates the duration of immunity is variable according to the challenging strains. Some workers reported that in field conditions, one primary infection invariably fails to protect against challenge and that reintroducing sheep or cattle to tick-infested areas after a removal of only 3 months resulted in febrile disease.[4,97] Other workers[80] reported solid immunity which may last for more than one year. It appears that in field conditions, the reported early breakdown of protective immunity is a reflection of the presence of different strains, while solid immunity reflects the presence of homologous or cross-protective strains.

Experimental studies indicate that sheep may resist homologous challenge for a period which may vary from a few months to more than a year, depending on the level of antibodies at the time of challenge or the presence of a carrier state.[9,22,28]

Humoral Immune Responses

The presence of humoral immune responses in experimentally or naturally infected ruminants has been established using the complement fixation test (CFT), counter immunoelectrophoresis and by indirect immunofluorescence.[24,28–30] A study of the kinetics of antibody production in experimentally infected sheep, revealed that both IgM and IgG antibodies appear in the sera of experimentally infected sheep within two weeks of experimental infection.[28] The IgM antibodies are predominant for the first three weeks, the IgG being predominant thereafter. Nevertheless, the IgM class of antibodies persist in carriers.[28]

There appears to be a correlation between antibody levels and protection against homologous challenge.[28]

Although the various strains of *C. phagocytophila* share common antigens it is possible to establish degrees of relatedness among strains using the complement fixation test.[32] However, the nature of the group-specific or type specific antigens has not been characterized.

Cellular Immune Responses

There is no information on the role of T cells in the development of protective immunity but there is some evidence of the production of antigen-specific lymphokines as measured by the leucocyte migration inhibition test.[76]

Mechanisms of Immunosuppression

Infection with TBF is often followed by other bacterial or viral complications.[57,61,64] For example, lambs infected with TBF often succumb to tick-pyemia and to respiratory infections due to *P. haemolytica*.[63,98] Several workers have tried to explain the factors involved in immunosuppression. Foggie[64] found that experimentally infected lambs were more susceptible to experimental infections with *Staphylococcus aureus* particularly during the period of neutropenia. Leucocytes obtained from sheep experimentally infected with TBF were less effective in phagocytosing and killing *S. aureus*.[67] Other experiments presented evidence which suggested that infection with TBF may affect the functional integrity of polymorphonuclear cells (PMN). For example, it has been experimentally demonstrated that PMN bearing the organisms display less diapedetic capacity than normal PMN and that infected cells have reduced capacity to adhere to glass or plastic surfaces.[67,69]

Experiments have also been carried out to investigate whether or not infection with TBF affects specific or nonspecific immune responses. Experimental studies showed that the humoral immune responses of sheep to bacterial or viral antigens were significantly reduced following experimental infection with TBF.[61,66] Leucocytes obtained from sheep experimentally infected with TBF were less responsive to mitogens *in vitro*[68] and leucocytes obtained from sheep infected with TBF produced soluble factors which inhibited the *in vitro* migration of peripheral blood leucocytes of normal sheep.[76] The nature of these factors has not been investigated but recent work with other rickettsia indicate that rickettsial and PMN interactions may result in the production of the potent immunosuppressive prostaglandin PGE_2. For example, it was recently shown[99] that murine PMN incubated with *R. prowazekii* secreted higher quantities of PGE_2 than PMN incubated without rickettsiae.

Diagnosis

In sheep, the onset of very high fever in tick-infested areas during the spring and summer period in association with hematological changes and the presence of inclusions within granulocytes is diagnostic. In cases of abortions and tick-pyemias associated with TBF, blood smears should indicate its association, particularly when abortions occur after pregnant animals were moved from tick-free to tick-infested pastures. A retrospective investigation into the causes of abortions may be helped by demonstrating a rise in antibody titres by the indirect immunofluorescent test (Woldehiwet, unpublished observations).

In dairy cattle, the main clinical signs are a sudden drop in milk yield and abortions.[5,100] The other clinical sign commonly associated with TBF in cattle is respiratory illness after the herd had been introduced on to tick-infested pasture.[4] TBF must also be considered when abortions and stillbirths, particularly in heifers, occur soon after their introduction on to tick-infested pastures.[82,100] Therefore, in areas which are enzootic to TBF, blood smears must be examined for the presence of organisms in all cases of abortion in sheep and cattle and when milk yield is suddenly reduced soon after the animals had returned to pasture.

Treatment and Control

The short-acting oxytetracyclines are regarded as the most effective drugs.[37,38] Other antibiotics such as penicillin, streptomycin and ampicillin do not prevent relapses.[37]

In endemic areas regular dipping against ticks may be necessary. Alternatively, long-acting tetracyclines may be used as a prophylactive measure against TBF. A dose of 20 mg/kg of a long-acting tetracycline is reported to be sufficient to prevent the development of TBF when given as early as 5 days before experimental infection with *C. phagocytophila*.[39] When susceptible animals, particularly pregnant ewes and new-born lambs are to be moved from tick-free to tick-infested areas, it may be necessary to combine dipping with prophylactic therapy with long-acting tetracyclines. Alternatively, it may be sensible to deliberately infect the animals and treat them with oxytetracyclines before the onset of fever. This would allow multiplication of the organism and therefore stimulation of immune responses without uncontrolled clinical disease but it is reported that a minimum duration of parasitemia is required for protective immunity to develop.[37]

References

1. MacLeod, J. 1932. Preliminary studies in the tick transmission of louping ill. II. A study of the reaction of sheep to tick infestation. *Vet. J.* **88:** 276–284.
2. Gordon, W.S., Brownlee, A., Wilson, D.R. and MacLeod, J. 1932. Tick-borne fever (a hitherto undescribed disease of sheep. *J. comp. Path.* **45:** 301–312.
3. Gordon, W.S., Brownlee, A. and Wilson, D.R. 1940. Studies on louping ill, tick-borne fever and scrapie. *Proc. Third Int. Congr. Microbiol.* pp. 362–362.
4. Hudson, J.R. 1950. The recognition of tick-borne fever as a disease of cattle. *Br. vet. J.* **106:** 3–17.
5. Tuomi, J. 1966. Studies on the epidemiology of bovine tick-borne fever in Finland and clinical description of field cases. *Ann. Med. exp. Biol. Fenniae* **44:** (Suppl. 6) 1–62.
6. Hinaidy, H.K. 1973. Zwei neue infectione Blutkranheiten des Rindes in Ostereich. *Weijn. Tierartl. Mscht.* **12:** 364–366.
7. Juste, R.A., Scott, G.R., Paxton, E.A., Gelabert, J.L. and Jimenez, S. 1989.

Presence of *Cytoecetes phagocytophila* in an atypical disease of cattle in Spain. *Vet. Rec.* **124:** 636.
8. PFISTER, K., ROESTI, A., BOSS, P.H. and BALSIGER, B. 1987. *Ehrlichia phagocytophila* als Erreges des "Weidefiebes" in Bernes Oberland. *Schweiz. Arch. Tierleilk.* **129:** 343–347.
9. FOGGIE, A. 1951. Studies on the infectious agent of tick-borne fever in sheep. *J. Path. Bact.* **63:** 1–15.
10. FOGGIE, A. 1962. Studies on tick pyaemia and tick-borne fever. *Symp. Zool. Soc., Lond.* **6:** 51–58.
11. TYZZER, E.E. 1938. *Cytoecetes microti*, N.G.N. Sp., a parasite developing in granulocytes and infective to small rodents. *Parasitology* **30:** 247–257.
12. TUOMI, J. and VON BONDSDORFF, C.H. 1966. Electron microscopy of tick-borne fever agent in bovine and ovine phagocytizing leucocytes. *J. Bact.* **92:** 1478–1492.
13. RISTIC, M. and HUXSOLL, D.L. 1984. Tribe *Erhlichieae* (Philip 1957). In: *Bergey's Manual of Systematic Bacteriology,* pp. 704–710. N.R. KREIG and J.G. HOLT (Eds). Williams and Wilkins, Baltimore.
14. WEISBURG, W.G., DOBSON, M.E., SAMUEL, J.E., DASCH, L.P., MALLAVIA, L.P., BACA, O., MADELCO, L., SECHREST, J.E., WEISS, E. and WOESE, C.R. 1989. Phylogenetic diversity of the rickettsiae. *J. Bacteriol.* **171:** 4202–4206.
15. ANDERSON, B.E., DAWSON, J.E., JONES, D.C. and WILSON, K.H. 1991. *Erhlichia chaffeensis*, a new species associated with human ehrlichiosis. *J. clin. Microbiol.* **29:** 2838–2842.
16. MCEWEN, A.D. 1947. Tick-borne fever in young lambs. *Vet. Rec.* **59:** 198–201.
17. GORDON, W.S., BROWNLEE, A., WILSON, D.R. and MACLEOD, J. 1962. The epizootiology of louping ill and tick-borne fever with observations on the control of these sheep diseases. *Symp. Zool. Soc., Lond.* **6:** 11–27.
18. WOLDEHIWET, Z. and SCOTT, G.R. 1982. Stages in the development of *Cytoecetes phagocytophila*, the causative agent of tick-borne fever. *J. comp. Path.* **92:** 469–474.
19. WOLDEHIWET, Z., CARTER, S.D. and DARE, C. 1991. Purification of *Cytoecetes phagocytophila*, the causative agent of tick-borne fever, from peripheral blood of infected sheep. *J. comp. Path.* **105:** 431–438.
20. TUOMI, J. 1967. Experimental studies on bovine tick-borne fever. (1). Clinical and haematological data, some properties of the causative agent and homologous immunity. *Acta path. microbiol. scand.* **70:** 429–445.
21. THRUSFILED, M.V., SYNGE, B.A. and SCOTT. G.R. 1978. Attempts to cultivate *Ehrlichia phagocytophila in vitro. Vet. Microbiol.* **2:** 257–260.
22. WOLDEHIWET, Z. 1981. Observations on the immune responses of sheep infected with *Cytoecetes phagocytophila*. Ph.D. Thesis, University of Edinburgh.
23. WOLDEHIWET, Z. and SCOTT, G.R. 1982. *In vitro* propagation of *Cytoecetes phagocytophila*, the causative agent of tick-borne fever. *Vet. Microbiol.* **7:** 127–133.
24. JONGEJAN, F., WASSIX, L.A., THIELEMANS, M.J.C., PERIE, N.M. and UILENBERG, G. 1989. Serotypes of *Cowdria ruminantium* and relationship with *Ehrlichia phagocytophila* determined by immunofluorescence. *Vet. Microbiol.* **21:** 31–40.
25. FOGGIE, A. and ALLISON, C.J. 1960. A note on the occurrence of tick-borne fever in cattle in Scotland with comparative studies of bovine and ovine strains of the organism. *Vet. Rec.* **72:** 767–770.
26. TUOMI, J. 1967. Experimental studies on bovine tick-borne fever. (2)

Differences in virulence of strains of cattle and sheep. *Acta path. microbiol. scand.* **71:** 577–589.

27. SNODGRASS, D.R. and RAMACHANDRAN, S. 1974. Complement fixation test for tick-borne fever in sheep. *Br. vet. J.* **127:** xliv–xlvi.
28. WOLDEHIWET, Z. and SCOTT, G.R. 1982. Immunological studies on tick-borne fever in sheep. *J. comp. Path.* **92:** 457–467.
29. PAXTON, E.A. and SCOTT. G.R. 1989. Detection of antibodies to the agent of tick-borne fever by indirect immunofluorescence. *Vet. Microbiol.* **21:** 133–138.
30. WEBSTER, K.A. and MITCHELL, G.B.B. 1988. Use of counter immunoelectrophoresis in detection of antibodies to tick-borne fever. *Res. vet. Sci.* **45:** 28–30.
31. TUOMI, J. 1967. Experimental studies on bovine tick-borne fever. (3) Immunological strain differences. *Acta path. microbiol. scand.* **71:** 89–100.
32. WOLDEHIWET, Z. and SCOTT, G.R. 1982. Differentiation of strains of *Cytoecetes phagocytophila*, the causative agent of tick-borne fever, by complement fixation. *J. comp. Path.* **92:** 475–478.
33. TUOMI, J. 1967. Experimental studies on bovine tick-borne fever. (4) Immunofluorescent staining of the agent and demonstration of antigenic relationship between strains. *Acta path. microbiol. scand.* **70:** 429–445.
34. FOGGIE, A., LUMSDEN, W.H.R. and MCNEILLAGE, G.J.C. 1966. Preservation of the infectious agent of tick-borne fever in a frozen state. *J. comp. Path.* **76:** 413–416.
35. BOVARNICK, M.R., MILLER, J.C. and SNYDER, J.C. 1950. The influence of certain salts, amino acids, sugars and proteins on the stability of rickettsiae. *J. Bact.* **59:** 509–522.
36. TUOMI, J. 1967. Experimental studies on bovine tick-borne fever. (5). Sensitivity of the causative agent to some antibiotics and to sulphonamides. *Acta path. scand. microbiol. scand.* **71:** 109–113.
37. SYNGE, B.A. 1976. Chemotherapeutic studies on tick-borne fever and heartwater. M.Phil. Thesis, University of Edinburgh.
38. ANIKA, S.M., NOUWS, J.F.M., VAN GOGH, H., NIEUWENHUIJS, J., VREE, T.B. and VAN MIERT, A.S.P.A.M. 1986. Chemotherapy and pharmacokinetics of some antimicrobial agents in healthy dwarf goats and those infected with *Ehrlichia phagocytophila* (tick-borne fever). *Res. Vet. Sci.* **41:** 386–390.
39. EVANS, A.T. 1972. Preliminary observations on the chemotherapy of tick-borne fever of sheep and cattle. *Trans. Roy. Soc. trop. Med. Hyg.* **66:** 547.
40. BRODIE, T.A., HOLMES, P.H. and URQUHART, G.M. 1988. Prophylactic use of long-acting tetracyclines against tick-borne fever (*Cytoecetes phagocytophila*) in sheep. *Vet. Rec.* **122:** 43–44.
41. RAGHAVACHARI, K. and REDDY, A.M.K. 1959. *Cytoecetes ovis var. deccani* (n.sp.) as the cause of tick-borne fever in sheep in India. *Ind. J. Vet. Sci.* **29:** 69–86.
42. NEITZ, W.O. 1969. Cited by RETIEF, G.P., NEITZ, W.O. and MACFARLANE, I.S. 1971. Observations on the effect of tick-borne fever (*Cytoecetes phagocytophila*, Foggie, 1949) on the spermatogenesis of bulls. *J. S. Afr. vet. med. Ass.* **42:** 321–325.
43. TUTT, J.B. and LOVING, C. 1955. Tick-borne fever in dairy cattle. *Vet. Rec.* **67:** 866.
44. VENN, J.A.J. and WOODFORD, M.H. 1956. An outbreak of tick-borne fever in bovines. *Vet. Rec.* **68:** 67–73.
45. OVERAS, J. 1959. Tick-borne fever (sjodogg). Some arsak til abort hos sau. *Nord. Vet. Med.* **11:** 475–482.
46. VAN MIERT, A.S.P.J.A.M., VAN DUIN, C.T.M., SCHOTMAN, A.J.H. and FRANSSEN, F.F. 1984. Clinical, haematological and blood biochemical changes

in goats after experimental infection with tick-borne fever. *Vet. Parasit.* **16:** 225–233.
47. GRAY, D., WEBSTER, K. and BERRY, J.E. 1988. Evidence of louping ill and tick-borne fever in goats. *Vet. Rec.* **122:** 66.
48. MCDIARMID, A. 1965. Modern trends in animal health and husbandry. Some infectious diseases of free-living wild-life. *Br. vet. J.* **121:** 245–257.
49. FOSTER, W.N.M. and GREIG, J.C. 1969. Isolation of tick-borne fever from feral goats in New Galloway. *Vet. rec.* **85:** 585–586.
50. FOGGIE, A. and HOOD, C.S. 1961. Adaptation of the infectious agent of tick-borne fever to guinea pigs and mice. *J. comp. Path.* **76:** 414–427.
51. SNODGRASS, D.R. 1974. Studies on bovine petechial fever and ovine tick-borne fever. Ph.D. Thesis, University of Edinburgh.
52. MACLEOD, J. and GORDON, W.S. 1933. Studies on tick-borne fever of sheep. I. Transmission by the tick *Ixodes ricinus* and description of the disease produced. *Parasitology* **25:** 273–283.
53. MACLEOD, J. 1936. Studies on tick-borne fever of sheep. II. Experiments on transmission and distribution of the disease. *Parasitology* **28:** 320–329.
54. MACLEOD, J. 1962. Ticks and disease in domestic stock in Great Britain. *Symp. Zool. Soc., Lond.* **6:** 29–50.
55. MUNROE, R., HUNTER, A.R., MACKENZIE, G. and MCMARTIN, D.A. 1982. Pulmonary lesions in sheep following experimental infection by *Ehrlichia phagocytophila* and *Chlamydia psittaci*. *J. comp. Path.* **92:** 117–129.
56. WOLDEHIWET, Z. and SCOTT, G.R. 1981. Corticosteroid therapy of tick-borne fever. *Vet. Rec.* **110:** 151–152.
57. TAYLOR, A.W., HOLMAN, H.H. and GORDON, W.S. 1941. Attempts to reproduce the pyaemia of associated with tick-bite. *Vet. rec.* **53:** 339–344.
58. FOSTER, W.N.M. and CAMERON, A.E. 1968. Thrombocytopenia in sheep associated with experimental tick-borne fever infection. *J. comp. Path.* **78:** 251–254.
59. BATUNGBACAL, M.R., SCOTT, G.R. and BURRELLS, C. 1982. The lymphocytopenia of tick-borne fever. *J. comp. Path.* **92:** 403–407.
60. WOLDEHIWET, Z. 1991. Lymphocyte subpopulations in the peripheral blood of sheep experimentally infected with tick-borne fever. *Res. vet. Sci.* **51:** 40–43.
61. BATUNGBACAL, M.R. and SCOTT, G.R. 1982. Tick-borne fever and concurrent parainfluenza-3 virus infection in sheep. *J. comp. Path.* **92:** 415–428.
62. GRONSTOL, H. and ULVAND, M.J. 1977. Listeric septicaemia in sheep associated with tick-borne fever *(Ehrlichiosis ovis)*. *Acta vet. scand.* **18:** 575–577.
63. GILMOUR, N.J.L., BRODIE, T.A. and HOLMES, P.H. 1982. Tick-borne fever and pasteurellosis in sheep. *Vet. Rec.* **111:** 512.
64. FOGGIE, A. 1956. The effect of tick-borne fever on the resistance of lambs to staphylococci. *J. comp. Path.* **66:** 278–285.
65. FOGGIE, A. 1957. Further experiments on the effects of tick-borne fever infection on the susceptibility of lambs to staphylococci. *J. comp. Path.* **67:** 369–377.
66. BATUNGBACAL, M.R. and SCOTT, G.R. 1982. Suppression of immune response to clostridial vaccine by tick-borne fever. *J. comp. Path.* **92:** 409–413.
67. WOLDEHIWET, Z. 1987. The effects of tick-borne fever on some functions of polymorphonuclear cells of sheep. *J. comp. Path.* **97:** 481–485.
68. WOLDEHIWET, Z. 1987. Depression of lymphocyte response to mitogens in sheep infected with tick-borne fever. *J. comp. Path.* **97:** 637–643.
69. FOSTER, W.N.M. and CAMERON, A.E. 1970. Observations on the functional

integrity of neutrophil leucocytes infected with tick-borne fever. *J. comp. Path.* **80:** 487–491.
70. FOSTER, W.N.M. and CAMERON, A.E. 1970. Observations on ovine strains of tick-borne fever. *J. comp. Path.* **80:** 429–436.
71. GORDON, W.S. 1934. Recent advances in the control of certain diseases of sheep. *Vet. J.* **90:** 439–446.
72. WALTON, C.L. 1927. The control of tick infestation and a related disease of lambs. *Parasitology* **19:** 265–273.
73. STEWART, W.L. and PONSFORD, A.P. 1937. Lamb diseases coincident with louping-ill. *J. comp. Path.* **50:** 767–782.
74. MCDIARMID, A. 1946. Studies on enzootic staphylococcal infection in lambs associated wtih tick-bite. I. The nature of the disease, clinical findings and differential diagnosis. *Vet. Rec.* **58:** 103–104.
75. FOSTER, W.N.M. and CAMERON, A.E. 1968. Aetiology of enzootic staphylococcal infection (Tick pyaemia) in lambs. **78:** 243–250.
76. WOLDEHIWET, Z. and SCOTT, G.R. (1982). Tick-borne fever: Leucocyte migration inhibition. *Vet. Microbiol.* **7:** 437–455.
77. STEWART, W.L. 1936. Contributions to discussion. *Vet. Rec.* **48:** 1231.
78. HARBOUR, H.E. 1945. Abortion in cattle and sheep. *Trans. Roy. Highland Soc. Scot.* **57:** 16–40.
79. JAMIESON, S. 1950. Tick-borne fever as a cause of abortion in sheep. Part II. Vet. Rec. **62:** 468–470.
80. LITTLEJOHN, A. I. 1950. Tick-borne fever as a cause of abortion in sheep. *Vet. Rec.* **62:** 577–579.
81. STAMP, J.T. and WATT, J.A. 1950. Tick-borne fever as a cause of abortion in sheep—Part I. *Vet. Rec.* **62:** 465–468.
82. WILSON, J.E., FOGGIE, A. and CARMICHAEL, M.A. 1964. Tick-borne fever as a cause of abortion and still-births in cattle. *Vet. Rec.* **76:** 1081–1084.
83. WATSON, W.A. 1964. Infertility in the ram associated with tick-borne fever. *Vet. Rec.* **76:** 1131–1136.
84. RETIEF, G.P., NEITZ, W.O. and MACFARLANE, I.S. 1971. Observations on the effect of tick-borne fever *(Cytoecetes phagocytophila*, Foggie, 1949) on the spermatogenesis of bulls. *J. S. Afr. vet. med. Ass.* **42:** 321–325.
85. OVERAS, J. 1972. Studies on immunity to tick-borne fever. Disease in sheep kept on *Ixodes ricinus* infected pastures. *Nord. vet. Med.* **83:** 561–567.
86. BRODIE, T.A., HOLMES, P.H. and URQUHART, G.M. 1986. Some aspects of tick-borne fever of British sheep. *Vet. Rec.* **118:** 415–418.
87. MACLEOD, J. and GORDON, W.S. 1932. Studies in louping ill. II. Transmission by the sheep tick *Ixodes ricinus. J. comp. Path.* **42:** 240–256.
88. REID, H.W., BUXTON, D. and POW, I. 1986. Response of sheep to experimental concurrent infection with tick-borne fever and louping-ill virus. *Res. vet. Sci.* **41:** 56–62.
89. FOSTER, W.N.M., CAMERON, A.E. and NISBET. 1968. Haemorrhagic enteritis in sheep experimentally infected with tick-borne fever. *J. comp. Path.* **78:** 255–258.
90. ANGUS, K.W., RENWICK, C.C. and ROBINSON, G.W. 1971. Segmental necrosis of the ileum in a lamb associated with a phycomycete. *Vet. Rec.* **88:** 654–656.
91. NAERLAND, J. 1956. Cited by OVERAS, J. 1962. Studies on the immunity to tick-borne fever in Norway. *Nord. vet. Med.* **14:** 620–630.
92. GREIG, H., MACLEOD, N.S.M. and ALLISON, C.T. 1977. Tick-borne fever in association with mucosal disease and cobalt deficiency in calves. *Vet. Rec.* **100:** 562–564.

93. WOLDEHIWET, Z. 1983. Tick-borne fever: A review. *Vet. Res. Commun.* **6:** 163–175.
94. UNRUH, D.H.A. 1977. Disseminated intravenous coagulation; a study into the possible pathogenesis of tick-borne fever. M.Sc. Thesis, University of Edinburgh.
95. VAN MIERT, A.S.P.J.A.M., VAN DUIN, C.T.M., VERHEIJDEN, J.H.M. and SCHOTMAN, A.J.H. 1984. Staphylococcal enterotoxin B and *Escherichia coli* endotoxin: Comparative observations in goats on fever and associated clinical, haematologic and blood biochemical changes after intravenous and intramammary administration. *Am. J. vet. Res.* **44:** 955–863.
96. SCOTT, G.R. 1984. Tick-borne fever in sheep. *Vet. ann.* **24:** 100–106.
97. JAMIESON, S. 1947. Some aspects of immunity to tick-borne fever in hoggs. *Vet. Rec.* **59:** 201–202.
98. OVERAS, J. 1962. Studies on the immunity to tick-borne fever in Norway. *Nord. vet. Med.* **14:** 620–630.
99. WALKER, T.S. and HOOVER, C.S. 1991. Rickettsial effects on leucotrine and prostaglandin secretion by mouse polymorphonuclear leucocytes. *Infect. Immun.* **59:** 351–356.
100. CRANWELL, M.P. and GIBBONS, J.A. 1986. Tick-borne fever in a dairy herd. *Vet. Rec.* **119:** 531–532.

14

Bovine Petechial Fever

G. R. SCOTT AND Z. WOLDEHIWET

Introduction

Bovine petechial fever (BPF) occurs in the highlands of Kenya in imported cattle and their crosses with indigenous breeds. The illness begins with a sudden agalactia, high fever and massive petechiation of the visible mucous membranes. The case fatality rate approaches 50% and pregnant animals abort. The reservoir host is the bushbuck (*Tragelaphur scriptus*).[1] Cattle acquire infection when stockowners are forced to graze their animals in bushbuck habitats. Bovine petechial fever, however, is not contagious and is believed to be transmitted by an as yet unknown vector.[2]

The disease emerged in 1928 when a newly imported shipment of European cattle was held in the Nairobi quarantine station while they were being immunized against anaplasmosis and babesiosis. The episode was intensively studied by Mettam[3] who concluded that it was a condition new in animal pathology. He described it as an hemorrhagic diathesis, the outstanding pathological features being capillary haemorrhages and the delayed clotting time of the blood. A few years later Danks[4] demonstrated that it was transmissible by injecting blood from sick cattle intravenously into cattle, sheep and dogs. The etiology was then tentatively considered to be a virus.

Clinical Agent

Classification

Between 1953 and 1959 Plowright[6] carried out postmortems on 62 natural cases of BPF in the course of which he observed in a few cases morula-like rickettsial bodies in von Kupffer cells. Meanwhile Brocklesby[7] detected rickettsias in films of cattle blood which he considered to be *Cytoecetes phagocytophila*, the causal agent of tick-borne fever and pasture fever; he did not associate the organisms with

BPF. An intensive study mounted by Haig and Danskin[8] led to a guarded conclusion that BPF was caused by a pleomorphic rickettsia-like parasite of circulating leucocytes and large lymphocytes of the spleen. They considered that their organisms resembled ehrlichias and they postulated that wild ruminants might be reservoirs of infection. In 1972 Krauss and colleagues[9] published the definitive study and they suggested that the agent be placed in the genus *Cytoecetes*[10] within the tribe *Ehrlichieae*, together with the casual agent of tick-borne fever, the "equine ehrlichia" agent and Tyzzer's vole organism. Subsequently Mugera and Kiptoon[11] discovered that the agent also invaded capillary endothelial cells and suggested that it be placed in the genus *Rickettsia* and be tentatively known as *Rickettsia ondiri*.

Morphology

Cytoecetes (Rickettsia) ondiri(i) is primarily a cytoplasmic parasite of circulating neutrophils,[9] endothelial and liver sinusoidal cells.[11] It also parasitizes, but to a lesser extent, eosinophils, monocytes and tissue macrophages.[9] The inclusions stain blue, bluish-mauve or pinkish-mauve with Giemsa[8] and, when once appreciated, can be differentiated from nuclear chromatin, phagocytosed debris and cytoplasmic granules. They are very pleomorphic and occur as single small irregularly round or ovoid bodies about 0.3 μ in diameter; as single larger bodies that are triangular or comma-shaped; as loose colonies up to 3–4 μ in size of mixed small and larger bodies, called giant bodies by Krauss and his colleagues[9] (Fig. 14.1); and as similar-sized, mulberry-like clusters of small bodies.[8,9]

Ultrastructure

Electron microscopy has revealed the bacterial nature of the causal organisms of BPF.[9] They occur in single or multiple membrane-lined vacuoles within the cytoplasm of parasitized cells. The small roundish bodies contain a central irregular, slightly electron-dense nucleoid within a cytoplasm densely packed with ribosomes. The plasma membrane is clearly separated from the cell wall. The small bodies may be embedded in a ground substance within the vacuole but more often large spaces lie between them. In the giant bodies there is no clear separation between the nucleoid and the cytoplasm, the former being interspersed between the ribosomes. The cell wall of the giant bodies is usually rippled like that of the initial bodies of *C. phagocytophila*.[12]

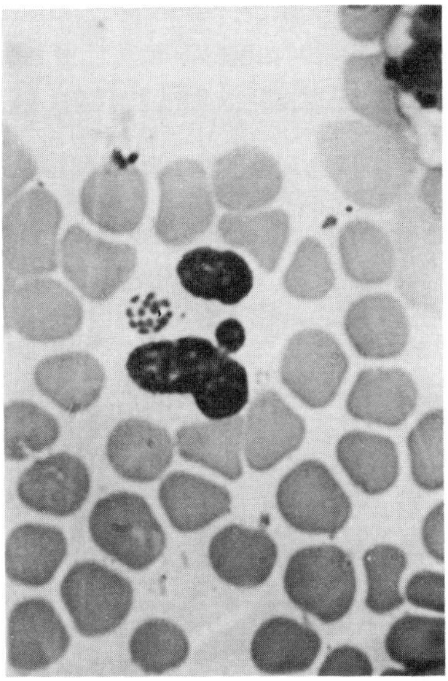

FIG. 14.1. Mixed colony of small and large bodies of *Cytoecetes ondiri* in the cytoplasm of a neutrophil (courtesy of D. Danskin).

Developmental Stages

Haig and Danskin[8] believed the small bodies present in the cytoplasmic vacuoles were elementary bodies that evolved into larger initial bodies. Binary fission occurred at any stage in this evolution.[9] Thereafter small bodies developed within the giant initial bodies and were released by the breakdown of the giant body or by budding from it.[9] Mugera and Kiptoon[11] described the process as multiple fission. Extension of the progeny small bodies from leucocytes was observed late in the developmental cycle.[9]

Cultural Characteristics

The causal organism is an obligate intracellular parasite and cannot be cultured on inanimate bacteriological media.[5] Similarly, early attempts to propagate the agent in embryonated hen eggs or unspecified cell cultures failed.[13,18] *In vitro* propagation in neutrophils is unlikely but the organism's predilection for tissue macrophages and endothelial cells suggests that culture in cell lines of these cells should be possible. Laboratory stocks of *C. ondiri* were maintained by serial passage in cattle and, more often, in sheep[8,9,13,15] until Snodgrass[14] preserved heparinized blood mixed with 10% dimethyl sulphoxide in ampoules immersed in liquid nitrogen.

Strain Differences

Strain differences between isolates of *C. ondiri* are recognized but have not been adequately studied. Isolates vary in their virulence for cattle[13] and sheep[14] and in their frequency of relapses.[13] Piercy[5] recorded that Danks had observed that virulence of the agent for cattle declined when infected blood was "needle-passaged" serially through 16 cattle. Some isolates readily infect cattle and sheep but others, pathogenic for cattle, do not regularly infect sheep.[13]

Antigenicity

Isolates of *C. ondiri* vary in antigenicity. Although most, but not all, isolates protect animals against challenge with the homologous isolate, protection against heterologous challenge is variable, being poor in sheep and better in cattle.[14]

Physico-Chemical Properties

Infective blood collected with anticoagulants such as heparin or EDTA retained its infectivity when stored in a refrigerator at 4–10°C for 9 days[8] but not for 10 days.[5] When stored at 37°C infectivity survived for 48 h.[8] Although storage at −20°C was lethal, portions of infected spleen retained their infectivity for 6 months at −60°C.[8] Lyophilization killed the agent.[8]

Both formalin and crystal violet inactivate infective blood.[15]

Sensitivity to Drugs

C. ondiri is unaffected by penicillin, streptomycin and chloramphenicol[6] whereas treatment of animals with oxytetracycline is effective if the drug is administered prior to or immediately at the onset of illness.[15] Snodgrass[16] later found that a single intravenous injection of alpha-ethoxyethylglyoxal at the rate of 5 mg/kg body weight was significantly more effective in cattle and sheep with overt parasitemias than two tetracycline formulations given intramuscularly on two successive days. Unfortunately alpha-ethoxyethylglyoxal is no longer commercially available.

Epidemiology

Geographical Distribution

Bovine petechial fever occurs sporadically only in exotic cattle and their crosses on farms in the highlands of Kenya at altitudes between 1500–2800 metres (5000–9000 feet).[5,8,15,17] A hyperacute form of the disease was reported from the highlands of Tanzania[18] but subsequently doubts were raised regarding the accuracy of the diagnosis.[19] The most striking epidemiological feature of BPF noted by Piercy[5] and Danskin and Burdin[15] was the localized restriction of the disease incidence; often only a particular small area of a farm or even part of an individual paddock appeared to harbor the infection. Walker and his colleagues[2] investigated in detail 14 sites where the disease had been confirmed during both the dry and the rainy seasons. The sites were in ecological Zones II, III and IV,[20] within the 510–760 mm mean annual rainfall isohyet and above the 1500 m contour. The only characteristic common to all sites was thick bush or undergrowth cover giving heavy shade where the soil had a thick litter layer with a high relative humidity. All had resident populations of bushbuck and duiker. There was a spurious seasonal prevalence which arose because the relationship between incidence and rainfall was confounded by the tendency of farmers to use known infected paddocks only when forced to at the end of the dry season when grazing was scarce. Clinical cases are rarer today than in the past because increasing human population pressure on the land has eliminated most of the dangerous sites.

Host Range

The natural host range of *C. ondiri* appears to be restricted to domestic cattle (*Bos taurus, Bos indicus* and their crosses) and wild bushbuck (*Tragelaphus scriptus*).[1] The few attempts to detect the organism in other wild ruminants failed.[1]

Nevertheless, other domestic and wild ruminants responded to experimental infection, *viz.* sheep,[5] goats,[8] impala (*Aepyceros melampus*), Thomson's gazelle (*Gazella thomsonii*) and wildebeest (*Connochaetes taurinus*).[1] In contrast, a single eland (*Taurotragus oryx*) failed to react when injected intravenously with infected sheep blood.[1] Similarly horses,[5] pigs and dogs[8] were refractory. Attempts to infect laboratory rodents gave equivocal results despite blind passages, splenectomy, irradiation or treatment with corticosteroids; disease was not induced although the organism was occasionally isolated from blood samples from guinea-pigs, hamsters and mice.[21] The response of rabbits was similarly equivocal.[3] Inoculation of embryonated hens' eggs of various ages by the standard routes neither induced lesions nor killed the embryos despite four blind passages.[15] Likewise the organisms failed to grow in calf kidney, sheep kidney and sheep testis cells[15] nor in a mixed culture of bovine lymphatic and hamster cells.[13]

Transmission

Although BPF is ordinarily not a contagion, transplacental infection has been observed in two cows whose fetuses had lesions mimicking those of their dams, the cardiac hemorrhages being most noticeable.[15] Transmission is readily achieved experimentally when exotic cattle and their crossbreds are injected intravenously, subcutaneously or intratracheally with large volumes of infected blood.[11,15] For example, serial passage of the agent in cattle was maintained up to the 27th passage level when the inoculum was about 300 ml but an inoculum of 3 ml failed to induce disease after one or two passages.[15] Snodgrass[22] found that a reproducible intravenous dose in cattle was the buffy coat fraction from 200 ml blood whereas 1 ml blood sufficed when sheep were being infected intravenously. In cattle blood is infective at the onset of fever and remains infective for 4 days after the disappearance of clinical signs.[15]

The epidemiology of BPF necessitates a vector being involved but fleas and lice are rare on cattle under Kenya range conditions. Moreover biting flies do not have habits or life cycles that fit in with the field picture of BPF. Nevertheless six genera of biting flies and three genera of ticks were tested for infection or transmission capability without success in 1937 and 1957 at the Veterinary Laboratory, Kabete.[2] In addition Walker and colleagues[2] tested the hypothesis that trombiculid mites might be the vector but found it wanting.

Animal Reservoirs

The only known reservoir of *C. ondiri* is the bushbuck. Attempts to implicate rodents were not successful; 11 species of rodents were trapped at the known sites of BPF infections and 54 rodent spleens were inoculated into test sheep in 15 pools with negative results.[2]

The prevalence of carriers among bushbuck appears to be high; for example, Snodgrass and his colleagues[1] isolated *C. ondiri* from 3 out of 4 bushbuck shot in an area where BPF in cattle was known to be common. The duration of the carrier state in an experimentally infected buffalo exceeded 2 months and in an experimentally infected impala was greater than one month.[1] The duration of the carrier state in experimentally infected sheep ranged from 1 to 12 weeks.[14] In a group of 4 experimentally infected cattle, 2 did not become carriers after recovery, 1 was a carrier for 1 but not 2 weeks, and 1 was a carrier for 4 but not 8 weeks.[14]

Pathogenesis

In experimentally infected sheep, *C. ondiri* was recovered from blood and spleen within 24 h of inoculation.[14] Within a further 48 h, but still in the prepatent period, the organism was also recovered from lung, liver and bone marrow. Peak titers of the pathogen assessed by titrations in sheep occurred on the third day of fever and ranged from $10^{3.5}$ ED_{50} ml^{-1} of blood to $10^{5.5}$ ED_{50} g^{-1} of spleen. The tissues were all still infective up to the 10th day after the onset of fever but, thereafter, were negative.[14]

The distribution, evolution and infectivity titers of *C. ondiri* in cattle tissues were similar to those in sheep except that the peak titers in the tissues of all but liver were attained at the onset of the clinical reaction.[14] Simultaneously overt parasitemia commenced and within 24 h the circulating organisms colonized and damaged capillary endothelial cells allowing erythrocytes to escape to form petechiae.[23]

Clinical Disease

Natural Infections

Incubation periods following movement of susceptible cattle onto pastures containing thick bush harboring *C. ondiri* range from 7 to 21 days.[8] The subsequent clinical reactions may be inapparent in indigenous zebu cattle, subacute in cross-bred stock reared in the Kenya highlands, acute or peracute in imported exotic cattle.

Subacute reactions in lactating cows are manifested by transient low-grade fevers and a transient fall in the milk yield. In steers subacute reactions are seldom noticed by the stockowners unless the steers become grossly anemic and lose condition. Affected animals continue to eat and behave normally.[15]

Acute reactions begin abruptly with a high prodromal fever.[15] Other signs are minimal except in lactating cows which are suddenly agalactic, lag behind the rest of the herd, and lie down instead of grazing.[13] Next day fine petechiae emerge in the hyperemic visible mucous membranes of the naso-oral and uro-genital tracts and the conjunctivae.[5] They are particularly common and prominent in the under-surface of the tip of the tongue.[6] Within hours the fine petechiae enlarge and suffuse into ecchymoses.[17] Although individual petechiae fade in about 48 h they are continually replaced and are observed for up to 10 days.[15] In cattle, fevers last three or four days and are accompanied after the prodromal period by muscular tremors, depression, anorexia, staring coat and profuse serous lachrimo-nasal discharges.[8,17,22] The blood is slow to clot and epistaxis and subcutaneous hemorrhages are not uncommon.[5,15] Some fatal cases develop a severe unilateral conjunctivitis colloquially known as a "poached-egg eye" in which the conjunctival sacs are grossly swollen and everted around a tense, protuberant eyeball that often contains free blood in the lower part of the anterior chamber.[15] Free blood also appears in the feces which turn tarry and fetid.[5] Sometimes the palpable lymph nodes are slightly swollen.[15] Affected animals cease to ruminate, grind their teeth, lose condition and stand motionless.[17] Although the case fatality rate is about 50%,[17] the severity of the initial signs is no guide to prognosis.[15] If respiratory distress develops as a result of pulmonary edema, affected animals collapse and die in two to three days.[5] Some animals that experience a severe loss of blood in the feces become profoundly anemic and die two to three weeks later.[15] The usual course, however, is 4–11 days, but recovery to full health is slow.[17] Pregnant animals abort.[8,15]

Cattle affected peracutely exhibit respiratory distress, collapse and die one to three days after the onset of fever.[22]

Experimental Infections

Cattle inoculated with infective blood had incubation periods between 4 and 10 days.[5,17,22] Thereafter the clinical picture was similar to that observed in field cases. The case mortality rate, however, was much lower; Haig[24] cited 20% and Snodgrass[22] 10%.

Incubation periods in experimentally infected sheep ranged from 2 to 7 days.[9,13,22] Ill-health was manifested by a sudden fever which reached a peak of about 42°C and lasted 3–5 days.[9,22] Dawe and colleagues[13] observed relapse fevers about one week after recovery from the primary fever in most sheep (65%). The relapse temperature was always lower. Other clinical signs were conspicuously absent apart from a few sheep that became dull and exhibited an increased respiration rate.[13,22] All recovered.

Wildlife successfully experimentally infected were: one bushbuck, that became febrile and dull and recovered; two Thomson's gazelle, that died one and two weeks after inoculation; and one impala and two wildebeest that showed no clinical reactions.[1] Postmortem examinations of the dead gazelles revealed enlarged lymph nodes, hemorrhages and edema.[1]

Pathology

Hematology

Leucocytic changes in BPF-affected animals are consistent and dramatic even in subclinical and inapparent cases. Depression of the total leucocytes begins before the end of the pre-patent period and the onset of fever.[6,9,17,22] The leucopenia is caused first by a profound lymphocytopenia that lasts 4–6 days, and secondly, by a persistent slow decline in neutrophil numbers to a low nadir after the fever has abated[9,22] (Fig. 14.2). Eosinophils fall precipitously and concurrently with the fall in lymphocytes, disappear and only re-emerge in the convalescent phase.[22] Monocyte numbers appear to be unaffected.[22]

The parasitemia is restricted to the neutrophils, eosinophils and a few monocytes.[9] In cattle parasitemias and fevers occur together and last 3–4 days[22] whereas parasitemias in sheep last longer, being patent 24 h before the onset of fever and persisting until the fever regresses[9] (Fig. 14.2).

During the prepatent period the packed cell volume and hemoglobin concentration rise slightly then fall together with erythrocyte numbers during and after the patent parasitemia.[6,15,17] Anemic changes are observable in blood films, basophilic stippling being particularly marked in the more severe cases.[15] Thrombocyte levels are severely depressed with resultant increases in clotting times.[15]

Clinical Pathology

Scant attention has been paid to the clinical pathology of BPF. Kiptoon *et al.*[17] found that serum proteins decreased while levels of serum glutamate oxaloacetic transaminase (SGOT) and serum alkaline phosphate increased. They also noted a marked increase in the clearance of bromosulphthalein.

Gross Pathology

In contrast to the clinical pathology, the gross pathology of BPF is well documented because it is so striking and characteristic. Animals dying in the acute stages of the disease are in good condition whereas the carcasses of dead chronic cases are emaciated, soiled and fetid.[15] Petechial hemorrhages are everywhere.[5] Profuse hemorrhages associated with slight gelatinous edemas are found over submucosal and subserosal surfaces, in subcutaneous tissues and intermuscular tissues.[17] Cardiac splash hemorrhages are particularly prominent both subepicardially and endocardially.[5,6,17] The wall of the gall bladder is so severely affected that it sometimes resembles a hematoma, a lesion that Plowright[6] considered did not occur in any other cattle disease. The liver in acute deaths appears normal but in chronic deaths it has a mottled yellow appearance.[6,15] Petechiae and splash hemorrhages are present in the serosa of the alimentary tract from the forestomachs to the colon.[6] A gelatinous edema swells the mucosal folds and wall of the abomasum and the mucosae of the fundic and pyloric areas are eroded and contain petechiae and splash hemorrhages.[6] Hemorrhages and petechiae are also found in the cortex of the kidney, kidney fat using bladder mucosa.[6,17] The

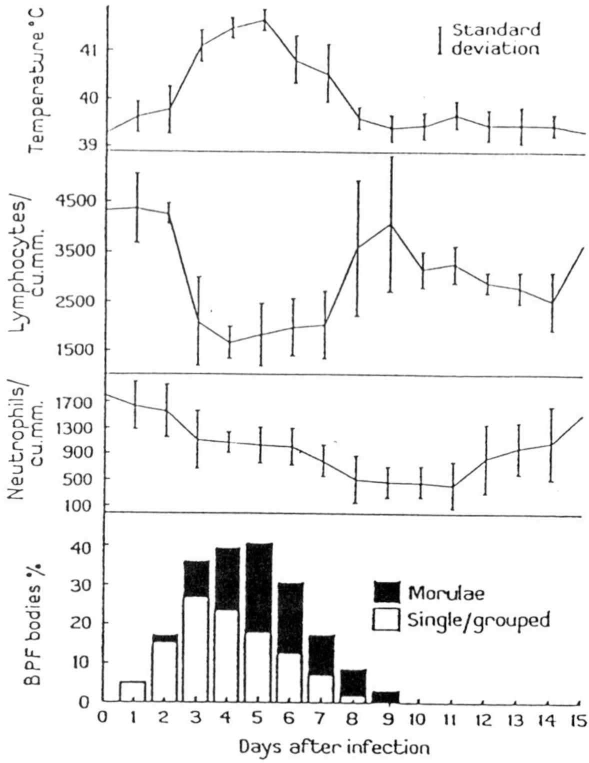

FIG. 14.2. Evolutions of fever, lymphocytopenia, neutropenia and parasitemia in sheep experimentally infected with *Cytoecetes ondiri* (courtesy of Krauss *et al.*[9]).

respiratory tract likewise has hemorrhages and ecchymoses throughout its length.[6] Lesions in the lungs are not extensive and consist, when present, as congestion and edema with small hemorrhagic foci.[6] The only lesion in the central nervous system is slight meningeal congestion and, occasionally, hemorrhages in the dura mater.[6,15]

Histopathology

The larger cells of the lymphoid series are hyperplastic and vascular endothelial cells are swollen.[6] Hemorrhages with accompanying mononuclear cell infiltrations into connective, muscular and epithelial tissues are extensive, infiltrations in the lungs and myocardium being especially prominent.[17] Microscopic changes in the liver are acute and severe with congestion and parenchymal necrosis of hepatocytes. Sinusoidal cells are swollen and often contain intracytoplasmic morulae.[6,17] Morulae are also present in the large splenic macrophages.

Immunity

Innate Resistance

Differences in innate resistance between races of cattle are conspicuous. Zebus indigenous to the Kenya highlands are susceptible but the clinical response is muted,[15] whereas cattle exotic to the Kenya highlands react severely and often die.[5] For example, Snodgrass[22] showed that Sahiwals from Pakistan and Borans from northern Kenya were uniformly susceptible while Ayrshire and Hereford cattle reared in the Kenya highlands were refractory. Danskin and Burdin[15] had earlier inoculated 1077 European-zebu crossbred cattle in a series of transmission experiments and reported that only half reacted. In the light of the fact that clinical BPF is most often observed in European-type cattle and, in the absence of any serological findings, it seems reasonable to conclude that the nonreacting European-type cattle were previously infected. Irrespective of breed or origin sheep possess a high degree of innate resistance such that when they are experimentally infected they develop fevers, parasitemias and characteristic leucocytic changes but exhibit no other clinical signs.[5,9,13,22]

Active Immunity

Piercy[5] emphasized that a noticeable feature of BPS on farms where the disease was endemic was the observation that clinical cases occurred less frequently in adult cows born and reared on the farm. He attributed the phenomenon to immunity acquired in calfhood that was either permanent or constantly reinforced by contact with the infective agent. Danskin and Burdin[15] tested the duration of the acquired immunity by needle challenge and concluded that most recovered animals were solidly immune for at least two years after primary exposure. Moreover animals immune to one strain resisted challenge with a heterologous strain. In contrast Dawe and his colleagues[13] found that experimentally infected sheep withstood homologous challenge for four weeks, but not for five weeks. Snodgrass[14] confirmed the strong homologous and heterologous strain immunities seen in cattle, but his findings refuted those of Dawe and his colleagues; he detected a strong homologous strain immunity in sheep, only one out of five sheep being susceptible after one year. The heterologous strain immunity, however, was poor.

Snodgrass[14] also observed in two cattle given a heterologous challenge low levels of parasitemia of one to two days duration only without other clinical signs.

Humoral and Cellular Immunity

Surprisingly there are no published reports on the presence or absence of humoral antibodies. Similarly the role and significance of cellular immune responses are unknown.

Immunosuppression

Despite the similarities that exist between the leucocytic changes in BPF and tick-borne fever/pasture fever caused by *Cytoecetes phagocytophila*, exacerbation of latent infections or superinfections as seen in tick-borne fever has not been described in BPF. The exceptionally high mortality rate in the original outbreak studied by Mettam[3] were perhaps linked to concurrent infection; all but one of the affected cattle that died were undergoing "immunising" infections against babesiosis and anaplasmosis.

Diagnosis

A presumptive diagnosis is based on the history, particularly a history of recent movement of animals onto rough grazing where pockets of infected scrub are known to exist, the clinical signs and postmortem lesions. Because the latter are not pathognomonic, a positive diagnosis depends on the demonstration of the causative rickettsia.[19] Giemsa-stained blood films and impression smears from a cut surface from the spleen taken within an hour or two of death should be searched for *C. ondiri* in the cytoplasms of granulocytes and spleen macrophages.[19,24] But direct observation of *C. ondiri* may not succeed because parasitemias are waning when severe signs of illness have developed. In such circumstances blood in heparin or EDTA and suspensions of lung and spleen should be inoculated intravenously into susceptible sheep or cattle blood films from which are examined daily for 10 days. It is not sufficient to rely on blood-sampling only in the event of a fever developing because some isolates of *C. ondiri* do not cause fevers on first passage.[19]

Bovine petechial fever has been confused in the past with several other hemorrhagic syndromes such as anthrax, arsenical poisoning, corridor disease caused by *Theileria parva lawrencii*, cowdriosis, hemorrhagic septicemia caused by *Pasteurella multocida*, plant poisoning by bracken and cestrum and Rift Valley fever.[5,15,19,24]

Treatment

Active multiplication of *C. ondiri* occurs before, and for shortly after, the onset of clinical signs. Treatment with oxytetracyclines at the onset of the parasitemia, therefore, is effective but once marked clinical signs have developed rickettsicidal drugs are of little value.[8,24] Sulphonamides also have some therapeutic value at that stage. Snodgrass[16] later showed that dithiozemicarbazone was more efficacious statistically than tetracycline formulations but the drug has been withdrawn from the market because of adverse side-effects.

Mettam[3] claimed to have saved the lives of advanced cases by administering massive doses of adrenaline hydrochloride as a vasoconstrictor. Others have treated advanced cases with drugs that encourage coagulation of the blood; examples were the slow intravenous injection of turpentine and the subcutaneous injection of gelatin.[5]

Control

The inoculation of cattle with infected tissues treated with formalin or crystal violet to inactivate the organism conferred no immunity against challenge.[15] An adapation of the serum-virus simultaneous method of vaccination, however, had some success but it was never taken up.[15] Haig[24] later suggested that a method of immunization based on that used to protect cattle in South Africa against cowdriosis whereby susceptible animals are infected and then treated at the onset of parasitemia could be developed. This also was not developed and the only available reliable prophylactic measure is to avoid grazing cattle in forest edges and in paddocks with patches of thick scrub.

References

1. Snodgrass, D.R., Karstad, L.H. and Cooper, J.E. 1975. The role of wild ruminants in the epidemiology of bovine petechial fever. *J. Hyg., Camb.* **74:** 245–250.
2. Walker, A.R., Cooper, J.E. and Snodgrass, D.R. 1974. Investigations into the epidemiology of bovine petechial fever in Kenya and the potential of trombiculid mites as vectors. *Trop. Anim. Hlth Prod.* **6:** 193–198.
3. Mettam, R.W.M. 1930. Nairobi quarantine disease. *Rep. Dept. Agric. Kenya,* 1929. Govt. Printer, Nairobi, pp. 243–293.
4. Danks, W.B.C. 1936. An undescribed virus disease of cattle. *Rep. Dept. Agric.* Kenya, 1935, Vol. 1, Govt. Printer, Nairobi, p. 146.
5. Piercy, S.E. 1953. Bovine infectious petechial fever. *E. Afr. Agric. J.* **19:** 65–68.
6. Plowright, W. 1962. Some notes on bovine petechial fever. (Ondiri disease) at Muguga, Kenya. *Bull. Epiz. Dis. Afr.* **10:** 499–505.

7. BROCKLESBY, D.W. 1958. The occurrence of *Eperythrozoon wenyoni, Bartonella bovis,* and *Anaplasma marginale* in an ox in Kenya. *J. Parasit.* **44:** 51.
8. HAIG, D.A. and DANSKIN, D. 1962. The aetiology of bovine petechial fever (Ondiri disease). *Res. Vet. Sci.* **3:** 129–138.
9. KRAUSS, H., DAVIES, F.G., ODEGAARD, O.A. and COOPER, J.E. 1972. The morphology of the causal agent of bovine petechial fever. (Ondiri disease). *J. comp. Path.* **82:** 241–246.
10. TYZZER, E.E. 1938. *Cytoecetes microti,* N.G., N.Sp, a parasite developing in granulocytes and infective to small rodents. *Parasitology* **30:** 242–257.
11. MUGERA, G.M. and KIPTOON, J.C. 1978. Some observations of the morphology and infection of the agent of bovine petechial fever. *Bull. Anim. Hlth. Prod. Afr.* **26:** 99–105.
12. TUOMI, J. and BONSDORFF, C.H.V. 1966. Electron microscopy of tick-borne fever agent in bovine and ovine phagocytozing leucocytes. *J. Bact.* **92:** 1478–1492.
13. DAWE, P.S., OHDER, H., WEGENER, J. and BRUCE, W. 1970. Some observations on bovine petechial fever (Ondiri disease) passaged in sheep. *Bull. Epiz. Dis. Afr.* **18:** 361–368.
14. SNODGRASS, D.R. (1975). Pathogenesis of bovine petechial fever. Latent infections, immunity, and tissue distribution of *Cytoecetes ondiri. J. Comp. Path.* **85:** 523–530.
15. DANSKIN, D. and BURDIN, M.L. 1963. Bovine petechial fever. *Vet. Rec.* **75:** 391–394.
16. SNODGRASS, D.R. 1976. Chemotherapy of experimental bovine petechial fever. *Res. Vet. Sci.* **20:** 108–109.
17. KIPTOON, J.C., MUGERA, G.M. and LUTU. W.Z. 1977. Studies on the pathogenesis of bovine petechial fever (Ondiri disease). *Bull. Anim. Hlth Prod. Afr.* **25:** 211–217.
18. JAFFERY, M.S. and MWANGOTA, A.V. 1974. Hyperacute bovine petechial fever. *Vet. Rec.* **85:** 212–213.
19. SNODGRASS, D.R. 1975. Diagnosis of bovine petechial fever. *Vet. Rec.* **96:** 132–133.
20. PRATT, D.J., GREENAWAY, P.J. and GWYNNE, M.D. 1966. A classification of East African rangeland, with an appendix on terminology. *J. appl. Ecol.* **3:** 369–382.
21. COOPER, J.E. 1973. Attempted transmission of the Ondiri disease (bovine petechial fever) agent to laboratory rodents. *Res. Vet. Sci.* **15:** 130–133.
22. SNODGRASS, D.R. 1975. Clinical response and apparent breed resistance in bovine petechial fever. *Trop. Anim. Hlth Prod.* **7:** 213–218.
23. KIPTOON, J.C. and MUGERA, G.M.1983. Invasion of capillary endothelial cells by *Ehrlichia ondiri. Vet. Rec.* **112:** 59–60.
24. HAIG, D.A. 1966. Petechial fever, bovine. In: *International Encyclopaedia of Veterinary Medicine,* pp. 2260–2264. DALLING, T., ROBERTSON, A., BODDIE, G.F. and SPREULL, J.S.A. (Eds), Green and Son, Edinburgh.

15

Other Ehrlichioses of Ruminants

G. UILENBERG

Introduction

Some members of the tribe *Ehrlichieae* multiply mainly in the granulocytes but others prefer mononuclear white blood cells. In ruminants, *Cytoecetes (Ehrlichia) phagocytophila* and *C. ondiri* occur in granulocytes and cause tick-borne fever and petechial fever respectively. However, there are also less well-studied members which invade mononuclear cells of ruminants. These are *Ehrlichia bovis* and *E. ovina*, named after their respective hosts, although there is no conclusive evidence that they are two separate species.

Their importance may be under-rated in many countries, especially for exotic and cross-bred stock. Knowledge of these microorganisms is limited and sketchy, and accounts of their pathogenicity in different areas are widely divergent, to the point where one wonders whether different authors are dealing with the same infectious agent.

Mononuclear Ehrlichiosis of Cattle and Sheep

Causal Agents

Ehrlichia bovis and *E. ovina* are found in cattle and sheep respectively in many tropical and subtropical parts of the world. They occur in mononuclear cells, particularly monocytes, not in the granulocytes as do *C. phagocytophila* and *C. ondiri*.

Morphology

They occur as round or irregular shaped intracytoplasmic structures, ranging from 2 to over 10 μm in diameter, consisting of numerous small granulations. They stain various shades of violet, quite different from bright red azurophilic granules, which are moreover not found in agglomerations. The development cycle described for *E. bovis*[1] includes "initial bodies" of 2–8 μm, "morulae", which are initial bodies disintegrating into elementary bodies, and "elementary bodies", 0.2–0.8 μm in diameter.

E. bovis was found to be most numerous in the lungs, and is also present in the capillaries of the meninges, in the kidneys, the liver, the spleen, the circulating blood, the lymph nodes and some other organs.[1,2] It occurs in monocytes or macrophages and rarely in lymphocytes,[3] but not in the endothelial cells of blood vessels.

Cultural Characteristics

E. bovis can be maintained in mononuclear cell cultures and antigen smears prepared from cultures gave positive results in the immunofluorescent test with sera from recovered cattle.[4,5,6]

There are no reports on the cultivation of *E. ovina* and the molecular biology of both organisms has not been investigated.

Antigenicity

Strong cross-reactions in various serological tests have been reported between *Cowdria ruminantium* and certain species of *Ehrlichia*, including *E. bovis* and *E. ovina* (see Chapter 17 in this book), and it is known that *Ehrlichia* and *Cowdria* are closely related.[7]

Epidemiology

Natural Transmission

Known vector ticks belong to the genera *Hyalomma, Rhipicephalus* and *Amblyomma*.

E. bovis has been transmitted trans-stadially with *Hyalomma* ticks (presumably *H. anatolicum anatolicum sensu*, see Hoogstraal and Kaiser)[8] *Rhipicephalus appendiculatus* and *Amblyomma cajennense*.[2,4,9,10]

Amblyomma variegatum may be a vector, as the infection was transmitted in Senegal by injecting homogenized ticks collected on local cattle.[1]

E. ovina has been transmitted trans-stadially by *Rhipicephalus evertsi*.[9] *R. bursa* may be a vector, as *E. ovina* was transmitted by injecting a suspension of homogenized ticks previously fed on infected sheep.[11] In Sri Lanka, *R. haemaphysaloides* is suspected to be a vector.[12]

Experimental Infection

Few experimental infections have been carried out. Cattle and sheep can easily be infected by intravenous inoculation of blood containing *E. bovis* or *E. ovina* respectively. Other parenteral routes can also be used. Generally, such infections are not fatal. The appearance of the rickettsiae in circulating monocytes, after an incubation period of 2 weeks or less, is associated with a rise in temperature which may last for more than a week. A stock of *E. bovis* from Kenya[6] caused moderate but prolonged fever in a Friesian calf at Utrecht. The animal recovered uneventfully and a few ehrlichia morulae were present in its blood (unpublished data, Fig. 15.1). A stock of *E. ovina* from Turkey, received from Prof. E. Schein in Berlin, caused prolonged fever in Dutch sheep, which eventually recovered spontaneously (G. Uilenberg, unpublished data). *E. bovis* has also been transmitted by injecting infected leucocyte cultures.[5]

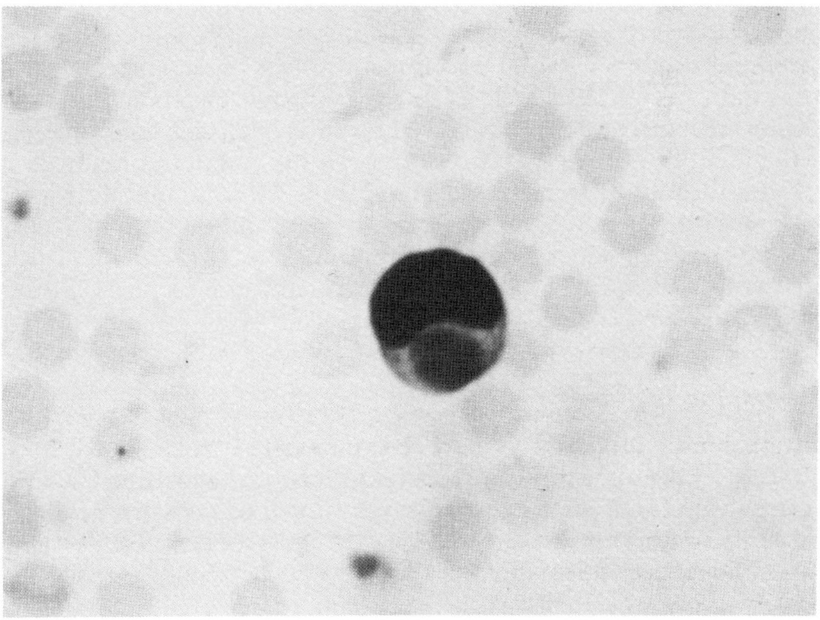

FIG. 15.1. *Ehrlichia bovis*. Morula in mononuclear cell of calf. Kiswani isolate.[6] Faculty of Veterinary Medicine, Utrecht.

After transmission by ticks, the incubation period is reported to be 22 days for *E. bovis*[2] and 15–18 days for *E. ovina*.[13]

Hosts Affected

Cattle and domestic buffalos[14] are natural hosts of *E. bovis*. Sheep are reported by all authors to be natural hosts of *E. ovina* but there are few reports on the occurrence of *E. ovina* in mononuclear cells of goats.[15,16]

Sheep have been infected with *E. bovis* experimentally. For example, intravenous injection of blood from a fatal case of bovine ehrlichiosis resulted in fever and rickettsiemia in sheep.[17] The few attempts to infect goats with *E. bovis* were unsuccessful.[1,4] There are no reports on experimental infection of cattle with *E. ovina*. Critical work is needed to prove whether *E. bovis* is indeed a separate species from *E. ovina*, or a different strain of the same species.

E. bovis may also infect pigs. In Senegal an *Ehrlichia* species in monocytes and less frequently in neutrophilic granulocytes was identified as the cause of an outbreak of fatal disease in European pigs.[18] No ticks were detected on any of the pigs but a calf died 12 days after it was subinoculated with the blood of a pig with the fatal disease. The injection of homogenized, pooled *Hyalomma* and *Rhipicephalus* ticks from cattle was followed by the appearance of monocytic rickettsiae in a piglet as well as in a calf, without disease symptoms. Subinoculation of brain or spleen material from fatal cases induced fatal ehrlichiosis in experimental piglets. This work has unfortunately not been followed up and conclusive confirmation of the identity of the organism as *E. bovis* has not been obtained.

E. bovis could be transmitted to monkeys (*Macaca inua*),[19] which reacted with fever and rickettsiemia, while 2 out of 3 animals also showed transient general disease symptoms.

Attempts to infect dogs, rabbits, mice and guinea pigs with *E. bovis*, using blood or cell culture, failed.[1,4,17]

Geographic Distribution

Infections with *E. bovis* have been reported from all parts of Africa,[6,19–22] Iran,[2,23] the Indian subcontinent[14,24] and Brazil.[25] The reported distribution of *E. ovina* covers much of the same ground: northern, southern and western Africa,[11,26,27] Turkey and Iran[11,13] and the Indian subcontinent and Sri Lanka.[12,28] It has not been reported from the Western Hemisphere.

It has been suggested[29] that a mysterious disease of cattle in Guadeloupe might be caused by *E. bovis* but it was later found to be heartwater. This suggestion may have been responsible for the reported occurrence of bovine ehrlichiosis in some Caribbean islands[30] but this remains to be confirmed.

Pathogenesis

The pathogenesis has not been studied.

Clinical Disease

In most countries *E. bovis* is not thought to cause serious disease in cattle[10,19,23,31,32] or buffalo.[14] In South Africa, affected animals were reported to be more susceptible to theileriosis and babesiosis and one animal developed severe and widespread hemorrhages and profound anemia.[33] In Brazil, reported symptoms include fever, enlargement of peripheral lymph nodes, apathy, anorexia and loss of weight, clinical signs being more evident in debilitated cattle.[4,5]

A very different picture has been presented in central and western Africa: *E. bovis* has been reported to cause serious disease in zebu cattle in Mali, Central African Republic and Ivory Coast. The disease is known by the Fulani name of "Nofel", meaning "ear".[17,22,34–36] The disease occurs mainly during the rainy season or the beginning of the dry season. In the most characteristic acute form one ear, less often both, is held down over the parotid region and the head is tilted towards that side. The animal shakes its head frequently, as if to get rid of a foreign body, does not eat and is indifferent to its surroundings. Finelle[35] mentions itching and swelling of the ears. There is moderate hyperthermia. Nervous symptoms similar to those seen in heartwater develop but there are no terminal convulsions. Few animals recover from this form. Death occurs 12 to 48 h after the first symptoms. Other symptoms include swelling of the lymph nodes, mucosal congestion and lachrymation.

Losses of 10 to over 20% have been reported but the infection is usually mild.[35,37] It becomes more severe in animals whose resistance has been lowered due to unfavorable climatic conditions or intercurrent disease.[35]

The parotid lymph node is markedly edematous, inflamed and painful, which may explain the "sign of the ear".

In Senegal, bovine ehrlichiosis has been described as a serious and often fatal disease of imported cattle.[1] Out of 12 Sahiwal cattle imported from Tunisia, 10 contracted the disease, 4 died and 6 recovered after chlortetracycline treatment. Two of the animals showed a peracute form and died in about 12 h, one with spectacular nervous symptoms. The acute form lasted for 5–8 days. The author observed the "sign of the ear" in only one fatal case. The animal was listless and indifferent and it did not eat or ruminate. It had accelerated respiration and heart rates and suffered from diarrhea. Often there were nervous symptoms, varying from a transient paralysis of the pharynx or hyperexcitability, to central nervous symptoms, resembling those of heartwater.

A 3 month old Ndama calf, kept in a stable since birth, contracted an inapparent form of the infection after having been put out to pasture. It should be noted that in the Ivory Coast the disease was reported in zebu cattle moved southward by their Fulani owners to escape drought conditions, while local taurine cattle were not clinically affected.[36]

Gueye[38] considers bovine ehrlichiosis in Senegal to be an important disease of exotic cattle, while it is generally subclinical in local animals. Severe losses occur in European and Asian dairy cattle, unless early treatment or tick control is applied.

Experimentally infected animals usually show subclinical or mild disease and no fatal cases of "ear disease" have been reproduced.

Infection of sheep with *E. ovina* is considered to be mild by several authors, while others present quite a different picture.

In North Africa, Lestoquard and Donatien[11] considered it to cause a mild disease with little mortality, but in southern Africa *E. ovina* has been associated with a very acute and fatal disease in sheep but not goats.[27] It was suggested that helminthiasis, tick infestation and nutritional factors may have contributed to the heavy mortality.

Neitz[13] did not consider *E. ovina* to be an important pathogen by itself but believed that intercurrent disease may enhance its pathogenicity. He reported that infected animals recovered after a mild clinical disease characterized by a febrile period lasting 3–10 days, with anemia, listlessness and anorexia.

E. ovina was reported to have caused a fatal disease in a small flock of cross-bred Astrakhan–Mauritian sheep, introduced from Mauritania into Senegal.[39] Eleven of the 13 sheep died with symptoms similar to heartwater. *C. ruminantium* was found only in one case but *E. ovina* was detected in all of the animals. The animals died within 2–4 days after showing the clinical signs of anorexia, weakness, muscular trembling, drunken gait and bulging eyes but were without the terminal convulsions typical of cowdriosis. Typical clusters of *Ehrlichia* were demonstrated in the blood of affected animals.[39]

In Senegal, numerous fatal cases of *E. ovina* infection were reported in sheep which were moved from the arid Sahel zone, to a more humid area.[40] In Mali infection was reported in a flock of sheep sent from a low rainfall area to a more humid zone. Over 50% died in less than 3 weeks.[41] There was a high fever and the lymph nodes were swollen. *E. ovina* was demonstrated in lung smears of some of the animals that were killed in extremis, but it is not clear whether the author attributed the mortality to ehrlichiosis. Later,[17] he considered that the high pathogenicity reported by others[26,27,39] had not been conclusively proven and that heartwater may well have been involved.

In Sri Lanka[12] *E. ovina* caused disease in a ram imported from Australia. Treatment with oxytetracycline for 4 days brought temporary improvement, but the animal later died with pneumonia and heavy *Haemonchus* infestation.

Hematology

Monocytosis and eosinopenia appear to be the main changes in bovine ehrlichiosis and are considered to be important for diagnostic purposes,[3,37] as the rickettsiae may be rare. Degenerative changes of leucocytes and thrombocytes have been reported.[3,33]

A monocytosis has also been reported in terminal *E. ovina* infections.[39]

Pathology

In Senegal, lesions in cattle resembled those of heartwater, including hydropericardium, hydrothorax, ascites, acute pulmonary edema and swollen lymph nodes. In addition, there may be congestion of subcutaneous conjunctive tissue and superficial skin muscles. A careful search in all fatal cases for cowdriosis gave negative results.[1] Striking histopathological lesions were limited to necrosis and lysis of the cells of the uriniferous tubules of the kidneys, while the glomeruli were not affected.[3]

The main macroscopical lesions of the "Nofel" disease syndrome are swelling of the superficial lymph nodes, particularly the parotid gland and an increase in the cerebrospinal fluid.[34,37] In fatal cases of *E. ovina* infections,[39] hydropericardium, hydrothorax, splenomegaly and swollen lymph nodes may be present.

Immunity

Animals which have recovered from acute infections remain as carriers for variable periods. The duration and nature of immunity is not known but splenectomy and possibly other immunodepressive factors may provoke a relapse.

Diagnosis

A tentative diagnosis of ehrlichiosis is justified only in cattle with typical clinical signs of the syndrome of "ear disease" or "Nofel" in West and Central Africa, and should be confirmed by demonstrating the organism in mononuclear blood cells, in conjunction with monocytosis and eosinopenia.

Otherwise, clinical signs of febrile disease in sheep or cattle only warrant suspicion of ehrlichiosis when associated with the presence of *Ehrlichia* in mononuclear cells, in areas where the organisms are known to occur. Presence of the organisms without clinical and hematological signs may mean no more than that the animal is a healthy carrier. Other possible causes of disease, in particular heartwater, should be carefully considered and eliminated.

The rickettsiae can be demonstrated by staining blood or organ smears with Giemsa. According to Neitz,[13] *E. ovina* may be found as soon as the temperature rises, but more readily so from the third day of fever.

Treatment

Sulfonamides do not appear to be effective against "Nofel".[17,34]

Daily doses of 4–5 mg/kg of chlortetracycline administered intravenously for 4–5 days was effective against the acute form of *E. bovis* infection, but intramuscular injections of penicillin–streptomycin or tetracycline intramuscularly had no effect.

Pierre[36] reported that treatment of the whole herd with 3–5 intramuscular injections of 750 mg of oxytetracycline may stop outbreaks of bovine ehrlichiosis. Treatment was not successful when the parotid lymph node was affected.

Compounds active against other members of the order *Rickettsiales*, including imidocarb and rifampicin, should be tried.

No data on the treatment of ovine ehrlichiosis are available.

Control

Apart from the method of herd treatment of cattle,[36] intensive tick control appears to be the only way of prevention. Local circumstances will determine the cost/benefit of such measures (value of the animals, virulence, other stress factors, presence of other tick-borne diseases, etc.).

Other Ehrlichia Infections of Small Ruminants

Manjrekar[42,43] reported a non-fatal rickettsial infection of monocytes of sheep and goats in India, resembling *E. ovina*. The organism was named *Rickettsia belgaumii* and considered to be different from *E. ovina*, as guinea pigs could be infected and the infection could be transmitted from guinea pigs to small ruminants. It could also be maintained in white rats. It was transmitted to small ruminants by injecting homogenized *Haemaphysalis bispinosa* ticks. Tests in guinea pigs suggested reciprocal cross-immunity with *R. typhi*, but recovered sheep and goat sera neutralized *R. belgaumii* but not *R. typhi*. It is difficult to reach conclusions in the absence of further evidence.

Another rickettsial organism described in India in sheep as *Cytoecetes ovis* var. *deccani*[44] occurred mainly in granulocytes. As there is no other ehrlichia with the specific name of ovis, the designation "var. *deccani*" is not justified. The organism caused no mortality. The infection could be transmitted by subcutaneous injection of homogenized *Rhipicephalus haemaphysaloides* ticks collected from recovered animals. Goats and cattle could also be infected, but not rabbits, guinea pigs or dogs. It is not known whether this organism is different from *Cytoecetes phagocytophila*.

References

1. Rioche, M. 1966. La rickettsiose générale bovine au Sénégal. *Rev. Elev. Méd. vét. Pays Trop.* **19:** 485–494.
2. Donatien A. and Lestoquard, F. 1936. *Rickettsia bovis,* nouvelle espèce pathogène pour le boeuf. *Bull. Soc. Path. Exot.* **29:** 1057–1061.
3. Rioche, M. 1967. Lésions microscopiques de la rickettsiose générale bovine à *Rickettsia (Ehrlichia) bovis* (Donatien & Lestoquard 1936). *Rev. Elev. Méd. vét. Pays Trop.* **20:** 415–427.
4. Massard, C. de A. 1984. *Ehrlichia bovis* (Donatien & Lestoquard, 1936). Diagnóstico, cultivo *in vitro* e aspectos epidimiológicos em bovinos no Brasil. Summary of Ph.D. Thesis, Universidade Federal Rural do Rio de Janeiro.
5. Araújo, T. 1985. Aspectos da infecçao experimental por *Ehrlichia bovis* (Donatien & Lestoquard, 1936) em bezerros. M.Sc. Thesis, Universidade Federal de Minais Gerais.
6. Morzaria, S.P., Irvin, A.D., Kocan, K.M. and Voigt, W.P. 1985. Isolation and characterization of an *Ehrlichia* sp. from cattle in Kenya. Workshop on diseases caused by leukcocytic rickettsiae of man and animals, University of Illinois, Urbana-Champaign: Abstr. 30.
7. Van Vliet, A.H.M., Jongejan, F. and Van Der Zeijst, B.A.M. 1992. Phylogenetic position of *Cowdria ruminantium* (Rickettsiales) based on analysis of amplified 16S rRNA sequences. *Int. J. Syst. Bact.* **42:** 494–498.
8. Hoogstraal, H. and Kaiser, M.N. 1959. Observations on Egyptian *Hyalomma* ticks (Ixodoidea, Ixodidae). 5. Biological notes and differences in identity of *H. anatolicum* and its subspecies *anatolicum* Koch and *excavatum* Koch among Russian and other workers. Identity of *H. lusitanicum* Koch. *Ann. Ent. Soc. Am.* **52:** 243–261.
9. Neitz, W.O. 1956. A consolidation of our knowledge of the transmission of tick-borne diseases. *Onderstepoort. J. Vet. Res.* **27:** 115–163

10. MATSON, B.A. 1966. Epizootiology and control of tick borne diseases of cattle in Rhodesia. *Rhod. Agric. J.* **63:** 118–122.
11. LESTOQUARD, F. and DONATIEN, A. 1936. Sur une nouvelle *Rickettsia* du mouton. *Bull. Soc. Path. Exot.* **29:** 105–108.
12. SENEVIRATNA, P. and JAINUDEEN, M.R. 1967. The presence of *Ehrlichia ovina*-like organisms in the mononuclear cells of sheep in Ceylon. *Ceylon vet. J.* **15:** 141.
13. NEITZ, W.O. 1968. *Ehrlichia ovina* infection. *Bull. Off. Int. Epiz.* **70:** 337–340.
14. MOHAN, R.N. 1968. Diseases and parasites of buffaloes. *Vet. Bull.* **38:** 567–576.
15. GUEYE, A., CAMICAS, J.L., DIOUF, A. and MBENGUE, M. 1987. Tiques et hémoparasitoses du bétail au Sénégal. II. La zone sahélienne. *Rev. Elev. Méd. vét. Pays Trop.* **40:** 119–125.
16. GUEYE, A., MBENGUE, M. and DIOUF, A. 1989. Tiques et hémoparasitoses du bétail au Sénégal. IV. La zone sud-soudanienne. *Rev. Elev. Méd. vét. Pays Trop.* **42:** 517–528.
17. ROUSSELOT, R. 1953. Notes de Parasitologie tropicale. Tome I. Parasites du sang des animaux. *Vigot Frères:* 152 pp.
18. RIOCHE, M. and BOURDIN, P. 1968. Rickettsiose des monocytes observée chez le porc au Sénégal. *Rev. Elev. Méd. vét. Pays Trop.* **21:** 455–461.
19. DONATIEN, A. and LESTOQUARD, F. 1940. Rickettsiose bovine algérienne à *R. bovis*. *Bull. Soc. Path. Exot.* **32:** 245–248.
20. DE KOCK, G., VAN HEERDEN, C.J., DU TOIT, R. and NEITZ, W.O. 1937. Bovine theileriasis in South Africa with special reference to *Theileria mutans*. *Onderstepoort J. Vet. Sci. Anim. Ind.* **8:** 9–125.
21. MALBRANT, R., BAYROU, M. and RAPIN, P. 1939. Protozooses sanguines des animaux domestiques en Afrique Equatoriale Française. *Bull. Soc. Path. Exot.* **31:** 953–950.
22. ROUSSELOT, R. 1942. Sur quelques hémocytozooses connues ou inconnues du Soudan Français. *Bull. Serv. Zootechn. Epizoot. Afr. Occid. Fr.* **5:** 210–224.
23. DELPY, L. 1937. Les theilériosis bovines en Iran. *Arch. Inst. Pasteur Algérie* **15:** 225–264.
24. EBENEZER, RAJA, E., JOSEPH, S.A. and LALITHA, C.M. 1980. Some observations on the mode of multiplication of intralymphoid stage of *Theileria annulata* in the bovine host. In: *Haemoprotozoan Diseases of Domestic Animals,* pp. 57–66. GAUTAM, O.P., SHARMA, R.D. and DHAR, S. (Eds), The Commonwealth Veterinary Association, Asian/Australian regions.
25. MASSARD, C. DE A. and MASSARD, C.L. 1982. *Ehrlichia bovis (Rickettsiales:* Rickettsiaceae) em Gado de Leite no Brasil. *Arq. Univ. Fed. Rur. Rio de J.* **5:** 237–239.
26. CURASSON, G. 1941. La rickettsiose générale ovine au Sénégal. (Première note.) (La maladie expérimentale.) *Bull. Serv. Zootechn. Epizoot. Afr. Occid. Fr.* **4:** 34–36.
27. SCHULZ, K. 1939. A rickettsiosis new to South Africa. *J. S. Afr. vet. Med. Ass.* **10:** 176–178.
28. RAY, H.N. 1950. In: RAO, V.N.A., PALANISWAMI, K.S., GHELLAPPA, D.J., JOSEPH, S.A. and GNANABARANAM, J.F. 1991. A report on concurrent haemoprotozon and rickettsial infections in sheep. *Indian Vet. J.* **68:** 487–488.
29. FLOCH, H., CAPPONI, M. and GIROUD, P. 1972. Une rickettsiose bovine probable en Guadeloupe; difficultés du diagnostic. *Bull. Soc. Path. Exot.* **65:** 194–198.
30. SCOTT, G.R. 1990. Diseases caused by rickettsia. In: *Handbook on Animal*

Diseases in the Tropics, pp. 227–256. SEWELL, M.M.H. and BROCKLESBY, D.W. (Eds), 4th edn. Baillière Tindall.

31. LEEFLANG, P. and ILEMOBADE, A.A. 1977. Tick-borne diseases of domestic animals in northern Nigeria. II. Research summary, 1966–1976. *Trop. Anim. Hlth Prod.* **9:** 211–218.
32. NORVAL, R.A.I. 1979. Tick infestations and tick-borne diseases in Zimbabwe–Rhodesia. *J. S. Afr. vet. Ass.* **50:** 289–292.
33. DE VOS, A.J. 1981. *Rhipicephalus appendiculatus*: cause and vector of diseases in Africa. *J. S. Afr. vet. Ass.* **52:** 315–322.
34. GIRARD, H. and ROUSSELOT, R. 1945. La rickettsiose bovine à *Rickettsia bovis* au Soudan Français. *Bull. Soc. Path. Exot.* **38:** 64–77.
35. FINELLE, P. 1958. Rickettsiose à *Rickettsia bovis* en Oubangui-Chari. *Rev. Elev. Méd vét. Pays Trop.* **11:** 291–292.
36. PIERRE, F. 1983. L'ehrlichiose bovine en Côte d'Ivoire. Epidémiologie–traitement–prophylaxie. *Rev. Elev. Méd. vét Pays Trop.* **36:** 337–341.
37. GIRARD, H. and ROUSSELOT, R. 1947. Les rickettsioses animales au Soudan. Rickettsioses bovine and ovine. Rickettiose canine and heartwater. *Encyclopédie vét. Périod.* **4:** 403–418.
38. GUEYE, A. 1988. Tiques et maladies transmises au Sénégal. Données actuelles. *Rev. Sénég. Rech. Agric. Halieut.* **1:** 30–35.
39. CURASSON, G. 1942. La rickettsiose ovine au Sénégal. (Deuxiéme note.) (Maladie naturelle.) *Bull. Serv. Zootechn. Epizoot. Afr. Occid. Fr.* **5:** 3–8.
40. GUEYE, A., MBENGUE, M., DIOUF, A. and VASSILIADÈS, G. 1989. Prophylaxie de la cowdriose et observations sur la pathologie ovine dans la région des Niayes au Sénégal. *Rev. Elev. Méd. vét. Pays Trop.* **42:** 497–503.
41. ROUSSELOT, R. 1943. Sur quelques hémocytozooses connues ou inconnues du Soudan français. (Deuxième note.) *Bull. Soc. Zootechn. Epizoot. Afr. Occid. Fr.* **6:** 75–83.
42. MANJREKAR, S.L. 1951. Rickettsiosis in sheep and goats, in the State of Bombay. Thesis, Poona: 77 pp. (Summary in: *Vet. Bull.* **1954, 24:** 377–378).
43. MANJREKAR, S.L. 1954. Rickettsia of domesticated animals. (A short review.) *Ind. J. vet. Sci. Anim. Husb.* **24:** 217–222.
44. RAGHAVACHARI, K. and REDDY, A.M.K. 1959. *Cytoecetes ovis* var. *deccani* (n.sp.) as the cause of tick-borne fever in sheep in India. *Ind. J. vet. Sci. Anim. Husb.* **29:** 69–86.

16

Salmon Poisoning Disease

J. R. GORHAM AND W. J. FOREYT

Introduction

Salmon poisoning disease (SPD) or salmon disease, a highly fatal helminth-transmitted disease of domestic and wild Canidae, occurs indigenously on the western slopes of the Cascade Mountains from northern California to southwestern Washington (Fig. 16.1), with additional occurrences in southern Vancouver Island in British Columbia.[1] Occasionally, cases of SPD occur outside the indigenous range of the disease in areas where infected fish migrate or are transported. The disease is caused by two closely related rickettsiae, the salmon poisoning disease agent (*Neorickettsia helminthoeca*), and the Elokomin fluke fever agent that was designated as *Neorickettsia elokominica*. Rickettsia in the salmon disease complex are antigenically distinct from other pathogenic rickettsiae which infect dogs. Although SPD was first reported in Henry's Astoria Journal in 1814; the causative agent was not discovered until 1950.[2]

Causative Agent

The etiologic agent of clinical SPD, *Neorickettsia helminthoeca*, is classified in the Order, Rickettsiales, family Rickettsiaceae, and Tribe Ehrlichieae. The organism is a coccoid or coccobacillary rickettsia that is approximately 0.3 μm in size. Pleomorphic rods, up to 2 μm in length, sometimes bent in rings or crescents, have been observed. The gram-negative rickettsial organisms appear purple with Giemsa stain, red with Macchiavello's stain, black or dark brown with Levaditi's method, and pale blue with hematoxylin and eosin. The rickettsiae almost fill the cytoplasm of cells of the mononuclear phagocyte system (MPS) that they primarily infect. Initial attempts to grow the organism in embryonated chicken eggs, bacteriologic media and duck embryo tissue cultures, have been unsuccessful, but

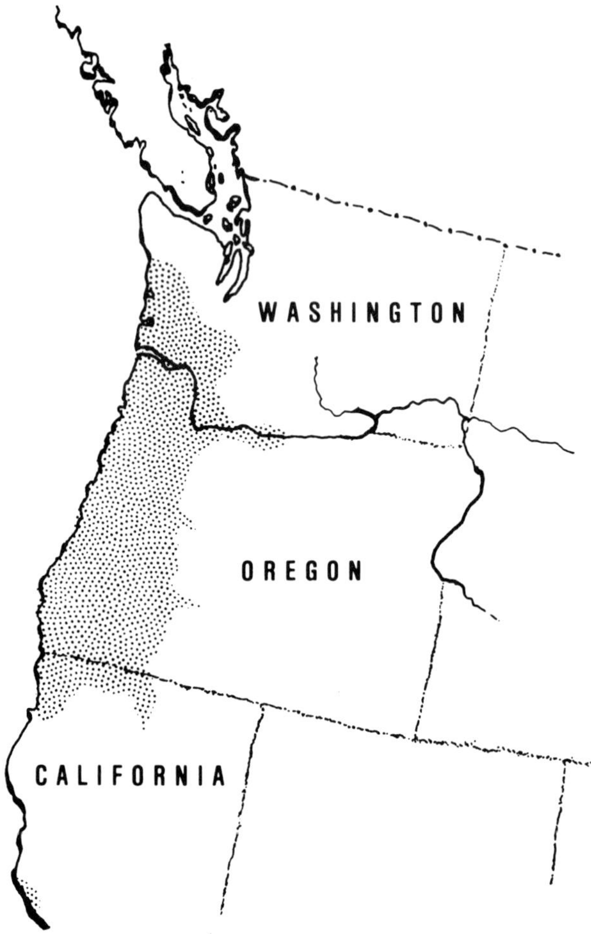

FIG. 16.1. Distribution of indigenous salmon poisoning disease. Area indicated by slashed lines represents the distribution of *Oxytrema silicula* and the usual distribution of salmon poisoning disease. Area indicated by dots represents occasional cases of salmon poisoning disease usually resulting from infected migrating fish (with permission from Dr Craig E. Greene and W. B. Saunders Company).

rickettsiae have been grown in canine monocytes,[3] in canine leukocytes and sarcoma cells and in mouse lymphoblasts.[4]

In live fish, rickettsiae in metacercariae (encysted trematode larvae) probably survive for more than a year, but in dead fish, rickettsiae in metacercariae do not ever survive for 30 days at 4°C.[5] In lymph nodes, organisms resist freezing at −20°C for 31 to 158 days;[6] they remain viable in leukocytes at 4.5°C for 48 h and at 52.5°C for

2 min, but not at 60°C for 5 min.[7] At −80°C, the agent can be maintained in cell culture fluid for up to 3 months.[8]

The Elokomin fluke fever (EFF) agent is often classified as *N. elokominica*,[9] but probably is another strain of *N. helminthoeca*, rather than a separate species.[3,10] The disease in dogs associated with the EFF agent results in high morbidity but a lower mortality than SPD. It appears that metacercariae can harbor both EFF and SPD agents simultaneously. The EFF agent was isolated from salmon in the Elokomin River in southwestern Washington, but is rarely recognized as a distinct entity in the naturally occurring disease. Histologically, EFF infections in dogs are similar to but less severe than those seen with SPD.

Epidemiology

The vector of SPD is a trematode, *Nanophyetus salmincola*, which harbors the rickettsiae throughout its life cycle stages from egg to adult.[11] Three different hosts, snails, fish and mammals or birds are required for the completion of the trematode life cycle (Fig. 16.2).

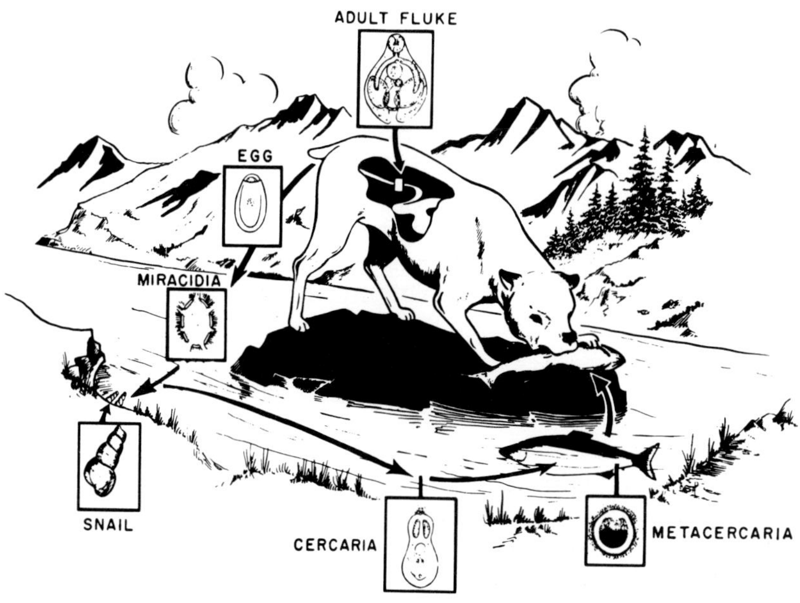

FIG. 16.2. Epizootiology of *Nanophyetus salmincola* and salmon poisoning disease (with permission from Dr Craig E. Greene and W. B. Saunders Company).

The snail intermediate host, *Oxytrema silicula*, is a pleurocerid that inhibits fresh or brackish stream water in coastal areas of Washington, Oregon, and northern California. Areas of trematode infection therefore depend on the distribution of *O. silicula*. Cercariae (free-swimming trematode larvae) leave the snail and penetrate the second intermediate host, which is usually a salmonid fish, certain species of nonsalmonid fish, or the Pacific giant salamander (*Dicamptodon ensatus*). The metacercariae usually localize in the kidneys of fish but can be found in any tissue or in the slime on the surface of the fish. Fish are infected in fresh water and retain the trematode and the rickettsial infection throughout their ocean migration before returning to fresh water up to 3 years later.[12]

Trematodes develop to the adult stage in the intestine approximately 6 days after the ingestion of metacercariae-infected fish by dogs and certain other fish-eating mammals, such as bears and raccoons, and birds, that serve as definitive hosts. Lists of intermediate and definitive hosts of the fluke can be found elsewhere.[11] Clinical signs of rickettsial disease occur in Canidae, primarily dogs and coyotes. However, two captive polar bears receiving long-term glucocorticoid therapy for skin conditions succumbed to an SPD-like disease after eating inadequately frozen salmon.[13] Cats are not susceptible to SPD, but trematide will develop when infected fish are ingested.[11]

SPD also has been transmitted by parenteral injection of infected blood, spleen and lymph suspensions, adult flukes, helminth-infected snail livers, and helminth eggs. Partial transmission success was obtained by transferring ticks (*Haemaphysalis leachi* and *Rhipicephalus sanguineus*) that had fed on infected dogs to susceptible dogs and by parenteral injection of suspensions of *R. sanguineus* into dogs.[14] Susceptible dogs have also been experimentally infected with aerosolized lymph node suspensions from infected dogs, and on rare occasions, by direct transmission of infection between dogs has been suspected.[7,15]

Pathogenesis

After ingestion of raw, metacercariae-infected salmonid fish by a susceptible dog, the fluke matures, and the adult stage attaches to the mucosa of the intestine and by some unknown mechanism inoculates the rickettsiae. Initial replication of rickettsiae probably takes place in the epithelial cells of the villi or in the intestinal lymphoid tissue. Inflammation of the solitary lymphoid follicles and Peyer's patches along the intestinal tract contributes to enteritis. Mild enteritis and diarrhea may be observed in dogs infected only with the flukes, without rickettsiae. In those cases, lymphadenopathy is not present and infected dogs and coyotes remain alert and active, but often have diarrhea or diarrhea with blood. Massive infection of a cougar (*Felis concolor*) kitten with approximately 650,000 flukes apparently resulted in its death due to malnutrition from impaired nutrient absorption.[16] Similar cases in dogs have not been observed.

Rickettsiae enter the blood early in the course of the disease and spread to the lymph nodes, spleen, tonsils, thymus, liver, lungs, and brain.[10] Although secondary bacterial infections often occur, the exact cause of death in SPD is unknown. Definitive investigations to demonstrate a toxin have been limited.

Clinical Disease

The signs of infection are consistent in all Canidae infected with SPD. The usual incubation period following the ingestion of parasitized fish is 5–7 days, although some dogs have incubation periods as long as 19–33 days. The first sign usually is a sudden febrile response, which typically reaches a peak of 40–42°C (104–107.6°F) (Fig. 16.3). The temperature gradually decreases to

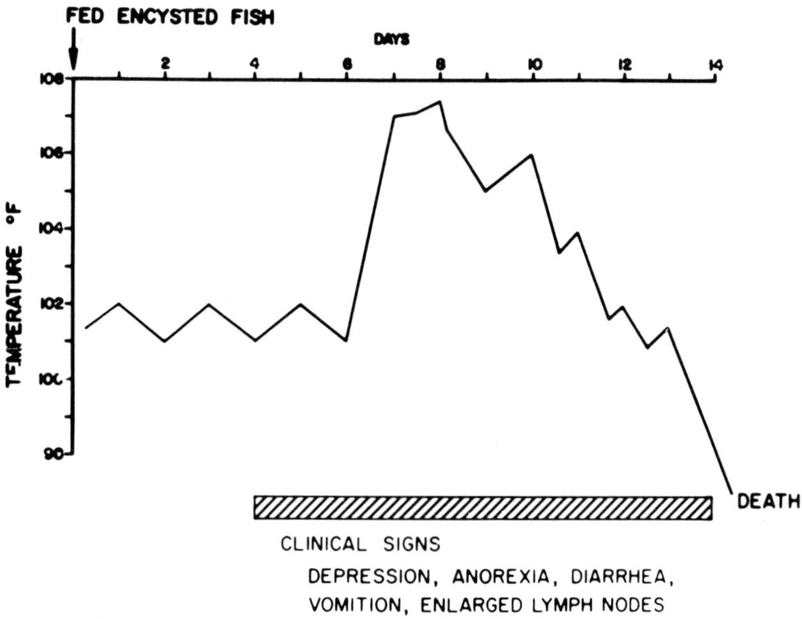

FIG. 16.3. Clinical course of salmon poisoning disease in a dog (with permission from Dr Craig E. Greene and W. B. Saunders Company).

normal or below normal over the next 4–8 days. Dogs are frequently hypothermic when death occurs 7 to 10 days after the initial clinical evidence of infection. Some animals show only a slight increase in temperature or a shortened febrile period; however, they may still die if left untreated. In untreated cases of SPD, the mortality rate is approximately 90%.

Anorexia frequently accompanies or follows the onset of fever and may be marked and complete. Affected animals often continue to have inappetence throughout the course of the disease. Marked weight loss, weakness and depression usually follow. Within 14 days of eating infected fish, coyotes on a controlled experiment lost approximately 58% of their body weight when compared with uninfected coyotes.[5] Diarrhea and vomiting may occur, the diarrhea becoming progressively worse and often consisting primarily of blood at the time of death. The animal will occasionally exhibit extreme thirst and will drink copious quantities of water. A serous nasal discharge may be recorded early in the febrile period. Later, a mucopurulent conjunctival exudate may be seen. Enlarged cervical and prescapular lymph nodes can be palpated as early as 5 days p.i., and are present throughout the infection period.[20]

SPD-infected dogs may show severe GI signs that are often clinically indistinguishable from canine parvovirus enteritis. Distemper, canine parvovirus and SPD can occur concurrently, and appropriate laboratory tests can be conducted to determine which agent is involved in a particular animal.

Elokomin Fluke Fever

The incubation period for Elokomin fluke fever is generally 5–12 days. The febrile period, which differs from that of SPD, is marked by a plateau of elevated temperature lasting 4–7 days, followed by a decline, usually to subnormal temperature.[9] Other signs are similar to those of SPD.

Pathology

The principal gross findings at necropsy are changes in lymphoid tissues. The tonsils, thymus and visceral and somatic nodes are markedly enlarged. The most pronounced swelling occurs in the ileocecal, colic, mesenteric, portal and lumbar nodes. The nodes are usually yellowish, with prominent white foci representing the cortical follicles. Occasionally, nodes show diffuse petechiae, and edema is often observed.

The spleen frequently ranges from slightly swollen to nearly twice the normal size. Splenic follicles, which often appear as grayish white nodules in foxes, are not observed in dogs. The spleens of animals that die of SPD are typically a dark bluish red, smooth, soft, and bloodfilled. Livers of dogs are usually normal, although those of foxes are usually soft and pale yellowish brown. Hemorrhages may appear in the gallbladder wall. Petechiae may be the only change in the pancreas. The kidneys of dogs are grossly normal, whereas those of foxes may have a slight color change toward a pale yellowish brown. The mucosa of the urinary bladder may show petechiae.

Along the intestinal tract, petechiae may be apparent in the mucosae of the lower esophagus, large intestine, ileocolic valve, distal colon, rectum, and gastric serosa. There may be bleeding ulcers in the pylorus. Intussusception of the ileum into the colon may also occur. The intestinal contents frequently contain free blood. Some blood may also appear in the colon and rectum. The intestines are typically empty except for some bile-stained mucus. Flukes can be observed in the small and large intestine, primarily in the duodenum, and cause some tissue damage. Adult flukes are very small (0.5–1.2 mm) and are often difficult to observe, even though thousands are often present.

Microscopically, a characteristic pattern is observed in lymphocytic tissues. The lymph nodes show a marked and consistent depletion in the number of mature lymphocytes, with hyperplasia of the MPS cells in the cortex and medulla. In most foxes and dogs, there are foci of necrosis in the MPS cells. The central nervous system is occasionally involved with nonsuppurative meningitis or meningoencephalitis.[17]

Hematologic and biochemical findings of SPD infected domestic dogs are often nonspecific and total leukocyte counts have ranged from leukopenia to leukocytosis.[18] Laboratory results of 45 dogs representing 17 breeds and various mixed breeds that were naturally infected with SPD are presented in Table 16.1. Thrombocytopenia (in 88% of the dogs tested), lymphopenia (77%), eosinopenia (77%), increased alkaline phosphatase values (64%) and reduced serum albumin values (49%) were the consistent findings.[19] In experimentally infected coyotes, significantly higher numbers of band cells, lower numbers of eosinophils and lower concentrations of creatinine, glucose, calcium, inorganic phosphorus, albumin, and activity of alkaline phosphatase were detected when compared to uninfected coyotes.[5]

Immunology

There is a marked immunological response to *N. helminthoeca*. This is based on anecdotal observations that dogs that have recovered

TABLE 16.1. *Results of Initial Laboratory Tests in Dogs with Salmon Poisoning* (n=45)

	Normal range	Maximum	Minimum	Mean	SD	No. above NR*	No. below NR*	No. of dogs
Leukocytes/μl	6,000–17,000	66,000	4,200	12,800	10,600	6	6	44
Mature neutrophils	3,000–11,500	62,604	1,792	10,908	10,296	13	1	44
Band neutrophils	0–300	2,548	0	168	430	8	0	44
Lymphocytes	1,000–4,800	3,776	92	791	667	0	34	44
Eosinophils	100–1,250	891	0	77	202	0	34	44
Monocytes	150–1,350	4,137	0	824	811	10	0	44
Packed cell volume (%)	37–55	54	25	43	7	1	8	43
Platelet counts $\times 10^3$/dl	200–500	377	16	113	108	0	14	16
Fibrinogen (mg/dl)	200–400	700	100	400	160	14	3	38
Serum sodium (meq/L)	145–154	159	126	141	8	1	13	16
Serum potassium (meq/L)	4.1–5.3	5.3	3.4	4.4	0.5	0	3	16
Serum chloride (meq/L)	105–116	134	84	106	12	1	4	14
Total CO_2	16–26	24	15	18	3	0	4	10
Serum calcium (mg/dl)	9.9–11.4	10.8	7.3	9.1	0.9	0	30	37
Serum phosphorus (mg/dl)	3.0–6.2	7.9	3.0	4.8	1.5	7	0	36
Creatinine (mg/dl)	0.8–1.6	1.7	0.5	1.1	0.5	2	2	17
Blood urea nitrogen (mg/dl)	8–31	90	9	22	19	6	0	37
Serum glucose (mg/dl)	70–118	133	44	92	17	4	2	37
ALT (IU/L)	19–102	499	21	92	83	9	0	37
AST (IU/L)	15–66	274	24	90	60	17	0	35
Alkaline phosphatase (IU/L)	15–150	2,098	60	254	339	23	0	36
Total protein (g/dl)	5.4–7.4	8.2	3.9	5.9	1.1	4	11	37
Albumin (g/dl)	2.5–3.5	3.3	1.6	2.5	0.4	0	18	37
Total bilirubin (mg/dl)	0–0.4	2.0	0	0.4	0.6	4	0	37
Globulins (mg/dl)	2.9–3.9	5.8	1.9	3.4	0.9	9	10	37
Cholesterol (mg/dl)	135–300	408	99	215	85	8	6	37
Age (years)		12	0.3	5.0	3.7			45

*NR = Normal range.
From MACK, BECOVITCH, LING, TOBINGER, MELLI,[19] reprinted with permission.

from the disease are immune to reinfection for several years. Indeed, dog owners in SPD indigenous areas have an occasion intentionally fed their dogs fish containing the fluke vector. They waited for 4 to 6 days until the dog developed the early signs of SPD, and then treated the dog with effective antibiotics. These dogs were considered to have solid immunity to natural challenge infections. This hazardous immunization procedure caused the death of dogs that were treated too late in the course of the disease.

Diagnosis

In the enzootic area of transmission, SPD should always be included as a diagnostic possibility when signs compatible with SPD such as anorexia, depression, diarrhea, or vomiting are present. Operculated trematode eggs appear in dog feces 5 to 8 days following the ingestion of infected fish. The light brown egg is approximately 87–97 μm, with a small, blunt point on the end opposite the indistinct operculum. Eggs can be detected on direct smears or by a washing–sedimentation technique.[20] In addition, the authors routinely recover *Nanophyetus salmincola* eggs with the Sheather's sugar flotation technique (specific gravity, 1.27), and recommend this effective diagnostic technique. Eggs recovered by this latter method are somewhat deformed but recognizable. Fecal flotation tests are more reliable than sedimentation tests or direct fecal smears, and should be used for the diagnosis of the fluke vector. Diagnosis of the rickettsial disease cannot be made entirely on the presence of trematode eggs in feces, because trematode infection does not necessarily indicate rickettsial infection. In addition, animals that have recovered from the rickettsial disease may still shed trematode eggs since adult flukes are not killed by antibiotic therapy, or may be reinfected with the trematode. The trematode infection can remain patent for 60 to 250 days,[5] and dogs or coyotes can be reinfected with flukes.

For rickettsial diagnosis, fluid aspirated from enlarged lymph nodes can be air dried on a microscope slide, fixed, defatted for 1 min with a mixture of equal parts of ether and absolute alcohol, and than stained by Giemsa or Macchiavello's stain. In addition, a rapid-staining Giemsa technique that involves staining the fixed smears for 2 min with equal parts of stock Giemsa and buffered water at pH 7.2 and then washing the slides can be used.[20] Typical intracytoplasmic rickettsial bodies are characteristically seen in MPS cells. Extracellular organisms are not easily separated from artifacts and should not be considered diagnostic for SPD.

Treatment and Control

All patients should be hospitalized so that they receive adequate monitoring and nursing care. Control of the infectious agent, *N. helminthoeca,* can be achieved with oral or parenteral sulfonamides, penicillin, chlortetracycline, chloramphenicol, or oxytetracycline. Aminoglycosides are ineffective. The preferred treatment schedule is oxytetracycline given for at least 3 days (Table 16.2). Oral

TABLE 16.2. *Therapy for Salmon Poisoning Disease**

Drug	Dose† (mg/kg)	Route	Interval (h)	Duration (Days)
Oxytetracycline‡	7	i.v.§	8	3–5
Tetracycline‡	22	p.o.	8	3–5
Praziquantel‖	10–30	p.o., s.c.	Once	

* i.v. = intravenous, p.o. = oral, s.c. = subcutaneous.
† Dose per administration at specified interval, expressed as mg/kg unless otherwise stated.
‡ For rickettsial infection.
§ Parenteral therapy preferred because of GI signs.
‖ For fluke infection.

tetracycline therapy, used for most rickettsial disease, may be difficult and may not be indicated because of the severe vomiting and diarrhea that is usually present.

Relief of dehydration, emesis and diarrhea is also important. Fluid therapy with appropriate electrolytes should be administered i.v. In cases of hemorrhagic diarrhea, transfusion of whole blood may be necessary. Other antidiarrheal treatments include fasting followed by gradual introduction of a bland, high-calorie diet. In addition, the most supportive treatment consists of keeping the dog dry, clean, and warm.

Praziquantel, when given orally or subcutaneously as one dose at 5 mg/kg of body weight is highly effective against *N. salmincola* in coyotes and dogs.[21] Elimination of *N. salmincola* from infected animals will minimize the diarrhea associated from fluke infections alone and will minimize or eliminate fluke eggs from feces.

Vaccines have not been developed against SPD, and therefore, keeping dogs from eating infected fish is the best means of preventing infection. Since fluke metacercariae also occur in the slime of fish, licking fish can also result in infection. Because metacercariae can remain viable for months in rotting fish carcasses, dogs will become infected with the fluke if they eat decomposed fish; however, they may not develop SPD. Also, in many areas, metacercariae apparently contain nonpathogenic rickettsiae.[22] Freezing fish at $-20°C$ for 24 h or thoroughly cooking infected fish will kill both the metacercariae and rickettsiae.[23] Supplemental prevention methods include isolation of dogs with SPD and sterilization of equipment used in association with infected dogs.

Infection of fish in hatcheries, that use natural stream water can be prevented experimentally by passing incoming water through an elecronically charged grid or past an ultrasonic generator and thereby destroying free-living cercariae.[24] These methods have not been utilized on a large scale. Other control techniques such as snail elimination or reduction in wild animal hosts such as raccoons and bears are impractical. In areas of high metacercaria concentrations in fish, supplemental water pumped from wells will reduce the level of fish infection.

References

1. BOOTH, A.J., STOGDALE, L. and GRIGOR, J.A. 1984. Salmon poisoning disease in dogs on southern Vancouver Island. *Can. vet. J.* **25:** 2–6.
2. CORDY, D.R. and GORHAM, J.R. 1950. The pathology and etiology of salmon poisoning disease in the dog and fox. *Am. J. Path.* **26:** 617–637.
3. FRANK, D.W., MCGUIRE, T.C., GORHAM, J.R. and DAVIS, W.C. 1974. Cultivation of two species of *Neorickettsia* in canine monocytes. *J. infect. Dis.* **129:** 257–262.
4. NOONAN, W.E. 1973. *Neorickettsia helminthoeca* in cell culture. Ph.D. diss., Oregan State University, Corvallis, OR.
5. FOREYT, W.J., GORHAM, J.R., GREEN, J.S., LEATHERS, C.W. and LEAMASTER, B.R. 1987. Salmon poisoning disease in juvenile coyotes: clinical evaluation and infectivity of metacercariae and rickettsiae. *J. Wildlife Dis.* **23:** 412–417.
6. PHILIP, C., HADLOW, W.J. and HUGHES, L.E. 1954. Studies on salmon poisoning disease of canines. 1. The rickettsial relationships and pathogenicity of *Neorickettsia helminthoeca*. *Expl. Parasit.* **3:** 336–350.
7. SIMS, B.T. and MUTH, O.H. 1934. Salmon poisoning: transmission and immunization studies. *Proceedings 5th Pacific Sci. Cong.* (1933), pp. 2949–2960.
8. BROWN, J.L., HUXSOLL, D.L., RISTIC, M. and HILDEBRANDT, P.K. 1972. *In vitro* cultivation of *Neorickettsia helminthoeca*, the causative agent of salmon poisoning disease. *Am. J. vet. Res.* **33:** 1695–1700.
9. FARRELL, R.K. 1974. Canine rickettsiosis. In: *Current Veterinary Therapy V*, pp. 985–987. KIRK, R.W. (Ed.), W.B. Saunders Co., Philadelphia.
10. FRANK, D.W., MCGUIRE, T.C., GORHAM, J.R. and FARRELL, R.K. 1974. Lymphoreticular lesions of canine rickettsiosis. *J. infect. Dis.* **129:** 163–171.
11. KNAPP, S.E. and MILLEMANN, R.E. 1981. Salmon poisoning disease. In: *Infectious Diseases of Wild Mammals*, pp. 376–387. DAVIS, J.E. (Ed.), Iowa State University Press, Ames.
12. WEISETH, P.R., FARRELL, R.K. and JOHNSTON, S.D. 1974. Prevalence of *Nanophyetus salmincola* in ocean-caught salmon. *J. Am. vet. Med. Ass.* **165:** 849–850.
13. SCHMIDT, M. 1982. Personal communication. Portland, OR.

14. PHILIP, C.B. 1985. There's always something new under the "parasitological sun" (the unique story of the helminth-borne salmon poisoning disease). *J. Parasit.* **41:** 125–148.
15. BOSMAN, D.D., FARRELL, R.K. and GORHAM, J.R. 1970. Non-endoparasite transmission of salmon poisoning disease of dogs. *J. Am. vet. Med. Ass.* **156:** 1907–1910.
16. KISTNER, T.P., WYSE, D. and SCHMITZ, J.A. 1979. Pathogenicity attributed to massive infection of *Nanophyetus salmincola* in a cougar. *J. Wildlife Dis.* **15:** 419–420.
17. HADLOW, W.J. 1957. Neuropathology of experimental salmon poisoning in dogs. *Am. J. Vet. Res.* **18:** 898–908.
18. SCHALM, O.W. 1978. Leukocyte counts and lymph node cytology in salmon poisoning of dogs. *Canine Pract.* **5:** 59–63.
19. MACK, R.E., BECOVITCH, M.G., LING, G.V., TOBINGER, R.T. and MELLI, A.C. 1990. Salmon disease complex in dogs—A review of 45 cases. *Cal. Vet.* **44:** 42–45.
20. FARRELL, R.K., OTT, R.L. and GORHAM, J.R. 1955. The clinical laboratory diagnosis of salmon poisoning. *J. Am. vet. Med. Ass.* **127:** 241–244.
21. FOREYT, W.J. and GORHAM, J.R. 1987. Evaluation of praziquantel against induced *Nanophyetus salmincola* infections in coyotes and dogs. *Am. J. Vet. Res.* **48:** 563–565.
22. GREEN, J.S., LEAMASTER, B.R., FOREYT, W.J. and WOODRUFF, R.A., 1986. Salmon poisoning disease: research on a potential method of lethal control for coyotes. *Proceedings Twelfth Vertebrate Pest Conference,* pp. 312–317, University of California, Davis, CA.
23. FARRELL, R.K., SOAVE, O.A. and JOHNSTON, S.D. 1974. *Nanophyetus salmincola* infections in kippered salmon. *Am. J. publ. Hlth* **64:** 808–809.
24. FARRELL, R.K., WATSON, R.E. and LLOYD, M. 1973. Effect of ultrasound on trematode cercariae. *J. Parasit.* **59:** 747–748.

17

Heartwater (Cowdriosis)

G. UILENBERG AND E. CAMUS

Introduction

Heartwater is an African tick-borne disease affecting cattle and small ruminants in areas were the vector ticks, *Ambylomma* spp., are present. It was probably encountered as early as 1838 in South Africa.[1] The name heartwater was used because hydropericardium was regarded as a pathognomonic lesion of the disease. However, this lesion is not always present and a more appropriate name would be "cowdriosis". We will use both names indifferently. Cowdry[2] recognized heartwater as the first rickettsial disease of domestic animals and named the causal agent *Rickettsia ruminantium,* later assigned to a new genus *Cowdria,* as *Cowdria ruminantium.*

There seems to be little doubt that it originated in Africa. Its only known natural vectors are African *Amblyomma* ticks, and reports on its occurrence outside the area of distribution of these ticks have never been confirmed.[3] A long-held belief in South Africa that it may have been introduced from Iran was based on the mistaken view about the origin of the resistant blackheaded "Persian" breed of sheep. In fact, this breed is the blackheaded Somali sheep which originates from heartwater-endemic regions of East Africa and not from Iran.[4]

Heartwater is one of the main obstacles to the improvement of livestock productivity in Sub-Saharan Africa. It was first recognized as a major disease in southern Africa after the introduction of exotic breeds. Its importance depends to a very large extent on the type of livestock present. There are very few reliable figures about its importance in local breeds in endemic areas. However, there is no doubt that in endemic areas indigenous cattle are far more resistant than exotic or cross-bred cattle, presumably because of natural selection. In contrast, small ruminants in general, and goats in particular, are not always very resistant. In Guadeloupe an estimated 10% of local Creole goats succumb to the disease annually.[5]

At present it is considered to be the most important disease of cattle in Swaziland, as it prevents the introduction of exotic stock. There is actually a tendency to "downgrade" to the less productive but more resistant local Nguni cattle. Another example of loss of potential production is the situation in Guadeloupe, where the cattle population is almost entirely limited to the Creole zebu, because the disease prevents the introduction of more productive breeds.

For a long time it has remained a poorly known disease, relatively unnoticed and neglected even in Africa itself, except for areas where exotic breeds of cattle and small ruminants were introduced. Heartwater was thought to be restricted to Africa and the surrounding islands until it was reported in the Western Hemisphere in 1980, in Guadeloupe.[6] This discovery created renewed interest in the disease and coincided with the availability of better research tools. For instance, the first useful serological test was developed in 1981[7] and *C. ruminantium* was first successfully cultured *in vitro* in 1985.[8] Further developments in modern biotechnology have recently accelerated research on the subject.

In this chapter, the more recent literature on cowdriosis will be reviewed in some detail, but for a more complete coverage of the literature the reader is referred to earlier reviews.[3–5,9–13]

Causal Agent

Classification

In a series of remarkable studies, Cowdry,[2,14,15] showed that cowdriosis is due to a rickettsial organism, found in the ruminant host in groups or clusters in the cytoplasm of endothelial cells of blood vessels, as well as in epithelial cells of the gut and the gut lumen of the *Amblyomma* vector. The organism was originally named *Rickettsia ruminantium*,[2] and subsequently renamed *Cowdria ruminantium.*[16]

In *Bergey's Manual of Determinative Bacteriology*[17] it is assigned to the Order Rickettsiales, Family Rickettsiaceae, Tribe Ehrlichieae as the only member of the Genus *Cowdria*. Previous suggestions of a close relationship between *Cowdria* and *Chlamydia* have recently been shown to be erroneous.[18–20] Studies on the phylogenetic position of *C. ruminantium*, based on analysis of amplified 16S ribosomal nucleic acid sequences indicated that it is closely related to *Ehrlichia canis* and to the recently discovered human pathogen *E. chaffeensis*. It is also related to other *Ehrlichia* species and to *Anaplasma marginale.*[19,20]

Morphology and Developmental Stages

The diameter of individual organisms in a given cluster is rather uniform, but differs greatly from cluster to cluster, ranging from

0.5–3 μm (Figs 17.1–17.4). This indicates a developmental cycle.[21] It has become possible to assign a sequence to the cycle since the organism can be cultured in endothelial cells and observed over time. *C. ruminantium* divides by binary fission in intracytoplasmic vacuoles, resulting in large groups of "reticulate" bodies. After 3–4 days these develop into smaller intermediate bodies with an electron-dense core, which then condense into electron-dense elementary bodies. The latter are released into the culture medium after the rupture of the host cell. Elementary bodies invade other cells, initiating a new cycle lasting 5–6 days.[22]

Cultural Characteristics

Less than 10 years ago, the numerous attempts to grow *C. ruminantium* in cell culture systems could be summarized in one sentence: "So far *C. ruminantium* has not been cultured *in vitro* and has only survived for 2 weeks".[3]

A real breakthrough occurred in 1985 when workers at Onderstepoort, South Africa, succeeded in cultivating the organism in a bovine endothelial cell line.[8] It was at first thought that irradiation of the cells and centrifugation of the inoculum onto the cells were necessary to initiate cultures but it was later shown that this is not essential.[23,24] Primary endothelial cells from ruminants can also be used. The organism can now be cultured routinely for various research purposes. The cultures may also constitute a laboratory model for screening potential drugs against heartwater.

Molecular Biology

The breakthrough achieved in the cultivation of *C. ruminantium* has made it possible to obtain relatively pure DNA of *C. ruminantium*. Specific diagnostic probes have recently been developed.[25,26,27]

Antigenicity

Immunodominant, conserved proteins have been identified in all of the various stocks tested. Jongejan and Thielemans[28] identified an immunodominant 32 kDa antigen, common to 9 stocks. Rossouw *et al.*[29] also found a common immunodominant (31 kDa) protein and a minor 27 kDa one in 9 stocks. The overall antigenic profile detected by immunoblotting varied considerably between stocks.[28,29]

Antigens inducing protective immunity and their corresponding genes have not yet been identified.

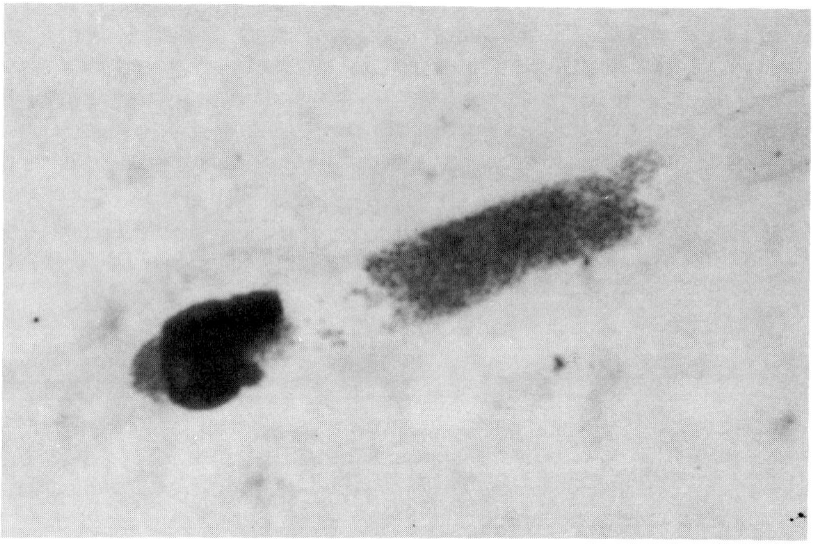

FIG. 17.1. *Cowdria ruminantium*. Elementary bodies in brain capillary of goat. Giemsa staining. Original photograph.

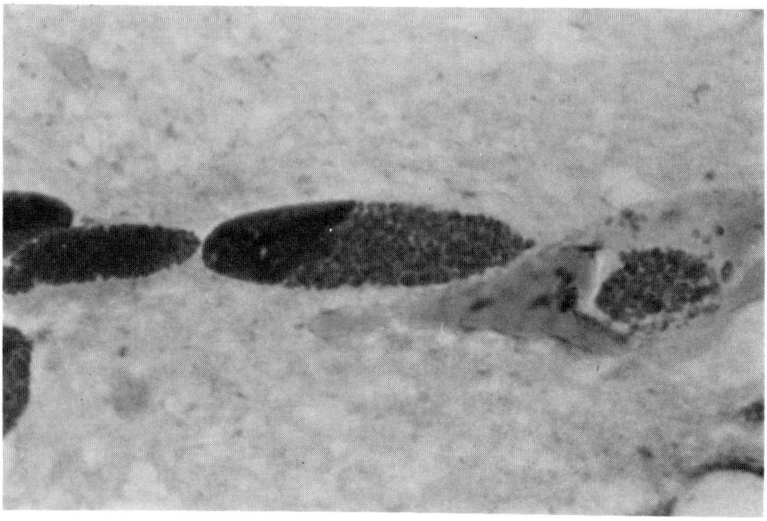

FIG. 17.2. *Cowdria ruminantium*. Intermediate and reticulate bodies in brain capillary of goat. Giemsa staining. Original photograph.

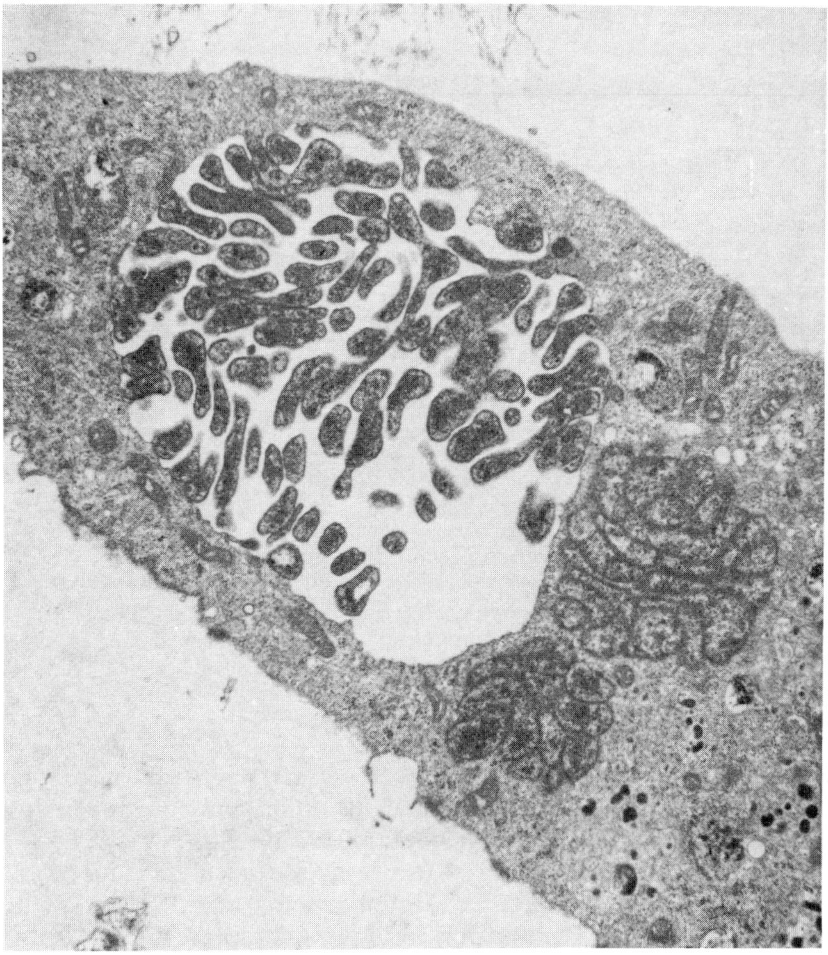

FIG. 17.3. *Cowdria ruminantium*. Elementary bodies in vacuole in cultured bovine umbilical cord endothelial cell. Electron microscope. (Courtesy of F. Jongejan, Utrecht.)

Physico-chemical Properties

C. ruminantium does not survive long outside the host, except when stored at low temperatures. Few figures are available because until recently infectivity could be tested only in ruminants. At room temperature, the infectivity of blood may be lost in less than 12 h,[9] but blood kept on ice retains its infectivity for at least 8 h.[13] The survival of the mouse-pathogenic Kwanyanga stock in different diluents was tested by inoculating mice with diluted infected mouse

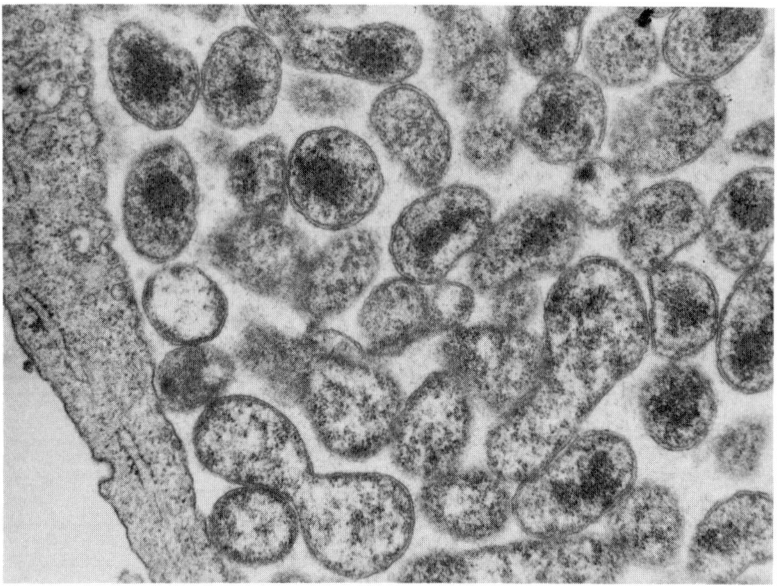

FIG. 17.4. *Cowdria ruminantium*. Intermediate and reticulate bodies in vacuole of cultured bovine umbilical cord endothelial cell. Electron microscope. (Courtesy of F. Jongejan, Utrecht.)

liver kept at 21°C. Sucrose–phosphate–glutamine medium (Snyder I) maintained infectivity best, but with other common diluents or media, infectivity declined considerably within 3 h.[30]

The organism can be stored in the deep-frozen state for years. From a review of the literature,[3] it appears that rapid freezing with dimethylsulphoxide, but not glycerol, as a cryoprotectant is favorable. However, large-scale infectivity assays comparing various methods of cryopreservation have not been carried out. In one study, lyophilized blood remained infective for at least 7 months at −28°C and for at least 3 months at 4°C.[31]

Sensitivity to Drugs

Sulfonamides were the first group of compounds shown to have a certain curative effect.[32] Later, tetracyclines were found to be active[33] and are now practically the only useful drugs for the treatment of the disease. Chlortetracycline, oxytetracycline, rolitetracycline and doxycycline have all been found to be effective.

Many other antibiotics, including penicillin, ampicillin, streptomycin, gentamycin, trobamycin, netilmycin, neomycin, amikacin, kanamycin, polymixin, spectinomycin and chloramphenicol have no effect.[34] Apart from the tetracyclines, the only other antibiotic known to be active is rifampicin.[35]

Now that *C. ruminantium* grows successfully in culture and certain strains are known to be pathogenic to mice, it should be easy to screen compounds in these laboratory models. However, the potential market is very limited and the pharmaceutical industry is not likely to be interested in developing drugs specifically for heartwater. However, any compound shown to be active against related rickettsial organisms should be tested in these laboratory models. Imidocarb has a curative action on anaplasmosis but not on heartwater (N. McHardy, in Ref. 3). Compounds other than sulfonamides and antibiotics are also worth looking at. For instance, a thiosemicarbazone (alpha-ethoxythylglyoxal dithiosemicarbizone = Gloxazone), known to be active against anaplasmosis, was shown to be active on heartwater but it never reached the market because of toxicity problems (B. A. Synge, in Ref. 36).

Epidemiology

Geographic Distribution

As far as is known, the disease is confined to most parts of Sub-Saharan Africa, the neighboring islands of Madagascar, La Reunion, Mauritius, Zanzibar, the Comores and São Tomé and to the Lesser Antilles region of the Carribbean.

The known distribution of the 10 experimentally proven African vectors in the Old World is given in Fig. 17.5. It is likely that the distribution of heartwater covers roughly the same area. It is not known whether it occurs in those parts of the Arabian Peninsula where African *Amblyomma* vectors are present.

The known distribution of the disease and its introduced African vector in the Caribbean region is given in Fig. 17.6. The presence of heartwater in the Antilles was first suspected in 1966 and finally confirmed in 1980.[6] For details, the reader is referred to several historical reviews.[3,37–40] The infection was almost certainly introduced in the 19th century, together with its vector *Amblyomma variegatum*, with cattle from Senegal. In Guadeloupe, the tick is popularly called "la tique senegalaise". Further transports of Senegalese cattle to the French Antilles took place as late as the 1950s (J. P. Marty and P. C. Morel, personal communications). Thus the vector tick and/or infected animals may have been introduced on more than one occasion.

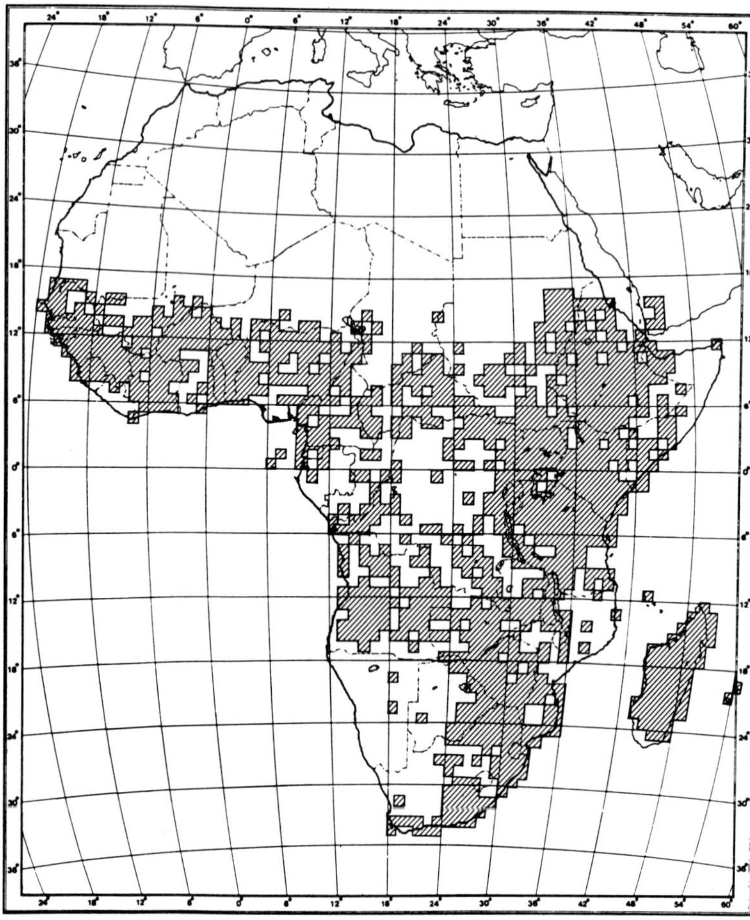

FIG. 17.5. Distribution of *Amblyomma* vectors of heartwater in Africa. (Based on Walker and Olwage.[150]).

However, the known distribution of the disease in the Caribbean is more restricted than that of its introduced vector. The presence of the infection has been confirmed only in Guadeloupe, Marie-Galante and Antigua. Nevertheless, there is serological evidence that the infection may be more widely distributed. Despite the absence of clinical evidence of the disease, antibodies were detected in bovine sera from Dominica, Grenada, Martinique, Montserrat, St. Kitts, St. Lucia, St. Martin and St. Vincent, by various serological tests.[41] Nevertheless, only the actual isolation of the micro-organism on

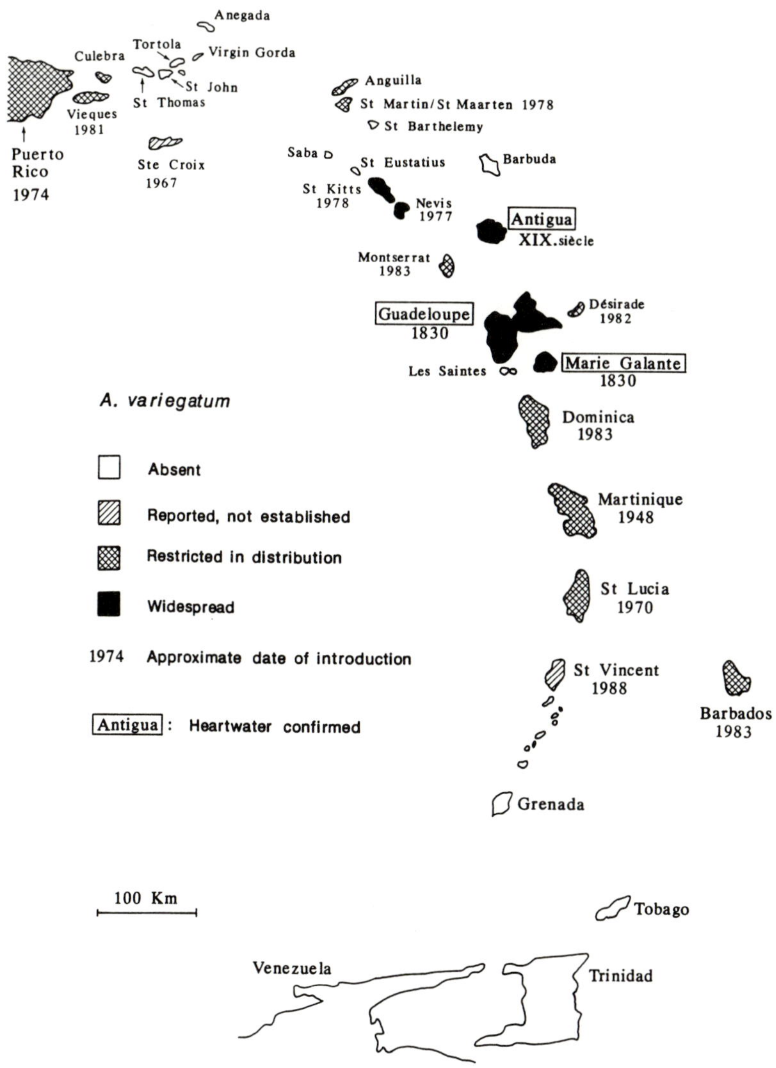

FIG. 17.6. Distribution of *Amblyomma variegatum* and heartwater in the western hemisphere. (Updated from Barré *et al.*[42])

these islands can provide conclusive evidence of the disease because of the possible cross-reactions of *C. ruminantium* with *Ehrlichia* species (Du Plessis *et al.*, unpublished observations). It should also be noted that the vector tick has not been reported from Grenada.

The presence of the disease in the Caribbean constitutes a major threat for the American mainland. This is particularly important for parts of the mainland where *A. variegatum* would be able to maintain itself and areas in which *Amblyomma* ticks capable of experimental transmission are already present.[42] Cowdriosis is, however, not the only serious threat that *A. variegatum* in the Caribbean presents to livestock on the mainland. Severe dermatophilosis is also associated with this tick and is responsible for enormous losses when it first appears.[40]

The threat appears to have greatly increased in recent years. Since 1967, when the tick was discovered on St. Croix, it has spread rapidly, for no apparent reason, until it was found on almost all of the islands from Puerto Rico to Barbados and St. Vincent. It is becoming more and more likely that the spread of the tick is associated with that of the African cattle egret (*Bubulcus ibis*), which invaded the Antilles in the 1950s and started to breed in large numbers shortly after that. In Guadeloupe infestation of the egret by immature *A. variegatum* is light[42,43] but large numbers of birds may be present in one island and are able to move extensively between islands (J. Corn, G. I. Garris, B. Thiébot and N. Barré, unpublished data).

If the role of the egret in the spread of the tick is confirmed, it would be only a matter of time before the tick appears in Trinidad, Venezuela, Hispanolia, Jamaica, Cuba and possibly Florida. Eradication of the tick from the Western Hemisphere must be considered and, if deemed feasible, should be undertaken in the shortest possible time. The invasion of the American continent would be a real disaster for its livestock industry.

Host Range

Cowdriosis is a disease of ruminants. It occurs in cattle, sheep, goats, domestic Asian buffalo and domesticated Java deer in Mauritius. One report on a case in a camel[44] remains unsubstantiated.

Naturally acquired fatal heartwater also occurs in African antelopes (springbuck, eland, sitatunga, Kafue lechwe). Experimental clinical infection has been demonstrated in a number of other African antelopes; African buffalo (*Syncerus caffer*) and the giraffe can be infected subclinically.

Several other species of *Bovidae* and *Cervidae*, not normally present in heartwater areas, have been shown to be susceptible to experimental infection, or have contracted natural infection in zoological gardens in endemic regions.[3,45]

Using a competitive ELISA,[46] preliminary indirect evidence of infection in rhinoceros and elephant was obtained in Zimbabwe (N. Kock and F. Jongejan, personal communication, 1990). There is, however, some doubt as to the significance of these results because certain species of *Ehrlichia* may cross-react with *C. ruminantium*.

Other vertebrates may also be infected experimentally. These include a carnivore, the ferret.[47,48] In 1941, it was demonstrated that *C. ruminantium* could survive in rodents.[48] Thirty years later, the first stock (Kümm) pathogenic to laboratory mice was isolated.[49] Apart from African Muridae (*Rhabdomys pumilio* and *Mastomys coucha*) and laboratory mice and rats, the guinea fowl (*Numida meleagridis*), the leopard tortoise (*Geochelone pardalis*) and the scrub hare (*Lepus saxatilis*)[13,45,50] have also been infected, in most cases subclinically.

A critical list of domestic and wild natural and experimental hosts is given by Oberem and Bezuidenhout.[45] Additional hosts include the scrub hare (*Lepus saxatilis*)[50] and Kafue lechwe (*Kobus leche kafuensis*).[51] Fatal cases of heartwater were recently observed in translocated lechwe in Zambia.[51]

Natural Transmission

Amblyomma ticks are the only known natural vectors of *C. ruminantium*. Transmission is normally trans-stadial, but there is one report of transovarial transmission.[52] Trans-stadial transmission may occur from the larval to the nymphal stage, or from the nymphal to the adult stage. Infection acquired in the larval stage may persist even if the nymph is fed on a nonsusceptible animal and be transmitted by the adult.

Males are considered to be important in the epidemiology of the disease. Uninfected males can acquire infection and transmit to another host.[53] Infected males may repeatedly transmit the disease when transferred from one host to another.[53]

Presently 10 African *Amblyomma* species are proven vectors, and there are 3 American species which can transmit infection experimentally.[54,55]

The African species are: *A. hebraeum, A. variegatum, A. pomposum, A. gemma, A. lepidum, A. tholloni, A. sparsum, A. astrion, A. cohaerens* and *A. marmoreum*.

The American species are: *A. maculatum, A. cajennense* and *A. dissimile*.

C. ruminantium can survive in the soft tick *Ornithodoros coriaceus* for at least 2 years[56] but no ticks other than *Amblyomma* spp. are known to transmit the organism. However, *Hyalomma truncatum* has been implicated in transmitting an *Ehrlichia*-like organism which on further passage appeared to be *C. ruminantium* or a very similar organism.[57]

Not all *Amblyomma* species are equally important in the field.

Some species appear to be more effective at transmitting the infection than others. There is some evidence to suggest that *A. hebraeum* is probably more effective in transmitting disease than *A. variegatum*. Infection rates of *A. hebraeum* reported from Zimbabwe[58] are higher than infection rates of *A. variegatum* in Guadeloupe.[5] Furthermore, higher percentages of domestic ruminants living in southern areas of Mozambique infested with *A. hebraeum* were seropositive by indirect immunofluorescent antibody test compared to the number of seropositive domestic ruminants in northern Mozambique infested with *A. variegatum*.[59] *A. hebraeum* may also be more aggressive than *A. variegatum* and occurs in greater numbers, but *A. variegatum* is globally more important because of its wider distribution. There may even be differences in vector capability between strains of one species.[60] Furthermore, host preferences are of great importance. Some efficient vectors have a limited geographical distribution.[3,61]

Concepts of the cycle of development of the organism in its vector host have recently changed. The hypothesis of Cowdry[14] that transmission might occur by regurgitation from the gut during feeding, had not been seriously challenged until 1982 when groups of *C. ruminantium* were demonstrated in tick salivary glands.[62] It now appears likely that *C. ruminantium* is injected into the host with the tick's saliva and develops in epithelial gut cells in a cycle similar to that in mammalian endothelial cells. The rickettsiae have been reported to occur in the Malpighian tubules, hypodermis and the rectal ampullae of infected females. Tick saliva has been reported to be infective to sheep.[50]

Experimental Infection

Susceptible animals can be experimentally infected by intravenous injection of infected blood, organ homogenates, tick homogenates, or endothelial cells infected *in vitro*.[63]

The infective dose and the route of inoculation are important. In ruminants, blood given subcutaneously will not usually cause infection.[3] In mice intravenous inoculation of certain stocks causes higher mortality than intraperitoneal inoculation.[64] A stock from Senegal caused inapparent infection in mice when infected blood was injected intravenously, but large doses of elementary bodies obtained from endothelial cell infected with the same stock *in vitro* were pathogenic (F. Jongejan, personal communication, 1989).

The discovery of stocks of *C. ruminantium* which are pathogenic for mice[49] was a significant breakthrough. The mouse laboratory model is useful for investigating the effects of potentially curative drugs[65] and to study the pathogenesis, immunology, the carrier state, innate resistance and other aspects of the disease.[56,66–71] Not all stocks of *C. ruminantium* are infective to mice and those which are infective do not always cause clinical disease.[3,64] Some can be serially passaged by intravenous inoculation and the organism may persist in infected mice for over a year.[67] In mice too, the outcome of experimental infection may be influenced by the route of inoculation and the dose of infective material.

Animal Reservoirs and Carrier Status

African wild ruminants were considered to be the wild reservoirs and natural hosts of *C. ruminantium.*

However, it has been shown that immatures of the tortoise tick *Amblyomma marmoreum* can acquire infection from experimentally infected tortoises, guinea fowls and scrub hares, and transmit the infection to ruminants.[13,50] The carrier state in tortoises can last for at least 3 months (P. T. Oberem, personal communication, 1990). Immatures of *A. marmoreum* are also found on wild and domestic ruminants and on guinea fowl and scrub hare, while immatures of *A. hebraeum* are found on large ungulates, guinea fowls, scrub hares and tortoises.[61,72] The role of these wild vertebrates could thus be potentially significant.

The possible role of free-living rodents in the epidemiology of heartwater has been the subject of speculation. *C. ruminantium* can survive for at least 2 weeks in the back-striped mouse (*Rhabdomys pumilio*)[48] and the multimammate mouse (*Mastomys coucha*) can also be infected.[73] However, a recent study[74] showed that low percentages of *R. pumilio* were infested with *A. hebraeum* and none were infested with *A. marmoreum*. The *A. hebraeum* recovered were either larvae (5 of 6) or nymphs.[74] Because transovarial transmission is exceptional, it is highly unlikely for this rodent to play any role in the epidemiology of heartwater.

Cowdriosis persists in domestic ruminants in the absence of wild reservoir hosts. In the past, it was generally accepted that a recovered animal loses its infection soon after recovery. Blood loses its infectivity 2–3 weeks after recovery but the organism is present in the brain for up to 9 weeks.[75] However, Donatien and Lestoquard[76] may have transmitted the disease with homogenized blood vessels of a sheep which had recovered 105 days earlier. Recently cattle, sheep and African buffalo in Zimbabwe (*Syncerus caffer*) were shown to be intermittently infective to nymphal *A. hebraeum* for 8 months.[77] In Guadeloupe, recovered goats failed to infect tick larvae,[78] but it was recently shown that they can remain intermittently infective to the nymphal stages of *A. variegatum* for 11 months (E. Camus, unpublished data, 1991).

Certain stocks of *C. ruminantium* may survive in mice for more than a year.[67]

Other Aspects

Tick activity influences the occurrence of the disease. In regions with a pronounced dry season, most infections tend to occur during the rains and appear to be particularly associated with the adult stage of the vector. In laboratory experiments, the transmission from larvae to nymphs is quite efficient. Nymphs are found in abundance during the dry season and in Senegal field challenge is very high during that time (A. Gueye, personal communication, 1992). In areas with less pronounced seasonal variation, such as Guadeloupe, adult tick activity and clinical cases of the disease occur throughout the year. *C. ruminantium* can survive in the tick vector for at least 15 months.[75] The organism may be transported over considerable distances by birds carrying nymphs infected during the larval stage.

Pathogenesis

The initial stages of infection in the vertebrate host are not clearly known. It has been suggested that the micro-organism may develop initially in the macrophages of lymph nodes.[79] It occurs in typical clusters in endothelial cells of blood vessels, where it apparently undergoes a developmental cycle. It also occurs in blood plasma, presumably as a result of lysis of the host cell. More recently, it has been shown to circulate in granulocytes,[80] but recognizable clusters are absent. In mice, one particular isolate multiplies in macrophages.[7] Some workers have reported microscopic evidence of the organism in other organs and cell types, but this requires further confirmation.[3] The mode of entry into the host cell has not yet been studied.

The pathogenesis of the disease is far from clear.[3,81–87] Transudates are ascribed to an increase in capillary permeability, but it is unknown how this is caused.

Hydropericardium might lead to cardiac insufficiency and hydrothorax and pulmonary edema to respiratory difficulties. Lung edema is often so pronounced in peracute heartwater that it may be responsible for the sudden death by asphyxia.

It remains difficult to explain death when lesions are not present. The occasional sudden fall in plasma volume preceding death has been associated with the development of the transudates.

The number of rickettsiae found in brain capillaries is not correlated with the intensity of central nervous symptoms. Brain lesions are often believed to be insufficiently consistent to explain the nervous symptoms; this is probably true when the macroscopical picture is considered, but not necessarily on the microscopical level. Toxins have been suggested as an explanation but have never been demonstrated convincingly. The demonstration of lipopolysaccharide (LPS) peaks in acute heartwater have led to the suggestion that the endotoxic activity of LPS may play a role in the pathogenesis of cowdriosis.[88]

Clinical Disease

Incubation Period

In controlled tick-transmitted infections, the incubation period varies from less than 10 days to more than a month.[9,10,89] The average incubation period is 2 weeks after nymphal transmission but is usually longer when adult ticks are used. This can partly be explained by the longer "pretransmission feeding period" between attachment and transmission (between 27 and 38 h in the case of nymphal and between 51 and 75 h in the case of adult *A. hebreum*).[50] For *A. variegatum*, minimum feeding periods of 2–3 days for nymphs and 4 days for adults have been reported.[5]

After intravenous inoculation of infected blood, the average incubation period is 9–10 days in small ruminants and 12–13 days in cattle.[3,90] The incubation period can be influenced by the stock of *C. ruminantium* and the dose of infective material. It may be as short as 4 days when highly infected cultures are used.[8]

In mice, the average incubation period and time of death may vary according to the stock of *C. ruminantium*, the infective dose, the route of inoculation and even the strain of mice used.[64,68]

Clinical Signs

The disease usually starts with a sudden rise in body temperature. In exotic breeds of cattle and small ruminants, it commonly exceeds 41°C within 2 days and usually remains high until shortly before death. In indigenous breeds, the temperature is usually lower.

Hyperthermia is followed by loss of appetite, listlessness and gradual development of nervous symptoms. These characteristic clinical signs of the disease are not always present. Tremors of superficial muscles may be seen before more pronounced, but very variable, symptoms start. In cattle, there may be trembling of the head and neck, irregular or staggering gait, circling movements, other manifestations such as kneeling (Fig. 17.7) or leaning or pushing against a wall and occasional aggressive behavior. Often the animal has an anxious and haggard facial expression, is hypersensitive, and has exaggerated responses to touch or sound. Blinking of the eyes is reported to be one of the most common symptoms.[10] Respiration and heart rates are increased. In a typical case the animal finally falls down in convulsions, exhibiting pedalling movements in lateral recumbency, and shows opisthotonus, nystagmus, dilated pupils and chewing movements (Fig. 17.8). There may be temporary remissions of such attacks, but the animal usually dies in the course of one of these crises, often in a position similar to tetanus, with limbs extended and head thrown back (Fig. 17.9).

It is common to see profuse, fetid and often hemorrhagic diarrhea in cattle but not in small ruminants. Dyspnea, wet bronchial rales and a moist cough, indicative of edema of the lungs, may be present. Pregnant animals often abort.

The nervous symptoms and diarrhea are usually followed by death within a few days and recovery is rare and prolonged.

Apart from the typical acute case, subacute cowdriosis also occurs, with less pronounced symptoms and a higher recovery rate. On the other hand, peracute cases may occur in imported breeds of cattle, goats and, less commonly, sheep. The animal suddenly collapses in convulsions and dies, sometimes within minutes, without premonition or with very short periods of nervous signs which went unnoticed.

The clinical symptoms may vary according to the stock of *C. ruminantium*.[90] For instance, the Kwanyanga and Kumm stocks do not usually cause nervous symptoms in goats.[91,92]

Mortality and Morbidity

Mortality rates vary according to the stock of *C. ruminantium* and the species, breed and age of the host. For example, subclinical and mild cases without nervous signs are common in local indigenous domestic ruminants and in very young animals of all breeds.

In untreated cases, mortality is usually in the region of 50% in exotic breeds of cattle, somewhat higher in exotic breeds of sheep and much higher in exotic goats (>90% in Angora goats). In endemic areas, indigenous cattle rarely die from heartwater but losses in indigenous small ruminants, particularly goats, may be considerable. The virulence of the stock of *C. ruminantium* is also important. For instance, European breeds of goats are highly susceptible to most

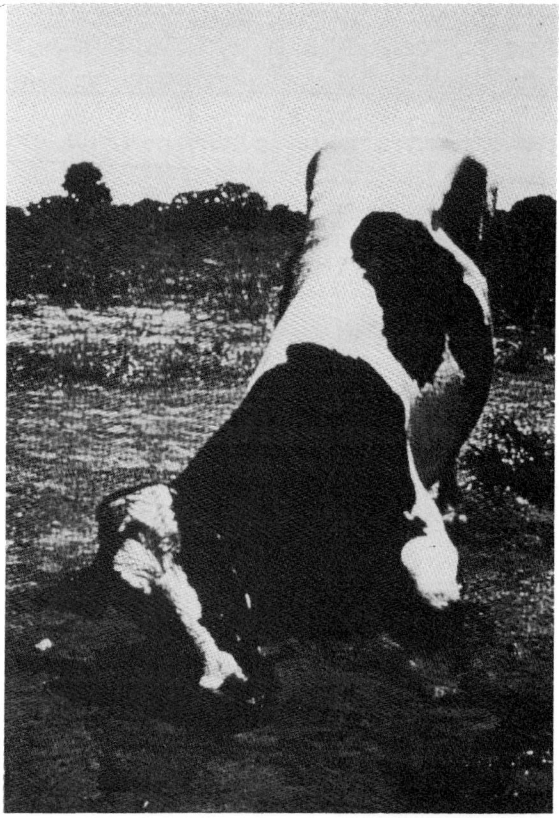

FIG. 17.7. Heartwater. Friesian cross-bred in abnormal posture. (Courtesy of A. A. Ilemobade, Zaria, Nigeria.)

stocks of *C. ruminantium* but the Kwanyanga stock appears to cause variable mortality rates.[91–93]

Cases of heartwater may occur at irregular intervals during seasons of tick activity but morbidity rates vary according to the number of infected ticks. Cases may continue to occur months and even years after field exposure.[3]

Pathology

Hematology and Clinical Pathology

Hematological changes are not spectacular. There is usually a degree of anemia and eosinopenia.[81,83–85] Among other changes, there is an acute terminal rise in blood levels of glucose,[81,85] pyruvate

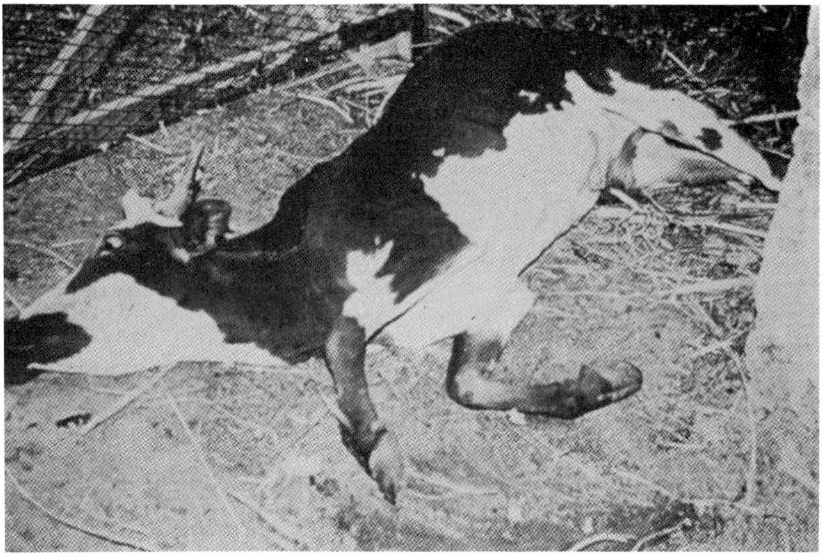

FIG. 17.8. Heartwater. Zebu cow in terminal stage. (Courtesy of A. A. Ilemobade, Zaria, Negeria.)

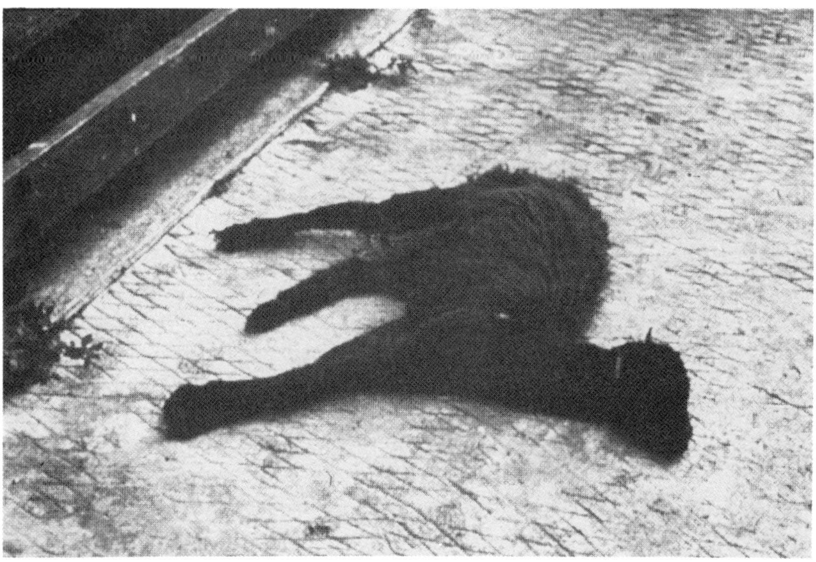

FIG. 17.9. Heartwater. Red Sokoto goat in tetanus-like state. (Courtesy of A. A. Ilemobade, Zaria, Nigeria.)

and lactate.[85] Particularly in Angora goats, the colour of the plasma may become deep orange-yellow, apparently due to increased levels of bilirubin.[94]

Gross Pathology

The postmortem picture is quite variable. Transudates are frequently present in the pericardium, and in the thoracic and peritoneal cavities. The liquid frequently clots on exposure to the air, indicating that fibrinogen molecules pass through the capillary wall. Edema of the lungs is one of the most common findings. Froth may be found in the respiratory passages, often spilling from the nostrils. Lung edema is usually very marked in peracute heartwater and may be the only visible lesion in such cases.[3,95] Other frequent lesions include edema of the mediastinal and perirenal tissues, congestion of the liver, distension of the gall-bladder, degeneration of heart muscles and kidneys, moderate splenomegaly and swelling of the lymph nodes. Often petechiae and hemorrhages are present in various organs. The mucosa of the abomasum often shows hyperemic patches. In cattle, enteritis, often hemorrhagic, is common.

Macroscopic changes in the brain are usually inconspicuous and limited to congestion of the meningeal blood vessels, edema of the meninges and petechiae in various parts of the brain.[82]

In spite of the marked clinical signs postmortem lesions are not always present, particularly in goats.

As is the case with the clinical picture, the lesions vary to some extent with the particular stock of *C. ruminantium* involved.[9] In experimental infections with two Malagasy stocks one of us (GU) rarely noticed enlargement of the spleen, which is frequently observed in animals that have died from certain other stocks. The Kümm stock commonly causes pronounced hydrothorax in goats.

Histopathology

Apart from the presence of typical intracytoplasmic clusters of rickettsiae in endothelial cells, histopathological and ultrastructural lesions are usually limited.[3] However, some workers have reported acute hemorrhagic encephalitis and brain swelling.[82,95,96] Histological findings in 27 cases included leucostasis, cell infiltration in the perivascular and subarachnoid spaces, swollen axis-cylinders, micro-cavitation, focal necrosis of the cerebellar cortex, degenerative and necrotic changes in the neuroglia with periodic acid-schiff (P.A.S.) positive intracytoplasmic granules and globules and accumulation of

P.A.S. positive globules in the Virchov–Robin spaces, choriomeningeal edema, fibrinous choriomeningitis, hemorrhages, edema and vascular changes.[82]

Immunity

Innate Resistance

Calves possess an age-linked resistance to bovine babesiosis and anaplasmosis, independent of the immune status of the dam, which may last for 9 months or more. Because of this phenomenon, a state of endemic stability is possible if the infection rate is sufficiently high to ensure that all calves develop active immunity before their innate resistance wanes.

An age-linked resistance also occurs in cowdriosis, but it is of a shorter duration. Calves of all breeds, usually resist infection until they are at least 3 weeks old, but individual animals may succumb.[66,97,98] Seven Merino lambs aged 3–9 days, born to susceptible uninfected dams, survived experimental infection, but two, 10–16 days old, died.[98] Creole goat kids are resistant until they are 2 weeks old (E. Camus, unpublished data).

Differences between breeds are not apparent in very young calves, because of the age-linked resistance, but can be significant in older animals. There is no difference between zebu and taurine breeds.[3] In endemic regions local zebu and taurine breeds, such as the N'Dama and Baoule, are usually very resistant,[37] presumably by long natural selection. In contrast, imported zebu breeds, such as the Brahman or Sahiwal, are as susceptible as European taurine breeds. Even African zebu populations from cowdriosis-free areas may pay a heavy toll when introduced into *Amblyomma*-infested zones.[99,100]

However, even in endemic areas, there may be very high mortality in local breeds of goats.[3,5] Goats are not preferential hosts of *Amblyomma* ticks, and are presumably less exposed to them[101] but one would imagine that even moderate disease pressure over the centuries would have made goat populations in endemic areas highly resistant. Sheep are less susceptible than goats[102] but in heartwater-free areas, even African breeds may suffer severe losses.[100,103]

In Guadeloupe, recent studies on Creole goats[104,105] indicate that the percentage of goats surviving experimental infection is related to the degree of previous exposure to heartwater, varying from 20% in a population which had not lived in an endemic area for decades, to over 75% in a flock which was continuously exposed. Resistance appears to be genetically controlled, with an estimated heritability of 0.26 for paternal half-sibs and 0.55 for full-sibs. A sex-linked gene could be involved. Further work is needed before valid conclusions can be drawn.

Acquired Immunity

Knowledge on the nature of immunity to heartwater is still limited. By themselves, circulating antibodies do not seem to affect the outcome of the disease. Immune serum or gamma-globulins administered together with the infective material, during the incubation period, or during the clinical phase had no effect.[71] Immune serum had no neutralizing effect on the infectivity of *C. ruminantium* to endothelial cells *in vitro*.[71,106]

Passive immunity has not been demonstrated, and the short-lived resistance of newborn animals is not related to the immune status of the dam. Colostrum-derived specific antibodies are found in calves and lambs born to immunized dams but are apparently not protective.[107]

The inability of athymic nude mice to mount an immune response and a degree of adoptive transfer of immunity with spleen cells of immune mice suggest that immunity in heartwater is largely cell-mediated.[71]

Lyt-2+ (CD8+) T cells were necessary for passive transfer of immunity and depletion of L3T4+ (CD4+) T cells had no effect on the protective effects of immune spleen cells.

Interferons and other cytokines may be involved in the resistance of cattle to cowdriosis.[108] There is a positive correlation between resistance of cattle and early interferon production. Bovine α- and especially γ-interferon showed a direct effect on the propagation of *Cowdria* in bovine endothelial cells of brain capillaries (but not in endothelial cells of umbilical artery origin) (P. Totté, personal communication, 1992). In contrast, γ-interferon appeared to potentiate penetration of *C. ruminantium* into bovine brain capillary endothelial cells in culture (P. O. Couraud, unpublished data, 1991).

There are conflicting reports on the duration of immunity and further studies are required.

Earlier experiments which indicated a rather variable immunity were probably confounded by other intercurrent infections.[3,98,109] Immunological strain diversity may well be responsible for some breakdowns of immunity in the field, and stress or intercurrent disease might cause relapses in subclinical carriers.

In the absence of reinfection, homologous protective immunity in sheep lasts for at least 4 years.[110] In Guadeloupe, Creole goats resisted homologous challenge for at least 2 years,[5] but immunity may be significantly shorter in the more susceptible Angora goat.[111] A period of 2 years has also been reported for cattle in South Africa but natural reinfections could have reinforced immunity.[112] Results of later experiments using calves immunized before the age of one month were much less convincing but the challenge used was not homologous.[113] Antibiotic treatment may also influence subsequent development of immunity, at least in Angora goats.[111]

Immunological Strain Diversity

Except for the South African mouse-pathogenic stocks, until recently it was thought that there was only one antigenic type affecting ruminants.[3,91,109] However, work in various countries has now conclusively shown that strains of *C. ruminantium* are immunologically heterogeneous irrespective of infectivity or pathogenicity for mice.[92,114–116]

Cross–protection between stocks may be complete, partial or virtually absent. Cross-protection may be unilateral, one stock protecting completely or partially against the other, but not, or to a lesser degree, vice versa. It has not been possible so far to detect a pattern in the diversity and the degree of cross-protection between various stocks is not clearly defined.[115,116]

The animal species influences the outcome of cross-protection tests. The expression of antigenic differences may be considerably greater in (European) goats than in sheep,[92] and this may partly explain reports of high numbers of immunized goats succumbing to field challenge.

Recent studies on rodents are also relevant. Laboratory mice immune to the Kwanyanga stock resisted challenge with the Welgevonden and Nonile stocks. Welgevonden protected against Nonile but not against Kwanyanga, and Nonile protected against Welgevonden but not against Kwanyanga. Susceptibility tests in laboratory mice and the multimammate mouse (*Mastomys coucha*) with four stocks pathogenic to laboratory mice and two which at most induce inapparent infection in laboratory mice are shown in Table 17.1 (modified from Stewart,[117] to incorporate data also known on ruminants). The Kwanyanga, Nonile and Mali stocks caused fatal disease in *Mastomys coucha* but the Kümm and Welgevonden stocks caused infections without mortality. Therefore cross-immunity tests in *Mastomys* would have given very different results from those obtained in laboratory mice. There may be differences too between breeds of one and the same host species. For example, the Welgevonden stock is pathogenic for one (inbred) strain of *M. coucha* (C. G. Stewart, unpublished data).

TABLE 17.1. *Comparison of stocks of* C. ruminantium *in different hosts*

Stock	Sheep	Cattle	Laboratory mice	*M. coucha*
Kümm	P	NP	P	NP
Kwanyanga	P	P	P	P
Nonile	P	P	P	P
Welgevonden	P	P	P	NP
Mali	P	P	NP	P
Ball 3	P	P	NP	NP

P = pathogenic; NP = nonpathogenic.

Diagnosis

Clinical Signs and Postmortem Lesions

Symptoms are often atypical and even when the most characteristic nervous signs are present, there is a long list of diseases to be considered in the differential diagnosis. These include rabies, cerebral babesiosis, cerebral theileriosis, tetanus, cerebral listeriosis, plant poisoning and other conditions, including infection with *Ehrlichia bovis* and *E. ovina*. Hemorrhagic diarrhea also occurs in coccidiosis and some types of plant poisoning and arsenical intoxications. In acute cases, pulmonary signs may resemble hemorrhagic septicemia and peracute cases must be differentiated from anthrax. On occasions, acute hemonchosis and peracute trypanosomiasis may be confused with heartwater.

When the animal is found dead, marks of pedalling movements on the ground may arouse suspicion. Postmortem findings may allow a tentative diagnosis if lesions such as hydropericardium and other transudates are present but even these are not pathognomonic and microscopic confirmation is essential. Even in cases with pronounced nervous signs, macroscopic lesions are not always present.

Direct Laboratory Diagnosis

Stained blood smears are of no use for the diagnosis of heartwater. Although the organisms occur in the granulocytes of affected animals, they are not present in recognizable clusters. However, their presence in granulocytes can be demonstrated within 1–2 days by maintaining separated granulocytes at 37°C *in vitro*. Clusters develop in the cytoplasm of granulocytes depending on the speed of multiplication of the particular stock of *C. ruminantium*.[80,118] The method is not suitable for all strains and, therefore, only positive results are conclusive.

A faster method of diagnosing the disease in the live animal is microscopic examination of brain cortex smears obtained by biopsy.[119] Although the operation is practically harmless for the animal and is useful for experimental studies, it is not suitable for routine diagnosis.

Heartwater can usually be diagnosed with certainty after death. It is possible to demonstrate the organism in histological sections of various organs but smears of the brain cortex which is rich in capillaries is by far the best material. Clusters of *C. ruminantium* are sometimes very scanty and prolonged examination is essential before pronouncing the result as negative. Satisfactory (cerebellar) material can be obtained with a sharp spoon through the foramen magnum after removing the head.[120] Cerebral cortex can be obtained in a more simple and safe way with a syringe and needle inserted through a hole in the skull made with a hammer and a large nail (Malika, J., Lawrence, J. A., Whiteland, A. P. and Kafuwa, P., unpublished data, 1991).

Although the old myth that *C. ruminantium* loses its staining properties after death has been laid to rest,[98] microscopic diagnosis may be difficult in animals which died 48 h or more after treatment with tetracyclines, as the elementary bodies tend to disappear and the larger forms in a cluster tend to fuse.[121]

Giemsa's stain is generally used and is probably the best. Fast stains such as Diff-Quick, CAM's Quick-stain, Field's stain and RAL 555 have the advantage of giving an acceptable result in minutes but they are inferior to Giemsa's especially in difficult cases.[121] Castañeda's stain is also satisfactory. Acridine orange has been used successfully for fast staining but it requires an immunofluorescence microscope.[122]

Use of Susceptible Ruminants

This is a useful method for showing conclusively the presence of heartwater in a particular area or in a particular animal species. Several approaches are possible:[123]

(1) A pool of randomly collected blood is intravenously inoculated into susceptible ruminants.

(2) Susceptible sentinel ruminants are introduced into the area of investigation and monitored for the development of disease.

(3) Pooled supernatant of homogenized *Amblyomma* ticks collected at random from animals are injected into susceptible animals.

(4) *Amblyomma* nymphs or adults collected from the ground or

collected as engorged larvae or nymphs from animals are allowed to feed on susceptible ruminants.

Serology

The first workable serological test was developed in 1981. The antigen for this indirect fluorescent antibody test (IFAT) consisted of peritoneal macrophages of mice infected with the Kümm stock.[7] Another IFAT uses the granulocyte fraction of the blood of reacting animals, in which clusters become visible when maintained *in vitro* at 37°C.[80,118] Infected bovine endothelial cell cultures, or their supernatants containing free elementary bodies, constitute the antigen for a third IFAT.[24] The endothelial cell culture antigen can be produced in large quantities at low cost, the reaction can be read easily and quickly. With the notable exception of the Kümm stock, almost all stocks can be grown in endothelial cell cultures.[124] In contrast, not all stocks are suitable for preparing antigens from infected granulocytes. Antigens from infected mouse macrophages can only be prepared from the Kümm stock. Antigens prepared from infected endothelial cells and granulocytes appear to be more reliable than antigens prepared from mouse macrophages infected with the Kümm stock. Antibody titers may be affected by the homologous or heterologous nature of the antigen prepared from infected granulocytes and, to a lesser degree, from infected endothelial cells.[24] We do not know whether such differences are detected with the Kümm antigens. This phenomenon introduces an element of uncertainty in serological surveys.

A murine monoclonal antibody reacting with the conserved immunodominant 32 kDa protein[28] was used for a competitive enzyme-linked immunosorbent assay (CELISA).[46] The CELISA may be especially useful for sera from free-living animals for which there are no specific conjugates. It was also hoped that it would solve the problems of serotypes and cross-reaction associated with the other tests.

A classical indirect ELISA and a dot-ELISA, using endothelial cell culture antigen have also given promising results (D. Martinez, unpublished, 1991, 1992). An earlier antibody-detecting ELISA used antigen obtained from infected ticks[125] and the detection of *C. ruminantium* in blood fractions using the ELISA was reported at the same time. It may be possible to develop an antigen-capturing ELISA for the detection of infected animals, using monoclonal antibodies against common antigens while other monoclonal antibodies might be useful for detecting antigenic strain differences.[46]

While the tests mentioned above are useful, serious doubts have been raised as to their applicability in the field. Because there are strong cross-reactions in the IFAT with *Ehrlichia* spp.,[126] it may make the interpretation of results from field surveys difficult and could be responsible for false positive reactions in areas where the disease is not known to occur. It has been suggested that the *C. ruminantium* antigen can be used for the serological diagnosis of canine ehrlichiosis.[127] Recently, blind studies were carried out in 4 laboratories, using the 3 types of IFAT, the CELISA, Western blotting and the indirect ELISA. A number of sera from animals, previously infected with various stocks of *C. ruminantium* and sera originating from a cowdriosis-free region, but which had been found positive in an IFAT and were therefore suspected of *Ehrlichia* infections were tested.[57] The most surprising result was that bovine and ovine sera suspected of having antibodies to *Ehrlichia* reacted with *C. ruminantium* not only in the 3 types of IFAT and ELISA but also in the CELISA and Western blotting (J. L. Du Plessis, J. D. Bezuidenhout, M. S. Brett, E. Camus, F. Jongejan, S. Mahan and D. Martinez, unpublished data, 1992). If confirmed, it would seriously detract from the value of these various tests in areas where *Ehrlichia* infections occur in ruminants, which probably cover most of the cowdriosis-endemic regions of Africa and beyond. This could explain why there were positive serological results in areas of Malawi and other parts of southern Africa regarded as heartwater-free (S. M. Mahan, L. A. Wassink and F. Jongejan, personal communications, 1991) and in areas of the Caribbean in which heartwater has not been previously diagnosed.[41] However, the presence of ehrlichial infections in the Caribbean is not yet known.

Nucleic Acid Probes

Specific nucleic acid sequences have been obtained and are being evaluated as diagnostic probes.[25–27] Because radioactive probes are not suitable for field use, nonradioactive probes are being developed (S. M. Mahan, personal communication, 1991). The signal obtained by DNA hybridization in plasma of infected sheep was greatly improved with the polymerase chain reaction (PCR).[27] Use of PCR may be necessary for the reliable detection of carrier animals in which the level of rickettsiemia appears to undergo cyclical variations indicated by intermittent infectivity to ticks and is probably too low for detection with DNA probes.[27]

Detection in Ticks

Detection of *C. ruminantium* in ticks is possible but not very practical. This is usually done by feeding the ticks and examining stained gut smears microscopically.

Du Plessis[128] demonstrated the presence of *C. ruminantium* in ticks by injecting individual homogenized specimens into individual mice and by subsequently demonstrating specific antibodies in the injected mice. It is not clear whether this method is suitable for all the stocks. In Guadeloupe, antibody response was induced only by 3 out of 200 ticks collected from 200 cattle.[5]

The use of DNA probes to detect the organism in ticks is particularly promising[26] and is likely to supersede other methods.

Treatment

There have been no new development during the past decade and the reader is referred to earlier reviews.[3,10,11,34]

As the course of the disease is rapid, treatment must be given on the basis of clinical signs without waiting for laboratory confirmation.

Sulfonamides have now been virtually abandoned and tetracycline antibiotics (chlortetracycline, oxytetracycline, rolitetracycline and doxycycline) are practically the only drugs in use for the effective treatment of the disease. Long-acting preparations have the advantage that one injection may suffice. In contrast, at least two injections, given at 24–48 h intervals, are required when ordinary formulations are used. These drugs are effective only when given during the early course of the disease. Once marked nervous symptoms and/or hemorrhagic diarrhea have developed, the animal usually dies irrespective of treatment. This limits the usefulness of chemotherapy in field situations because cowdriosis is not suspected until the nervous or other clinical manifestations are apparent. Certain stocks of *C. ruminantium* may be practically impossible to treat even if the disease is recognized early, particularly in goats of European breeds.[129] Little has been heard about the possible use of rifampicin after it was first reported to be effective against heartwater.[35]

It has been suggested that it may be useful to give anti-inflammatory and diuretic drugs in addition to specific treatment with antibiotics.[34] There was an abatement of nervous symptoms after experimentally infected goats were given dexamethasone and oxytetracycline but the fatal outcome was not affected (M. A. Asselbergs, unpublished data). Tranquillizers and muscle relaxants might possibly reduce convulsions but we are not aware of any work in this connection.

Control

Control methods have recently been reviewed and possible methods and strategies discussed.[130] There are several ways by which cowdriosis can be controlled or prevented.

Vector Control

In principle vector control systems which either eliminate *Amblyomma* ticks or at least block them from transmitting the disease are very attractive but they have many drawbacks. In most circumstances, total eradication is not possible and should only be attempted in isolated small islands.

Prevention of transmission requires treatment with acaricides at short intervals because *Amblyomma* spp. are three-host ticks. They can complete their cycle on free-living ungulates and they are indiscriminate feeders as immatures.

Intensive use of acaricides leads to lack of herd immunity and a vulnerable cattle population. When acaricide resistance develops or tick control breaks down because of other causes, heavy losses will occur.[131] The recent development of pour-on formulations offers the advantage of avoiding the use of expensive dipping or spraying installations. It is also possible to intervene less frequently through the use of the new pyrethroids which have long residual activity but they may well increase the risk of acaricide resistance.

Other Means of Vector Control

Immune resistance to ticks as a result of natural exposure does not provide a good basis for attempting to control heartwater. The practical feasibility of immunization against *Amblyomma* ticks with internal antigens derived from the vector ticks remains to be explored. This is in contrast with the situation concerning *Boophilus* ticks.[132,133]

Other possible methods of control include the use of attraction–fixation phermones[134,135] and measures of pasture and herd management.[136]

Immunization

The "infection and treatment" method of vaccination, first used half a century ago,[137] remains the only practical and effective means of immunization against heartwater.

The method is essentially crude, unsuitable for application to large numbers of animals and reasonably safe only under close supervision. Care should be taken to use a stock which is not unduly virulent. In southern Africa the Ball 3 stock is routinely used. Infective material is injected intravenously and the temperature is monitored daily.

Specific antibiotic treatment is then given as soon as hyperthemia starts. Alternatively, very young animals may be immunized without temperature monitoring because of their age-linked resistance. However, it is essential that they are closely watched because without treatment a small percentage may die.

The usual infective inoculum is blood from a reacting donor animal but material prepared from homogenized prefed infected ticks[138] may offer certain advantages. It is cheaper and the material is highly infective, making it feasible to store large numbers of effective doses in small volumes. It is also less likely to transmit contaminating infections. However, because it may cause serious shock in kids and lambs, the tick-derived "vaccine" has been withdrawn from use.[139] Preliminary experiments show that infected endothelial cell cultures are good candidates to replace infected whole blood.[140] For more detailed reviews we refer to other publications.[139,141]

Because it is necessary, to inject the animals intravenously and to monitor the temperature daily, infection and treatment is unsuitable for mass immunization. Furthermore, the intravenous inoculation of blood and tick-derived material may cause shock and some losses due to vaccine-induced clinical heartwater may occur. These losses are common in peracute cases because deaths occur before the rise in temperature is detected. The infective material is very fragile and has to be stored at $-70°C$ or below. After thawing, it should be kept on ice and used within a few hours. Moreover, even intravenous injection of proven infective material may not always infect all animals; a second injection sometimes produces a reaction. As with all live blood vaccines, the danger of transmitting other infective agents is real and a high standard of quality control is essential.

In spite of all the disadvantages, exotic stock cannot be maintained in endemic areas without immunization, unless excellent tick control can be sustained.

A number of strategies have been tried to reduce the problems associated with the blood vaccines.

In South Africa a slow-release preparation of doxycycline (Doximplant^{R}) subcutaneously implanted at the time of intravenous injection of infective material is reported to make monitoring of the immunized animals unnecessary[142] but its efficacy and safety have not been sufficiently documented.

To avoid the need to monitor individual temperatures, large numbers of animals can be immunized by the "block" method. All animals are then simultaneously and indiscriminately treated after a certain number of days, depending on the average incubation period of the immunizing stock of *C. ruminantium* used.[143] This method does not take individual variations in incubation period into account and if blocking treatment is carried out too early, the resulting immunity may be insufficient and sometimes the incubation period is simply prolonged. If it is too late, animals react before treatment and may die. Lyophilized infective materials have given encouraging results[31] but details of the optimal freeze-drying procedures have not been worked out. It would mean a considerable step forward and would eliminate the need to preserve live vaccines at very low temperatures.

Under field conditions the duration of protective immunity generated and the efficacy of vaccination is not clearly known because it is often difficult to diagnose accurately the cause of death in suspected failures. The Ball stock does not afford complete protection against field challenge and antigenic strain differences are likely to be responsible for some of the reported failures. Sheep appear to resist natural challenge better than goats. Immunological strain differences seem to be more apparent in goats,[93] but satisfactory results of immunization of Angora goats have been reported.[144] In immunized cattle, resistance to field challenge is not always satisfactory[3] and in particular, immunization of young calves is reported to give unreliable results.[113]

It has been reported that cattle given weekly injections of long-acting tetracyclines during the first exposure to high natural challenge will not develop disease but will acquire effective immunity.[145]

Other Approaches

One of the most important developments is the recent attenuation of a Senegalese stock of *C. ruminantium* by passages in bovine endothelial cell cultures. The attenuated material was not virulent to sheep and goats but induced solid immunity to homologous challenge.[146] Attenuation was attained after 69–229 days in culture. Another stock (Welgevonden) was not attenuated after 226 days. The Senegalese stock has since been similarly attenuated in Guadeloupe (D. Martinez, personal communication, 1991). Goats inoculated after 22–28 passages in bovine endothelial cell cultures, each lasting 10–15 days, reacted with hyperthermia at the most, but resisted homologous challenge a month later. In contrast, a stock from Guadeloupe remained virulent after 30 passages in culture.

However, this culture material is also fragile and is unlikely to solve the problem of antigenic diversity but it eliminates the dangers inherent in the use of virulent material and the need for monitoring the reaction. As cross-immunity studies between the Senegalese stock and several other stocks is incomplete,[92,114] this attenuated vaccine should first be tested only where it was originally isolated.

Recombinant vaccines would eliminate the risks associated with virulent material and solve the problem of inadvertent spread of contaminating disease agents. The problem of the fragility of *C. ruminantium* would also disappear or be reduced. It will first be necessary to determine the antigen or antigens inducing protection which is apparently mainly cell-mediated. Antigenic diversity may well be a bigger problem with this approach as individual antigens common to the various strains are unlikely to be as immunogenic as whole live organisms which do not always stimulate a satisfactory immune response.

Use of Resistant Animals

Indigenous populations in endemic regions show varying degrees of innate resistance to cowdriosis. The heritability of resistance and susceptibility has not been studied except for the preliminary work in Guadeloupe. If a genetic marker of resistance or susceptibility can be identified, it should be feasible to select for resistance to cowdriosis. Preliminary studies on the Caprine Lymphocyte Antigens of Creole goats indicate that certain specificities may be linked to resistance and others to susceptibility (P. C. Maillard, G. Ruff and E. Camus, unpublished data, 1991).

Use of Endemic Stability

Large numbers of *Amblyomma* ticks may be required to infect all young animals during the short period of age-linked resistance to heartwater. Two extreme types of epidemiological situation have been reported, depending on the species of vector involved.

In Zimbabwe, infection rates of *A. hebraeum* are high but the tick numbers necessary to maintain endemic stability can cause secondary abscesses, loss of teats, dermatophilosis and infestation with screw-worms, especially in exotic breeds.[37,147,148]

In Madagascar and in Guadeloupe the low infection rates of *A. variegatum* appear to be responsible for an endemically unstable situation[5,98] but this is expressed clearly only in susceptible exotic stock.

Vaccination during the period of peak larval and nymphal activity might help to create endemic stability by increasing the percentage of infected ticks.[149]

In spite of much progress in research on heartwater, the concluding sentence of a review which is more than a decade old[4] is still valid: "Because of the present unsatisfactory state of immunization and treatment, introduction of susceptible exotic breeds into heartwater areas must be strongly advised against unless strict, efficient acaricidal control can be guaranteed."

In areas where tick control and veterinary care are inadequate at present the only reasonable way of living with heartwater and its vectors is the use of indigenous breeds originating from endemic regions.

Acknowledgements

We thank the various persons quoted in allowing us to present their unpublished results. We are grateful to Dr Jane B. Walker for allowing us to use her maps[150] to compile (Fig. 17.5) to Prof. A. A. Ilemobade for the use of his photographs (Figs 17.7–17.9) and Dr F. Jongejan for the electron micrographs (Figs 17.3 and 17.4).

References

1. PROVOST, A. and BEZUIDENHOUT, J.D. 1987. The historical background and global importance of heartwater. *Onderstepoort J. vet Res.* **54:** 165–169.
2. COWDRY, E.V. 1925. Studies on the etiology of heartwater. I. Observation of a rickettsia, *Rickettsia ruminantium* (n.sp.), in the tissues of infected animals. *J. exp. Med.* **42:** 231–252.
3. UILENBERG, G. 1983. Heartwater (*Cowdria ruminantium* infection): current status. *Adv. vet. Sci. comp. Med.* **27:** 427–480.
4. UILENBERG, G. 1981. Heartwater disease. In: *Diseases of Cattle in the Tropics,* pp. 345–360. RISTIC, M. and MCINTYRE, I. (Eds), Martinus Nijhoff Publishers.
5. CAMUS, E. 1989. Etude épidémiologique de la cowdriose à *Cowdria ruminantium* en Guadeloupe. Etudes et Synthèses de l'I.E.M.V.T. no. 33. IEMVT-CIRAD, Maisons-Alfort, 196 p.
6. PERREAU, P., MOREL, P.C., BARRÉ, N. and DURAND, P. 1980. Existence de la cowdriose (heartwater) à *Cowdria ruminantium* chez les petits ruminants des Antilles françaises (La Guadeloupe) et des Mascareignes (La Réunion et Ile Maurice). *Rev. Elev. Méd. vét. Pays Trop.* **33:** 21–22.
7. DU PLESSIS, J.L. 1981. The application of the indirect fluorescent antibody test to the serology of heartwater. In: *Tick Biology and Control,* pp. 47–52. WHITEHEAD, G.B. and GIBSON, J.D. (Eds), Rhodes University, Grahamstown, South Africa.
8. BEZUIDENHOUT, J.D., PATERSON, C.L. and BARNARD, B.J.H. 1985. *In vitro* cultivation of *Cowdria ruminantium. Onderstepoort J. vet Res.* **51:** 113–120.
9. ALEXANDER, R.A. 1931. Heartwater. The present state of our knowledge of the disease. 17th Report of the Director of Veterinary Services and Animal Industry, South Africa (Part I): 89–150.
10. HENNING, M.W. 1956. Animal diseases in South Africa. 3rd edn. *Onderstepoort, S. Afr. Central News Agency Ltd.* pp. 1115–1179.
11. CAMUS, E. and BARRÉ, N. 1988. La cowdriose (heartwater). Revue générale des connaissances. 2e édition. Etudes et Synthèses de l'I.E.M.V.T. no. 4. IEMVT-CIRAD, Maisons-Alfort, 152 p.

12. YUNKER, C.E. 1991. The epidemiology, diagnosis and control of heartwater. In: *CTA Seminar Proceedings: Cowdriosis and Dermatophilosis of Livestock in the Caribbean region,* pp. 87–96. 12–14 November 1990, St John, Antigua. CARDI/CTA.
13. BEZUIDENHOUT, J.D. 1990. Recent research findings on cowdriosis. In: *Ehrlichiosis. A Vector-Borne Disease of Animals and Humans,* pp. 125–135. J.C. WILLIAMS and I. KAKOMA (Eds). Kluwer Academic Publishers.
14. COWDRY, E.V. 1925. Studies on the etiology of heartwater. II. *Rickettsia ruminantium* (n.sp.) in the tissues of ticks transmitting the disease. *J. exp. Med.* **42:** 253–274.
15. COWDRY, E.V. 1926. Studies on the etiology of heartwater. III. The multiplication of *Rickettsia ruminantium* within the endothelial cells of infected animals and their discharge into the circulation. *J. exp. Med.* **44:** 803–814.
16. MOSHKOVSKI, S.D. 1947. Comments by readers. *Science* **106:** 62.
17. RISTIC, M. and HUXSOLL, D.L. 1984. Tribe II. Ehrlichieae Philip 1957, 948[AL]. In: *Bergey's Manual of Systematic Bacteriology,* pp. 704–711. KRIEG, N.R. and HOLT, J.G. (Eds), Williams and Wilkins, Baltimore.
18. MOULDER, J.W. 1990. Evolutionary history of *Chlamydiae*: answers for some old questions, no answers for some new ones. In: *Ehrlichiosis. A Vector-Borne Disease of Animals and Humans,* pp. 112–124. J.C. WILLIAMS and I. KAKOMA (Eds), Kluwer Academic Publishers.
19. DAME, J.B., MAHAN, S.M. and YOWELL, C.A. 1992. Phylogenetic relationship of *Cowdria ruminantium,* agent of heartwater, to *Anaplasma marginale* and other members of the order Rickettsiales determined on the basis of 16S rRNA sequence. *Int. J. Syst. Bact.* **42:** 270–274.
20. VAN VLIET, A.H.M., JONGEJAN, F. and VAN DER ZEIJST, B.A.M. 1992. Phylogenetic position of *Cowdria ruminantium* (Rickettsiales) determined by analysis of amplified 16S ribosomal DNA sequences. *Int. J. Syst. Bactl.* **42:** 494–498.
21. PIENAAR, J.G. 1970. Electron microscopy of *Cowdria (Rickettsia) ruminantium* (Cowdry, 1926) in the endothelial cells of the vertebrate host. *Onderstepoort J. vet Res.* **37:** 67–78.
22. JONGEJAN, F., ZANDBERGEN, T.A., VAN DE WIEL, P.A., DE GROOT, M. and UILENBERG, G. 1991. The tick-borne rickettsia *Cowdria ruminantium* has a *Chlamydia*-like development cycle. *Onderstepoort J. vet Res.* **58:** 227–237.
23. BYROM, B. and YUNKER, C.E. 1990. Improved culture conditions for *Cowdria ruminantium* (Rickettsiales), the agent of heartwater disease of domestic ruminants. *Cytotechnology* **4:** 285–290.
24. MARTINEZ, D., SWINKELS, J., CAMUS, E. and JONGEJAN, F. 1990. Comparaison de trois antigènes pour le sérodiagnostic de la cowdriose par immunofluorescence indirecte. *Rev. Elev. Méd. vét. Pays Trop.* **43:** 159–166.
25. WILKINS, S.C. and AMBROSIO. R.E. 1989. The isolation of nucleic acid sequences specific for *Cowdria ruminantium. Onderstepoort J. vet Res.* **56:** 127–129.
26. WAGHELA, S.D., RURANGIRWA, F.R., MAHAN, S.M., YUNKER, C.E., CRAWFORD, T.B., BARBET, A.F., BURRIDGE, M.J. and MCGUIRE, T.C. 1991. A cloned DNA probe identifies *Cowdria ruminantium* in *Amblyomma variegatum* ticks. *J. clin. Microbiol.* **29:** 2571–2577.
27. MAHAN, S.M., WAGHELA, S.D., MCGUIRE, T.C., RURANGIRWA, F.R., WASSINK, L.A. and BARBET, A.F. 1992. A cloned DNA probe for *Cowdria ruminantium* hybridizes with eight heartwater strains and detects infected sheep. *J. clin. Microbiol.* **30:** 981–986.

28. JONGEJAN, F. and THIELEMANS, M.J.C. 1989. Identification of an immunodominant antigenically conserved 32-kilodalton protein from *Cowdria ruminantium*. *Infect. Immun.* **57:** 3243–3246.
29. ROSSOUW, M., NEITZ, A.W.H., DE WAAL, D.T., DU PLESSIS, J.L., VAN GAS, L. and BRETT, S. 1990. Identification of the antigen proteins of *Cowdria ruminantium*. *Onderstepoort J. vet Res.* **57:** 215–221.
30. BIRNIE, E.F., ENDRIS, R.G. and LOGAN, L.L. 1986. Comparison of diluents for maintaining the viability of *Cowdria ruminantium*. *Am J. vet. Res.* **47:** 1225–1228.
31. DU PLESSIS, J.L., VAN GAS, L., LABUSCHAGNE, F.J. and WIJMA, S. 1990. The freeze-drying of *Cowdria ruminantium*. *Onderstepoort J. vet Res.* **57:** 145–149.
32. NEITZ, W.O. 1939. Die Wirkung von Uleron auf das Herzwasser (*Rickettsia ruminantium*) der Schafe. *Berl. Münch. Tierärztl. Wschr.* **9:** 134–136.
33. SIMPSON, R.M. and WILEY, A.J. 1951. Experiments with aureomycin hydrochloride. Ann. Report 1949, pp. 23–27. Vet. Department, Kenya.
34. VAN AMSTEL, S.R. and OBEREM, P.T. 1987. The treatment of heartwater. *Onderstepoort J. vet Res.* **54:** 475–479.
35. OBEREM, P.T. and MATTHEE, J. 1988. A new pour-on remedy for the treatment of heartwater and some other important stock diseases. Biennial Report, Veterinary Research Institute, Onderstepoort, 1986/87: p.43.
36. SCOTT, G.R. 1978. Tick-borne rickettsial diseases of domestic livestock. In: *Tick-borne Diseases and their Vectors*, pp. 451–473. WILDE, J.K.H. (Ed.), Centre for Tropical Veterinary Medicine, University of Edinburgh.
37. CAMUS, E. and BARRÉ, N. 1990. *Amblyomma variegatum* and associated diseases in the Caribbean: strategies for control and eradication in Guadeloupe. *Parassitologia* **32:** 185–193.
38. MOREL, P.C. 1967. Etudes sur les tiques du bétail en Guadeloupe et Martinique. II. Agents pathogènes transmis par les tiques. *Rev. Elev. Méd. vét. Pays Trop.* **20:** 292–299.
39. UILENBERG, G., BARRÉ, N., CAMUS, E., BURRIDGE, M.J. and GARRIS, G.I. 1984. Heartwater in the Caribbean. *Prev. vet. Med.* **2:** 255–267.
40. UILENBERG, G. 1991. Global importance of ticks and tick-borne diseases: Historical review of the problem in the Caribbean. In: *CTA Seminar Proceedings: Cowdriosis and Dermatophilosis of Livestock in the Caribbean Region*, pp. 19–28. 12–14 November 1990, St John, Antigua, CARDI/CTA.
41. MULLER KOBOLD, A., MARTINEZ, D., CAMUS, E. and JONGEJAN, F. 1992. Distribution of heartwater in the Caribbean determined on the basis of detection of antibodies to the conserved 32-kilodalton protein of *Cowdria ruminantium*. *J. clin. Microbiol.* **30:** 1870–1873.
42. BARRÉ, N., UILENBERG, G., MOREL, P.C. and CAMUS, E. 1987. Danger of introducing heartwater onto the American mainland: potential role of indigenous and exotic *Amblyomma* ticks. *Onderstepoort J. vet Res.* **54:** 405–417.
43. BARRÉ, N., GARRIS, G.I., BOREL, G. and CAMUS, E. 1988. Hosts and population dynamics of *Amblyomma variegatum* (Acari: Ixodidae) on Guadeloupe, French West Indies. *J. med. Ent.* **25:** 111–115.
44. KARRAR, G. 1960. Rickettsial infection (heartwater) in sheep and goats in the Sudan. *Br. vet. J.* **116:** 105–114.
45. OBEREM, P.T. and BEZUIDENHOUT, J.D. 1987. Heartwater in hosts other than domestic ruminants. *Onderstepoort J. vet Res.* **54:** 271–275.
46. JONGEJAN, F., THIELEMANS, M.J.C., DE GROOT, M., VAN KOOTEN, P.J.S., VAN DER ZEIJST, B.A.M. 1991. Competitive enzyme-linked immunosorbent assay

for heartwater using monoclonal antibodies to a *Cowdria ruminantium*-specific 32-kilodalton protein. *Vet. Microbiol.* **28:** 199–211.

47. MASON, J.H. and ALEXANDER, R.A. 1940. The susceptibility of the ferret to heartwater. *J. S. Afr. vet. Med. Ass.* **11(3):** 98–107.
48. HUDSON, J.R. and HENDERSON, R.M. 1941. Some preliminary experiments on the survival of heartwater "virus" in rats. *J. S. Afr. vet. Med. Ass.* **12(2):** 39–49.
49. DU PLESSIS, J.L. and KÜMM, N.A.L. 1971. The passage of *Cowdria ruminantium* in mice. *J. S. Afr. vet. Med. Ass.* **42:** 217–221.
50. BEZUIDENHOUT, J.D. 1988. Sekere aspekte van hartwateroordraging, voorkoms van die organisme in bosluise en *in vitro* kweking. (Certain aspects of the transmission of heartwater, the occurrence of the organism in ticks, and *in vitro* culture.) Doctor of Science Thesis, University of Pretoria.
51. PANDEY, G.S., MINYOI, D., HASEBE, F. and MWASE, E.T. 1992. First report of heartwater (cowdriosis) in Kafue lechwe (*Kobus leche kafuensis*) in Zambia. *Rev. Elev. Méd. vét. Pays Trop.* **45:** 23–25.
52. BEZUIDENHOUT, J.D. and JACOBSZ, G.J. 1986. Proof of transovarial transmission of *Cowdria ruminantium* by *Amblyomma hebraeum. Onderstepoort J. vet Res.* **53:** 31–34.
53. ANDREW, H.R., NORVAL, R.A.I. 1989. The role of males of the bont tick (*Amblyomma hebraeum*) in the transmission of *Cowdria ruminantium* (heartwater). *Vet. Parasit.* **34:** 15–23.
54. BEZUIDENHOUT, J.D. 1987. Natural transmission of heartwater. *Onderstepoort J. vet Res.* **54:** 349–351.
55. JONGEJAN, F. 1992. Experimental transmission of *Cowdria ruminantium* (Rickettsiales) by the American reptile tick *Amblyomma dissimile* Koch, 1844. *Expl appl. Acarol.* **15:** 117–121.
56. ENDRIS, R.G., HASLETT, T.M., BIRNIE, E.F. and HESS, W.R. 1989. A mouse lethal dose assay for detection and titration of *Cowdria ruminantium* (Kwanyanga strain) in goats and ticks. *Vet. Microbiol.* **19:** 151–165.
57. DU PLESSIS, J.L. 1990. Increased pathogenicity of an *Ehrlichia*-like agent after passage through *Amblyomma hebraeum*: a preliminary report. *Onderstepoort J. vet Res.* **57:** 283–285.
58. NORVAL, R.A.I., ANDREW, H.R. and YUNKER, C.E. 1990. Infection rates with *Cowdria ruminantium* of nymphs and adults of the bont tick *Amblyomma hebraeum* collected in the field in Zimbabwe. *Vet. Parasit.* **36:** 277–283.
59. ASSELBERGS, M., JONGEJAN, F., LANGA, A., NEVES, L. and AFONSO, S. Antibodies to *Cowdria ruminantium* in Mozambican goats and cattle detected by immunofluorescence using endothelial cell culture antigen. *Trop. Anim. Hlth Prod.*, in press.
60. HAHN, N.E., NORVAL, R.A.I., WAGHELA, S.D., SHAW, M. and KOCAN, K.M. 1990. Different gut infection rates with *Cowdria ruminantium* in two laboratory colonies of *Amblyomma variegatum* ticks. *Bull. Soc. Franç. Parasit.* **8 (2):** 1177.
61. PETNEY, T.N., HORAK, I.G. and RECHAV, Y. 1987. The ecology of the African vectors of heartwater, with particular reference to *Amblyomma hebraeum* and *Amblyomma variegatum. Onderstepoort J. vet Res.* **54:** 381–395.
62. KOCAN, K.M., BEZUIDENHOUT, J.D. and HART, A. 1987. Ultrastructural features of *Cowdria ruminantium* in midgut epithelial cells and salivary glands of nymphal *Amblyomma hebraeum. Onderstepoort J. vet Res.* **54:** 87–93.
63. PROZESKY, L. 1987. Heartwater. The artificial transmission of *Cowdria ruminantium* in domestic ruminants and mice. *Onderstepoort J. vet Res.* **54:** 277–279.

64. MacKenzie, P.K.I. and McHardy, N. 1987. *Cowdria ruminantium* infection in the mouse: a review. *Onderstepoort J. vet Res.* **54:** 267–269.
65. McHardy, N. and MacKenzie, P.I. 1987. Identification of drugs effective against *Cowdria ruminantium* using a mouse screening system. *Onderstepoort J. vet Res.* **54:** 481–484.
66. Du Plessis, J.L. and Malan, L. 1988. Susceptibility to heartwater of calves born to non-immune cows. *Onderstepoort J. vet Res.* **55:** 235–237.
67. Wassink, L.A., Jongejan, F., Gruys, E. and Uilenberg, G. 1990. Observations on mouse-infective stocks of *Cowdria ruminantium*: microscopical demonstration of the Kwanyanga stock in mouse tissue and the carrier-status of the Senegal stock in mice. *Res. vet. Sci.* **48:** 389–390.
68. McHardy, N. and MacKenzie, P.K.I. 1984. Virulence of two strains of *Cowdria ruminantium* in mice and their use to predict drug activity against heartwater. *Trop. Anim. Hlth Prod.* **16:** 56–62.
69. Wassink, L.A., Franssen, F.F.J., Uilenberg, G. and Perié, N.M. 1987. Observations on mouse-infective stocks of *Cowdria ruminantium*: attempts to demonstrate persistence of the organism in mice immune to the Kwanyanga stock. *Res. vet. Sci.* **42:** 65–67.
70. Du Plessis, J.L., Meyer, E.H.H. and Van Gas, L. 1990. An attempt to establish an inbred line of mice genetically resistant to *Cowdria ruminantium*. *Onderstepoort J. vet Res.* **57:** 283–285.
71. Du Plessis, J.L., Berche, P. and Van Gas, L. 1991. T cell-mediated immunity to *Cowdria ruminantium* in mice: the protective role of Lyt-2^+ T cells. *Onderstepoort J. vet Res.* **58:** 171–179.
72. Petney, T.N. and Horak, I.G. 1988. Comparative host usage by *Amblyomma hebraeum* and *Amblyomma marmoreum*, (Acari, Ixodidae) the South African vectors of the disease heartwater. *J. appl. Ent.* **105:** 490–495.
73. MacKenzie, P.K.I. and McHardy, N. 1984. The culture of *Cowdria ruminantium* in mice: significance in respect of the epidemiology and control of heartwater. *Prev. vet. Med.* **2:** 227–237.
74. Howell, D.J., Petney, T.N. and Horak, I.G. 1989. The host status of the striped mouse, *Rhabdomys pumilio*, in relation to the tick vectors of heartwater in South Africa. *Onderstepoort J. vet Res.* **56:** 289–291.
75. Ilemobade, A.A. 1976. Study of heartwater and the causative agent, *Cowdria ruminantium* (Cowdry 1925), in Nigeria. Ph.D. Thesis, Ahmadu Bello University, Zaria, Nigeria, p. 276. Diss. Abstr. Int. 1977, **38(2):** 2.
76. Donatien, A. and Lestoquard, F. 1937. Etat actuel des connaissances sur les rickettsioses animales. *Arch. Inst. Pasteur Algérie* **15:** 142–187.
77. Andrew, H.R. and Norval, R.A.I. 1989. The carrier state of sheep, cattle and African buffalo recovered from heartwater. *Vet. Parasit.* **34:** 261–266.
78. Barré, N. and Camus, E. 1987. The reservoir status of goats recovered from heartwater. *Onderstepoort J. vet Res.* **54:** 435–437.
79. Prozesky, L. and du Plessis, J.L. 1987. Heartwater. The development and life cycle of *Cowdria ruminantium* in the vertebrate host, ticks and cultured endothelial cells. *Onderstepoort J. vet Res.* **54:** 193–196.
80. Logan, L.L., Whyard, T.C., Quintero, J.C. and Mebus, C.A. 1987. The development of *Cowdria ruminantium* in neutrophils. *Onderstepoort J. vet Res.* **54:** 197–204.
81. Clark, R. 1962. The pathological physiology of heartwater (*Cowdria (Rickettsia) ruminantium*)—Cowdry, 1926. *Onderstepoort J. vet Res.* **29:** 25–33.
82. Pienaar, J.G., Basson, P.A. and Van Der Merwe, J.L. de B. 1966. Studies on

the pathology of heartwater (*Cowdria (Rickettsia) ruminantium*, Cowdry, 1926). I. Neuropathological changes. *Onderstepoort J. vet Res.* **33:** 115–138.

83. OWEN, N.C., LITTLEJOHN, A., KRUGER, J.M. and ERASMUS, B.J. 1973. Physiopathological features of heartwater in sheep. *J. S. Afr. vet. Med. Ass.* **44:** 397–403.
84. VAN AMSTEL, S.R., GUTHRIE, A.J., REYERS, F., BERTSCHINGER, H., OBEREM, P.T., KILLEEN, V.M. and MATTHEE, O. 1987. The clinical pathology and pathophysiology of heartwater: a review. *Onderstepoort J. vet Res.* **54:** 287–290.
85. ILEMOBADE, A.A. and BLOTKAMP, C. 1978. Clinico-pathological study of heartwater in goats. *Tropenmed. Parasit.* **29:** 71–76.
86. PROZESKY, L. and DU PLESSIS, J.L. 1985. The pathology of heartwater. II. A study of the lung lesions in sheep and goats infected with the $Ball_3$ strain of *Cowdria ruminantium*. *Onderstepoort J. vet Res.* **52:** 81–85.
87. DU PLESSIS, J.L., MALAN, L. and KOWALSKI, Z.E. 1987. The pathogenesis of heartwater. *Onderstepoort J. vet Res.* **54:** 313–318.
88. VAN AMSTEL, S.R., OBEREM, P.T., DIDOMENICO, M., KIRKPATRICK, R.D. and MATHEE, J. 1988. The presence of endotoxin activity in cases of experimentally-induced heartwater in sheep. *Onderstepoort J. vet Res.* **55:** 217–220.
89. NEITZ, W.O. 1968. Heartwater. *Bull. Off. Int. Epizoot.* **70:** 329–336.
90. VAN DE PYPEKAMP, H.E. and PROZESKY, L. 1987. Heartwater. An overview of the clinical signs, susceptibility and differential diagnoses of the disease in domestic ruminants. *Onderstepoort J. vet Res.* **54:** 263–268.
91. UILENBERG, G., CAMUS, E. and BARRÉ, N. 1985. Quelques observations sur une souche de *Cowdria ruminantium* isolée en Guadeloupe (Antilles françaises). *Rev. Elev. Méd. vét. Pays Trop.* **38:** 34–42.
92. JONGEJAN, F., THIELEMANS, M.J.C., BRIÈRE, C. and UILENBERG, G. 1991. Antigenic diversity of *Cowdria ruminantium* isolates determined by cross-immunity. *Res. vet. Sci.* **51:** 24–28.
93. BROWN, C.C. and SKOWRONEK, A.J. 1990. Histologic and immunochemical study of the pathogenesis of heartwater (*Cowdria ruminantium* infection) in goats and mice. *Am. J. vet. Res.* **51:** 1476–1480.
94. METELERKAMP, N.C., LITTHAUER, D., NAUDE, R.J., OELOFSEN, W. and GRUSS, B. 1986. The orange–yellow pigment of heartwater-infected Angora goats. *Comp. Biochem. Physiol.* **84B:** 299–304.
95. PROZESKY, L. 1987. The pathology of heartwater. III. A review. *Onderstepoort J. vet Res.* **54:** 281–286.
96. ISOUN, T.T., AKPOKODJE, J.U., IKEDE, B.O. and FAYEMI, O. 1974. Heartwater in imported Brown Swiss breed of cattle in Western Nigeria. *Bull. Anim. Hlth Prod. Africa* **22:** 331–334.
97. NEITZ, W.O. and ALEXANDER, R.A. 1941. The immunisation of calves against heartwater. *J. S. Afr. vet. Med. Ass.* **12(4):** 103–111.
98. UILENBERG, G. 1971. Etudes sur la cowdriose à Madagascar. Première partie. *Rev. Elev. Méd. vét. Pays Trop.* **24:** 239–249.
99. GUEYE, A., MBENGUE, M., KEBE, B. and DIOUF, A. 1982. Note épizootiologique sur la cowdriose bovine dans les Niayes au Sénégal. *Rev. Elev. Méd. vét. Pays Trop.* **35:** 217–219.
100. LOGAN, L.L., TEMBELY, S. and MILLER, D.K. 1988. The importance of heartwater (*Cowdria ruminantium*) in Mali. *Bull. Anim. Hlth Prod. Africa* **36:** 89–92.
101. ILEMOBADE, A.A. 1977. Heartwater in Nigeria. I. The susceptibility of different local breeds and species of domestic ruminants to heartwater. *Trop. Anim. Hlth Prod.* **9:** 177–180.

102. Camus, E. 1991. La cowdriose caprine et ovine en Guadeloupe. *Rev. Elev. Méd. vét. Pays Trop.* Special Issue: 139–143.
103. Gueye, A., Mbengue, M., Diouf, A. and Vassiliadès, G. 1989. Prophylaxie de la cowdriose et observations sur la pathologie ovine dans la région des Niayes au Sénégal. *Rev. Elev. Méd. vét. Pays Trop.* **42:** 497–503.
104. Matheron, G., Barré, N., Camus, E. and Gogue, J. 1987. Genetic resistance of Guadeloupe native goats to heartwater. *Onderstepoort J. vet Res.* **54:** 337–340.
105. Matheron, G., Camus, E., Barré, N. and Gogue, J.M. 1991. Résistance à la cowdriose de chèvres Créole en Guadeloupe. Bilan en 1988. *Rev. Elev. Méd. vét. Pays Trop.* Special Issue: 145–153.
106. Yunker, C.E. 1988. Current research on heartwater in Zimbabwe. *Zimbabwe vet. J.* **19:** 25–31.
107. Du Plessis, J.L. 1984. Colostrum-derived antibodies to *Cowdria ruminantium* in the serum of calves and lambs. *Onderstepoort J. vet Res.* **51:** 275–276.
108. Totté, P., De Gee, A.L.W., Jongejan, F., Vandenbussche, P. and Wérenne, J. 1990. Infections par la rickettsie *Cowdria ruminantium*: rôle des interférons et d'autres cytokines dans la pathologie et la résistance à la maladie. *6ème Réunion des Interféronistes de Langue Française,* pp. 77–78. Bruxelles, 13–14 Sept. 1990.
109. Neitz, W.O. 1939. The immunity in heartwater. *Onderstepoort J. vet Sci. Anim. Ind.* **13:** 245–283.
110. Neitz, W.O., Alexander, R.A. and Adelaar, T.F. 1947. Studies on immunity in heartwater. *Onderstepoort J. vet Res.* **21:** 243–252.
111. Du Plessis, J.L., Jansen, B.C. and Prozesky, L. 1983. Heartwater in Angora goats. I. Immunity subsequent to artificial infection and treatment. *Onderstepoort J. vet Res.* **50:** 137–143.
112. Du Plessis, J.L. and Bezuidenhout, J.D. 1979. Investigations on the natural and acquired resistance of cattle to artificial infection with *Cowdria ruminantium. J. S. Afr. vet. Ass.* **50:** 334–338.
113. Du Plessis, J.L., Bezuidenhout, J.D. and Lüdemann, C.J.F. 1984. The immunization of calves against heartwater: subsequent immunity both in the absence and presence of natural tick challenge. *Onderstepoort J. vet Res.* **51:** 193–196.
114. Jongejan, F., Uilenberg, G., Franssen, F.F.J., Gueye, A. and Nieuwenhuijs, J. 1988. Antigenic differences between stocks of *Cowdria ruminantium. Res. vet. Sci.* **44:** 186–189.
115. Du Plessis, J.L., Van Gas, L., Olivier, J.A. and Bezuidenhout, J.D. 1989. The heterogenicity of *Cowdria ruminantium* stocks: cross-immunity and serology in sheep and pathogenicity to mice. *Onderstepoort J. vet Res.* **56:** 195–201.
116. Du Plessis, J.L., Potgieter, F.T. and Van Gas, L. 1990. An attempt to improve the immunization of sheep against heartwater by using different combinations of 3 stocks of *Cowdria ruminantium. Onderstepoort J. vet Res.* **57:** 205–208.
117. Stewart, C.G. 1989. *Cowdria ruminantium* stocks: how significant are they? *Zimbabwe vet. J.* **20:** 149–154.
118. Jongejan, F., Wassink, L.A., Thielemans, M.J.C., Perié, N.M. and Uilenberg, G. 1989. Serotypes in *Cowdria ruminantium* and their relationship with *Ehrlichia phagocytophila* determined by immunofluorescence. *Vet. Microbiol.* **21:** 31–40.

119. SYNGE, B.A. 1978. Brain biopsy for the diagnosis of heartwater. *Trop. Anim. Hlth Prod.* **10:** 45–48.

120. SCHREUDER, B.E.C. 1980. A simple technique for the collection of brain samples for the diagnosis of heartwater. *Trop. Anim. Hlth Prod.* **12:** 25–29.

121. PROZESKY, L. 1987. Diagnosis of heartwater at post-mortem in ruminants and the confirmation of *Cowdria ruminantium* in mice. *Onderstepoort J. vet Res.* **54:** 301–303.

122. CAMUS, E. and BARRÉ, N. 1988. Le diagnostic de la cowdriose à partir d'écrasement de cerveau. *Rev. Elev. Méd. vét. Pays Trop.* **41:** 247–252.

123. BARRÉ, N., CAMUS, E., BIRNIE, E., BURRIDGE, M.J., UILENBERG, G. and PROVOST, A. 1984. Setting up a method for surveying the distribution of cowdriosis (heartwater) in the Caribbean. *Proceedings XIIIth World Congress on Diseases of Cattle,* Durban, **1:** 536–541.

124. BEZUIDENHOUT, J.D. 1987. The present state of *Cowdria ruminantium* cultivation in cell lines. *Onderstepoort J. vet Res.* **54:** 205–210.

125. NEITZ, A.W.H., VILJOEN, G.J., BEZUIDENHOUT, J.D., OBEREM, P.T., VISSER, L. and VERMEULEN, N.M.J. 1986. Detection of *Cowdria ruminantium* antigen and antibody during the course of heartwater disease in sheep by means of an enzyme-linked immunosorbent assay. *Onderstepoort J. vet Res.* **53:** 205–207.

126. LOGAN, L.L., HOLLAND, C.J., MEBUS, C.A. and RISTIC, M. 1986. Serological relationship between *Cowdria ruminantium* and certain ehrlichia. *Vet. Rec.* **119:** 458–459.

127. DU PLESSIS, J.L., FOURIE, N., NEL, P.W. and EVEZARD, D.N. 1990. Concurrent babesiosis and ehrlichiosis in the dog: bloodsmear examination supplemented by the indirect fluorescent antibody test, using *Cowdria ruminantium* as antigen. *Onderstepoort J. vet Res.* **57:** 151–155.

128. DU PLESSIS, J.L. 1985. A method for determining the *Cowdria ruminantium* infection rate of *Amblyomma hebraeum*: effects in mice injected with tick homogenates. *Onderstepoort J. vet Res.* **52:** 55–61.

129. UILENBERG, G. 1989. La cowdriose caprine. In: *African Small Ruminant Research and Development,* pp. 427–435. WILSON, R.T. and AZEB, M. (Eds), ILCA, Addis Ababa.

130. UILENBERG, G. 1990. Methods currently used for the control of heartwater: their validity and proposals for future control strategies. *Parasitologia* **32:** 55–62.

131. NORVAL, R.A.I. and LAWRENCE, J.A. 1979. The control of heartwater in Zimbabwe Rhodesia. *Zimbabwe Rhodesia Agric. J.* **76:** 161–165.

132. UTECH, K.B.W., WHARTON, R.H. and KERR, J.D. 1978. Resistance to *Boophilus microplus* (Canestrini) in different breeds of cattle. *Aust. J. agric. Res.* **29:** 885–895.

133. WILLADSEN, P. 1990. Perspectives for subunit vaccines for the control of ticks. *Parasitologia* **32:** 195–200.

134. PAVIS, C., BARRÉ, N., MALOSSE, C., DELOT, J. and BONIJOL, A. 1991. Etude des phéromones d'agrégation-fixation chez la tique du bétail *Amblyomma variegatum. Rencontres Caraïbes en Lutte Biologique,* pp. 247–256. PAVIS, C. and KERMARREC, A. (Eds), Les Colloques de l'INRA no. 58, INRA, Paris.

135. NORVAL, R.A.I., YUNKER, C.E., DUNCAN, I.M. and PETER, T. 1991. Pheromone/acaricide mixtures in the control of the tick *Amblyomma hebraeum*: effects of acaricides on attraction and attachment. *Expl appl. Acarol.* **11:** 233–240.

136. BARRÉ, N. 1988. Mesures agronomiques permettant une diminution des

populations de la tique *Amblyomma variegatum*. *Rev. Elev. Méd. vét. Pays Trop.* **41:** 387–393.

137. NEITZ, W.O. and ALEXANDER, R.A. 1941. The immunisation of calves against heartwater. *J. S. Afr. vet. Med. Ass.* **12(4):** 103–111.
138. BEZUIDENHOUT, J.D. 1981. The development of a new heartwater vaccine using *Amblyomma hebraeum* nymphae infected with *Cowdria ruminantium*. In: *Tick Biology and Control,* pp. 41–45. WHITEHEAD, G.B. and GIBSON, J.D. (Eds), Rhodes University, Grahamstown, South Africa.
139. BEZUIDENHOUT, J.D. 1989. Cowdria vaccines. In: *Veterinary Protozoan and Hemoparasite Vaccines,* pp. 31–42. WRIGHT, I.G. (Ed.), CRC Press, Boca Raton.
140. BRETT, S. and BEZUIDENHOUT, J.D. 1989. Mass production of *Cowdria ruminantium* in tissue culture with the aim to replace the current heartwater blood vaccine with a tissue culture vaccine. *Newslett. Onderstepoort vet. Res. Inst.* **7(3):** 9.
141. ANONYMOUS. 1984. Methods of immunization against *Cowdria ruminantium.* In: *Ticks and Tick-Borne Disease Control. A Practical Field Manual, Vol. II. Tick-borne disease control,* pp. 564–576. FAO, Rome.
142. OLIVIER, J.A., LÖTTER, A.P., SCHWULST, W.G.E. and MATTHEE, O. 1988. Chemoprofilakse van hartwater met behulp van 'n onderhuidse pil of pasta. *Newslett. Onderstepoort vet. Res. Inst.* **6(1):** 7–9.
143. DU PLESSIS, J.L. and MALAN, L. 1987. The block method of vaccination against heartwater. *Onderstepoort J. vet Res.* **54:** 493–495.
144. GRUSS, B. 1987. Problems encountered in the control of heartwater in Angora goats. *Onderstepoort J. vet Res.* **54:** 513–515.
145. PURNELL, R.E. 1987. Development of a prophylactic regime using Terramycin/LA to assist in the introduction of susceptible cattle into heartwater endemic areas of Africa. *Onderstepoort J. vet Res.* **54:** 509–512.
146. JONGEJAN, F. 1991. Protective immunity to heartwater (*Cowdria ruminantium* infection) is acquired after vaccination with *in vitro*-attenuated rickettsiae. *Infect. Immun.* **59:** 729–731.
147. NORVAL, R.A.I., SUTHERST. R.W., JORGENSEN, O.G., GIBSON, J.D. and KERR, J.D. 1989. The effect of the bont tick (*Amblyomma hebraeum*) on the weight gain of Africander steers. *Vet. Parasit.* **33:** 329–341.
148. ASSELBERGS, M.J. and LOPES PEREIRA, C.M. 1990. Damage by *Amblyomma hebraeum* in local (*Bos indicus*) cattle in Mozambique. In: *Livestock Production in the Tropics,* pp. 358–360. KUIL, H., PALING, R.W. and HUHN, J.E. (Eds), Proc. 6th Int. Conf. Inst. Trop. Vet. Med., Wageningen, 1989. Faculty of Veterinary Medicine, Utrecht.
149. BEZUIDENHOUT, J.D. 1985. The epizootiology and control of heartwater and other tick-borne diseases of cattle in South Africa. *Onderstepoort J. vet Res.* **52:** 211–214.
150. WALKER, J.D. and OLWAGE, A. 1987. The tick vectors of *Cowdria ruminantium* (Ixodoidea, Ixodidae, genus *Amblyomma*) and their distribution. *Onderstepoort J. vet Res* **54:** 353–379.

18

Avian Chlamydiosis

G. A. CULLEN

Introduction

Chlamydia psittaci infects many species of animals and birds. From early times, when the organism was still known as the Bedsonia agent, it became customary to refer to the infection as psittacosis. This was because of the frequency of infection in psittacine birds. Strictly speaking, the term psittacosis should be restricted to infection in birds of the family Psittaciformes. In practice it is also used to refer to the infection in people, whether or not it was acquired from a psittacine bird. The term ornithosis is used to describe the infection in nonpsittacine birds. Now that the organisms are well understood and classified, it is more appropriate to refer to these infections as chlamydiosis.

Infection of birds with *C. psittaci* is widespread geographically and occurs in many species. Psittacine birds such as parrots, in their natural habitat, have endemic infection, which is often present as a latent and symptomless carrier state. On transport to another country such infections may become active, often leading to clinical disease. Imported psittacines, whether or not they appear sick, can be a source of infection to other birds, animals or people.

Of greater economic importance is the occurrence of chlamydiosis in poultry, mainly in turkeys and ducks. Outbreaks of disease have caused heavy losses to turkey producers in the United States and have considerable public health importance, as the workers in slaughter houses, and other points in the production chain, may acquire the infection. Breeding turkeys may show few signs other than a drop in egg production. Ducks are also a possible hazard to the health of processing plant workers, due to chlamydia. The infection rarely causes disease in the ducks themselves, although young ducklings are susceptible to severe disease. Pigeons are another reservoir of infection, and potential threat to human health, although it is thought that the strains of *C. psittaci* isolated from pigeons are usually of low virulence. It is characteristic of *C. psittaci* that there are considerable differences in the virulence of different isolates, but the biochemical basis for this is not understood. Individual people are said to show much variation in their susceptibility to infection.

Chlamydiosis in domestic poultry is relatively uncommon in most countries, except for latent infections in ducks. When outbreaks of disease are suspected, diagnosis is based on clinical signs and postmortem lesions, confirmed by isolation of the organism, or its detection by antigen-capture techniques. Microscopic examination of impression smears from thoracic and abdominal organs, suitably stained, is also helpful. Serological tests, such as complement fixation (CF) and enzyme linked immunosorbent assay (ELISA), can be used to detect antibodies for diagnostic or epidemiological purposes. In birds there may be considerable variation in the severity of symptoms, in rates of mortality and in morbidity within the flock. Disease in people may resemble relatively mild influenza, but can be very acute and serious, with rapid development of encephalitis. Such cases may prove fatal unless diagnosed and treated rapidly, especially in the very old or very young. A chronic form of the disease can also occur in humans, causing heart valve lesions.

The disease in humans, poultry, pigeons or psittacine birds can be treated with antibiotics. Experimental work on vaccines has not yet led to the development of effective products. Control of the infection is by good hygiene and reduction of the reservoir of infected birds, for example by quarantine of imported birds. In many countries there is legislation which specifies the action to be taken when chlamydiosis is diagnosed (see Control).

Causal Agent

The causal agent of avian chlamydiosis is *Chlamydia psittaci*, which is an obligate intracellular organism with a complex life cycle. It is classified in the order Chlamydiales, family Chlamydiaceae, genus *Chlamydia*. Three species are recognized, *C. trachomatis, C. psittaci* and *C. pneumoniae*.[1] *C. trachomatis* is the cause of trachoma and other human diseases. *C. psittaci* causes infection and disease in many species of birds and mammals. *C. pneumoniae* is a more recently described human pathogen, known for a time as the TWAR agent. The species are mainly differentiated on the basis of intracellular colonial morphology. The inclusions of *C. psittaci* are dense and lack glycogen, whereas those of *C. trachomatis* are vacuolated and contain glycogen. Although *C. trachomatis* has been subdivided into numerous biovars and serovars, this has not yet been described for

C. psittaci of avian origin. Restriction endonuclease analysis has been used to compare chlamydia from various avian and mammalian sources.[2]

Morphology

C. psittaci may be observed in two distinct morphological forms, representing different stages in its intracellular life cycle. These are the elementary body (EB) and the reticulate body (RB). The EB is the infectious form of the organism. It is a small, dense, spherical body, 200–300 nm in diameter. A few hours after phagocytosis by the host cell it enlarges to produce a RB (also known as an initial body). The RB is the metabolically active form. It is very variable in size, ranging from 500–1500 nm in diameter. It divides by binary fission to produce large numbers of smaller units, which become the next generation of EBs. In avain chlamydia this whole cycle takes about 30 h, although there is variation between strains in the speed of reproduction. The characteristic morphology is also of value in examination of stained smears, by light microscopy, for diagnostic purposes. More details of the life cycle are given elsewhere in this book, and in other publications, for example see Ref. 3.

Cultural Characteristics

C. psittaci can be cultivated in the yolk sac of 7 day old chicken embryos, in various cell cultures, or by inoculation of mice. Culture of chlamydia must be done with great care to avoid laboratory acquired infection, because of the very dangerous nature of the human disease. A Class III biohazard cabinet should be used for all manipulations where live chlamydia are, or may be, present.

Chicken Embryos

Specific pathogen free, specific antibody negative and antibiotic free chicken eggs should be used. They should be incubated at 39°C for 7 days, then inoculated into the yolk sac, and incubation continued at 39°C for a few days.[4] Infected embryos show vascular congestion of the yolk sac, from which the organism can be harvested, 3–10 days after inoculation.

Cell Cultures

Monolayers of appropriate cells are produced: mouse L929 cells, treated with 5-iodo-2-deoxyuridine are very suitable.[5] Other cells which have been used include McCoy, HeLa, Vero and BHK 21. Cell monolayers are examined daily, and chlamydia recognized by suitable staining and identified by the fluorescent antibody test.

Mice

Mice can be inoculated by either the intracerebral or intraperitoneal route. This used to be a routine diagnostic procedure, but can hardly be justified now that effective cell culture methods are available.

Molecular Biology

The chlamydial genome is a closed circular DNA molecule with a molecule weight of 6.6×10^8 Da. Chlamydia contain DNA and RNA, which are present in both the EBs and RBs. All avian strains of *C. psittaci* so far exmined contain a 5 kb plasmid which, by endonuclease restriction analysis, appears to be the same, regardless of avian host,[6] although some mammalian isolates carry plasmids distinct to the host. It has also been observed that some avian isolates of *C. psittaci* contain a bacteriophage, which can be seen in crystalline array in electronmicrographs. It has been characterized as a unique, single-stranded, circular DNA bacteriophage.[7]

Antigenicity

The antigenic structure of chlamydia is complex. There is an immunodominant "Group antigen" which is found in all members of the genus. There are also numerous proteinaceous antigens which are not all present in all isolates.

The group antigen, which is common to *C. trachomatis* and *C. psittaci*, is a lipoglycoprotein, containing an acidic polysaccharide which is the antigenic determinant. It is thermostable at 100°C for 30 min. The antigen is also resistant to phenol (0.5%), trypsin and papain. It can be purified and separated into several fractions by ion-exchange chromatography.[8]

The numerous protein antigens can be analyzed using SDS-PAGE. Some of them appear to be species specific and others subspecies specific. The major outer membrane proteins (MOMP) of chlamydia are important in the antigenic grouping of these organisms. Cloning and sequence analysis of the MOMP gene of *C. psittaci* has recently been described.[9] Two serogroups of *C. psittaci* have been demonstrated using immunoblotting on 12 isolates and they correspond with differences in infectivity for cell-cultures.[10]

Chlamydia produce toxins, and this can be demonstrated by the intravenous inoculation of mice with yolk-sac cultures. The toxins can be neutralized by specific antiserum.

Epidemiology

Natural Transmission

Natural infections with *C. psittaci* occur in domestic poultry, and have been described in over 120 wild avian species.[11] They are common in pigeons and sea gulls, and have been isolated from blackbirds and house sparrows. The infection is endemic in parrots and other psittacine birds in South America and other tropical and subtropical areas. In many cases these natural infections produce no signs of disease in the host, which may remain latently infected for long periods. It is likely that there is frequent transmission of *C. psittaci* between various avian species, including domestic poultry. It is thought unlikely that mammalian hosts are responsible for infections of poultry. Infection is usually acquired through the inhalation of dust, laden with chlamydia, having originated from dried nasal or ocular discharges or feces. Excretion of *C. psittaci* is intermittent, thus the infectivity of these discharges will vary from day to day. The migratory movements of free-living birds, and their tendency to mingle with others when feeding, facilitates the spread of infection. In this context it is desirable for domestic poultry to be housed in bird-proof pens. Free-range poultry are exposed to greater risk of infection from wild birds. It is not known whether arthropods act as vectors for this infection. Studies with turkeys have failed to demonstrate transovarian transmission of *C. psittaci*.[12] In wild birds there is a natural parent to nestling transmission. This can also occur in pigeon lofts where hygiene is poor.

Experimental Infection

It is likely that any species of bird could be infected with *C. psittaci*, although individual variation in susceptibility has been observed. This is reflected in the infective dose required to establish infection, the severity of the disease produced and the length of time during which the organism is shed.

Mice and sometimes guinea pigs have been used for laboratory work with chlamydia. Rabbits can be useful for raising antisera, although they are relatively resistant to infection.

Hosts Affected

Psittacine birds are frequently infected, often without clinical signs, but can show severe and fatal disease. Of domestic poultry, turkeys are most likely to suffer from severe disease. Ducks are often infected, usually with mild chronic disease, but sometimes with severe, rapidly fatal disease. Chickens appear to be relatively resistant to the infection. Geese have similar disease susceptibility to ducks. Pheasants have been reported with the disease, but only in isolated cases. Pigeons are frequently infected, often with mild strains, but sometimes show signs of severe disease.[13]

Young birds are observed to be more susceptible to disease than older birds, although the mechanism for this is not known. The young bird is more likely to show clinical disease, with mature birds tending to have inapparent infections, only becoming clinically ill when subjected to adverse conditions.

Geographical Distribution

C. psittaci is found throughout the world, in many species of animals and birds. So far as birds are concerned, the natural infection in psittacines is mainly found in South America, but infection of pigeons is widespread. Infection of poultry, mainly turkeys, has been reported chiefly from the U.S.A. and E. Europe.

Numerical data on the incidence of chlamydiosis in birds in different countries is limited. A study lasting nearly 10 years, from 1974 until 1983, was carried out in Britain. Diagnostic samples submitted to a central laboratory were examined both by culture and serology. The percentage of serological reactors was variable in domestic poultry, ranging from 1.5 in chickens to 22.2 in geese, and was highest in pigeons, 47.3 and collared doves, 51.4. A moderate incidence was found in game birds, 29.0, wild ducks, 23.3, and imported birds of the Order Psittaciformes, 15.9. The highest titers were recorded in pigeons, collared doves and psittacines, indicating that infection was both frequent and active. During the period 1976–1984, 1,531 samples were examined by culture and 196 were positive, pigeons, collared doves and psittacines being most affected.[14]

Reservoirs of Infection

As stated above, the tropical rain forests of South America form a large reservoir of infection in psittacine birds and the town pigeons seen in so many cities form another large pool of this infection.

Zoonotic Aspects

Some strains of *C. psittaci* are dangerous human pathogens. Psittacosis was first described in man by Riter, in 1879. During the 1930s there were severe epidemics of psittacosis, with many fatal cases, mainly in the United States and Europe. Such epidemics have not been seen in recent decades, but a significant disease problem remains in the human population. Each year hundreds of cases are reported. Cases are not reported unless a four-fold rise in complement-fixing antibodies has been demonstrated. There may be additional, mild, undetected cases.

Infection in people is often of unknown origin, but in those cases where a likely source can be identified, psittacine birds are often implicated.[15] Freshly imported birds, housed in pet shops, are the most likely cause of severe human disease. There have also been severe cases due to infection of persons entering the slaughter houses where ducks or turkeys are being eviscerated.

Pigeon fanciers are also at risk of infection and in these individuals, acute allergic alveolitis may also be present. Another possible source of infection is of course laboratory acquired, through examination of infected tissues or cultures, with inadequate safety precautions. The human disease usually takes the form of a mild to severe influenza-like illness. A typical case might show shivering, chest pain, coughing, vomiting and diarrhea, with fever and mental confusion. Appropriate antibiotic treatment needs to be started quickly. In addition to the typical acute disease, there may be chronic human disease due to *C. psittaci*. Using the indirect immunofluorescence test *C. psittaci* antigen was detected in 7 of 27 biopsy specimens taken from cases of acquired valvular heart-disease.[16]

Pathogenesis

Mode of Entry and Sites of Primary Multiplication

Infection with *C. psittaci* is usually through the intestinal or respiratory tracts. First, the EBs attach to microvilli on the outer surface of susceptible epithelial cells.[17] They travel down to rest in folds in the plasma membrane, subsequently becoming ingulfed by a process resembling endocytosis. Further multiplication then follows, as the organisms pass through their complex life cycle. The inclusion which develops may contain from 100 to 500 progeny.

Modes of Dissemination

Infection is usually spread by the inhalation or the ingestion of organisms derived from drops of respiratory or nasal discharges, or feces. It is thought that infection may also occur through direct contact. Build up of infection in nests, or in badly cleaned lofts and pens helps to perpetuate the infection. It has been found that homogenates of mites from turkey nests contained chlamydia,[18] but the importance of arthropod vectors has not been established.

Target Cells

Experimental infection of turkeys by the airborne route has been described.[19] The infection began in the epithelial cells of the lungs, thoracic and abdominal air-sacs. After 48 h, low numbers of organisms were found in the spleen, kidney, blood and pericardial membrane.

Inflammatory Response

The acute disease is characterized by the production of much inflammatory exudate. The pleural cavity may contain a fibrinous exudate, and in severe cases the thoracic cavity is filled with a dark transudate. The heart and pericardium also show inflammatory changes, with a thickened pericardial membrane covered with fibrinous exudate. Inflammatory changes are seen in many organs, including the testes in male turkeys.

Carrier State and Latency

Chronic disease, or the establishment of a latent infection, are most likely to happen when birds are infected with strains of low virulence. The natural resistance of the bird will also be a factor. Infection of turkeys with a strain of low virulence led to mild disease of long duration and low mortality.[20]

Clinical Disease

Prepatent Period

Clinical disease in birds may be acute or chronic, and vary greatly in severity. Its appearance will depend on both the species of the host and the pathogenicity of the infecting strain. The incubation period is also very variable. In turkeys experimentally infected with a virulent strain, definite signs of disease are seen after 5–10 days. Where there is natural infection, often with lower doses of organisms, the period may be much longer.

Clinical Signs

Typical signs of this disease are that the birds begin to show loss of appetite and inactivity. There is a serous or purulent exudate from the eyes and nostrils. Nervous signs are seen in some species. A common feature is diarrhea, with greenish-grey feces, often of gelatinous consistency, which may be blood stained. Respiratory distress and hypothermia may also be observed. Egg production in severely affected birds drops rapidly, e.g. 60% down to 20% or less.

Turkeys show the signs described above. In ducks, specially young ducklings, the nervous signs are more pronounced. They will show trembling, with an unstable walk, and will die in convulsions. The discharges from the eyes and nostrils may be very severe, leading to encrustation of the head feathers. In pigeons there is typically a conjunctivitis, with swollen eyelids, rhinitis, anorexia and an unthrifty appearance. Psittacine birds frequently carry the infection without obvious signs of disease, but where resistance breaks down, the typical signs are nasal and ocular discharges, with diarrhea, lethargy and inappetence.

Morbidity and Mortality

The range of these is very variable, as would be expected from the complex host–parasite relationship in which the balance between the pathogenicity of the organism and resistance of the host is unpredictable. In flocks of turkeys experiencing infection with virulent strains, the morbidity can reach 80%, and the mortality can reach 30%.

Pathology

Gross Pathology

Once again, the lesions will vary with the severity of the infection. There is a diffuse congestion of the lungs and the pleural cavity may contain fibribinous exudate. The air sacs become thickened and cloudy. The pericardial membrane is thickened, congested and covered with fibrinous exudate. There is enlargement and discoloration of the liver and spleen, which may contain small necrotic foci and small hemorrhages. A sticky fibro-purulent exudate covers the serosal surfaces. Damage to the heart and lungs causes death in turkeys, but in other species neurological damage may be of greater importance.

Histopathology

The exudates which are prominent in this disease contain large numbers of mononuclear cells which have chlamydial inclusions in their cytoplasm. There is cellular proliferation and necrosis in the major organs. Peritonitis, pericarditis and myocarditis are seen, but arteritis is relatively uncommon. Most birds show hepatitis in which the sinusoids may show dilation and infiltration with mononuclear cells and lymphocytes. In parrots, focal necrosis of the liver is seen, but in turkeys necrotic hepatic cells are scattered throughout the organ. In pigeons, higher than usual amounts of urates may be seen in the cloaca, associated with catarrhal enteritis.

Immunity

Protective Immunity

In a survey of published work on avian immunity to chlamydia,[21] the author concluded that birds, particularly psittacines and turkeys and possibly pigeons, can acquire resistance to chlamydiosis. This may be as a result of recovery from infection or following vaccination. Acquired resistance varies between individuals, is relative rather than absolute, and is probably of limited duration.

Mechanism of Immunity

The Complement Fixation (CF) test has been widely used to demonstrate the production of antibodies in response to both natural and experimental infection with *C. psittaci*. Agglutination tests have been used, especially in experimental work, and more recently ELISA tests have also been used. In an experimental infection of turkeys,[22] agglutinating antibodies were detected 3–4 days after infection, and CF antibodies 7–8 days after infection. Both these tests remained positive until the end of the experiment, 104 days later. In another study of turkeys, naturally infected with an isolate of low virulence,[23] serum antibodies and skin sensitivity remained for up to 25 months. The agglutination test has been shown to detect 19S antibody, whereas the CF test detects both 19S and 7S antibodies.[24] Neutralizing antibodies can be stimulated experimentally, but only following hyperimmunization.[25] The importance of neutralizing antibodies in protection against natural disease in birds is unclear. Early studies showed that bursectomy of turkey poults at one day of age prevented an antibody response to an experimental antigen, but did not reduce the ability of the birds to develop resistance to experimental infection.[26] However, when turkeys were thymectomized at 10 days of age, protection was eliminated. This suggests that the cellular, lymphocyte, response is more important than humoral antibody for protection. It appears that latent infection of psittacine birds can confer a high level of immunity.

Diagnosis

Clinical Signs

These have been described above. The most important are the production of profuse gelatinous diarrhea together with nasal and ocular discharges, accompanied by prostration, anorexia and in some cases ataxia and other nervous signs. Clinical material for diagnosis can be taken from live birds. This includes feces, cloacal swabs, nasal and conjunctival discharges and blood.

Pathognomonic Postmortem Findings

The most helpful diagnostic feature is the production of copious inflammatory exudates. Thickening of the pericardial membrane and epicardial encrustation, airsaculitis, hepatomegaly, splenomegaly and peritonitis are seen in severe cases.

Microscopic Examination of Stained Smears

Tissues and exudates should be collected for examination by various methods. The tissues of choice are spleen, air sacs, pericardium, heart, liver and kidney. Histological preparations for diagnostic purposes are usually made from impression smears of affected tissues. These should be heat fixed and may be stained by a variety of methods such as the Ziehl–Nielsen (ZN) technique. They are examined microscopically using the high power objective, Using the ZN stain, inclusions appear as groups of small, discrete, pink, intracytoplasmic bodies. When viewed under dark-ground illumination, the pink inclusions became apple green in colour, which can be a useful way to distinguish them from artefacts. Other stains commonly used include Giemsa (purple inclusions), Castañeda (blue), Macciavello and Gimenez (red).[27]

Results of Serological Tests

The serological test of choice for diagnostic purposes has for a long time been the CF test, although ELISA tests are now being developed[28,29] and require evaluation.[30] The commercially available antibody detection ELISA kits are made with antigen from *C. trachomatis*, and rely on the cross reacting group antigen. There are several ways of doing the CF test, and for some species of bird an indirect CF will be required. Suitable antigens can be made from infected chicken embryo yolk, but better results are obtained by use of cell cultures. More details of methodology have been published.[29]

Low titers to *C. psittaci* antigens are common, and are not diagnostic unless higher than 1/64 in poultry. Ideally, paired serum samples should be taken, about 14 days apart, in which case a four-fold rise in antibody titer is diagnostic.

Results of Culture

A definitive diagnosis of chlamydiosis can be made by culture and identification of the organism. The tissues mentioned above may be cultured by a variety of methods. Fertile hens eggs have been used, but it is preferable to use treated cell cultures.[31]

Before inoculation, samples may need treatment to inactivate contaminating microorganisms. This is essential for feces. A suitable procedure is to homogenize the tissue in diluent containing 500–1000 μg/ml each of streptomycin, vancomycin and kanamycin, followed by centrifugation at 1000–2000 $\times$ g for 30 min. The supernatant can be filtered using 0.45 μm pore size. Improved cell culture results may be obtained by centrifugation of the suspect inoculum onto cell cultures which have been grown on microscope cover slips. It is usual to examine cell cultures daily for evidence of growth. At least three serial passages are required to indicate reliably that clinical material did not contain viable chlamydia. After growth, the cultures should be stained for identification. It is best to use a fluorescent antibody technique for this.

Other methods are now becoming available for the detection of chlamydial antigen, which are less dependent on the viability of the organism. ELISA tests have been developed for antigen capture, and commercial kits are available, although they are usually based on reagents made from *C. trachomatis*. More recently polymerase chain reaction (PCR) has been shown to have high sensitivity and specificity for detecting chlamydia in specimens from birds.[32,33]

Treatment

Chemotherapy

Chlortetracycline (CTC) is generally regarded as the most suitable drug for the treatment of *C. psittaci* infections in poultry and other birds. A suitable treatment for turkeys is CTC at a concentration of 400 g/tonne of pelleted feed. The medicated feed should be given for a period of two weeks, and withdrawal periods observed before birds are sent for slaughter. Treatment may not be effective in completely removing infection. In the case of turkey flocks, it is best to treat, slaughter and then thoroughly cleanse and disinfect before restocking. In other birds, salmonellosis may be a complicating infection which would require treatment with additional antibiotics. In pigeons and other pet birds, it may be desirable to have periods of treatment alternating with no treatment, to eliminate the infection. In the case of some exotic species, it can be difficult to persuade the bird to take the treatment in the drinking water. Fruit eating birds can be medicated in syrup, and there are proprietory brands of medicated seed available for cage birds. Valuable individuals can of course be given daily injections. Treatment of psittacine birds should be continued for 35 consecutive days, and blood levels of CTC should be at least 1 μg/ml of blood.

Control

Control of the disease depends on identification of infected birds and prevention of transmission.

Vaccines

Despite the experimental demonstration of immune responses to vaccines, there are no commercially available vaccines which will produce long lasting immunity to avian chlamydia. Two doses of a live chlamydia vaccine given to turkeys produced protection against severe challenge in 90% of a group of young turkeys,[34] but this has not been exploited commercially. As outbreaks of chlamydia in turkeys are sporadic, the practicability of applying mass live vaccination is doubtful, even if a vaccine was available.

Hygiene

Good hygiene is the best way to prevent the introduction and spread of *C. psittaci* infection. Unfortunately, pigeon lofts and pet shops are often deficient in this respect. The agent is very susceptible to formaldehyde and to phenolic disinfectants. It is important to avoid spread through infected dust. For pet birds kept in cages with solid floors, this can be minimized by keeping the floor of the cage damp. Contact with vectors such as wild and feral birds should be avoided. Care should be taken to avoid mechanical transmission of the agent and to protect human attendants from the disease. Postmortem examinations and laboratory work with *C. psittaci* should be done in a suitable biohazard cabinet. Cabinets can be fumigated between use, using hot formaldehyde.

Statutory Controls

Infection of birds with *C. psittaci* is subject to various legal regulations in different countries. In the United Kingdom, for example, the disease is not notifiable, but is subject to the control measures set out in the Psittacosis/Ornithosis Order 1953 (SI 1953, No. 38). This provides for the detention and isolation of affected or suspect birds and for other precautions to prevent the spread of disease, including the cleansing and disinfection of premises and equipment. The Importation of Birds, Poultry and Hatching Eggs Order, 1979 (SI 1979, No. 1702), provides for a 35 day quarantine period for imported birds. It was designed mainly for the control of Newcastle disease.[35]

References

1. MOULDER, J.W. 1984. Chlamydiales. In: *Bergey's Manual of Systematic Bacteriology*, Vol. 1, pp. 729–739. KREIG, N.R. (Ed.), Williams and Wilkins, Baltimore.
2. ANDERSEN, A.A. 1991. Comparison of avian Chlamydia psittaci isolates by restriction endonuclease and serovar-specific monoclonal antibodies. *J. clin. Microbiol.* **29:** 244–249.
3. MOULDER, J.W. 1985. Comparative biology of intracellular parasitism. *Microbiol. Rev.* **49:** 298–337.
4. PAGE, L.A. 1971. The influence of temperature upon the multiplication of chlamydiae in chicken embryos. *Excerpta Med. Proc. Trachoma Conf. Int. Conf. Ser.* **223:** 40–51.
5. BEVAN, B.J., CULLEN, G.A. and READ, W.M.E. 1978. Isolation of *Chlamydia psittaci* from avian sources using growth in cell culture. *Avian. Path.* **7:** 203–211.
6. LUSHER, M., STOREY, C.C. and RICHMOND, S.J. 1988. Characterization of plasmids from different Chlamydia psittaci strains. In: *First Conference of the European Society for Chlamydia Research*, p. 63. CEVENINI, R. (Ed.), Societa Editrice Esculapio, Bologna, Italy.
7. STOREY, C.C., LUSHER, M. and RICHMOND, S.J. 1988. Characterization of a bacteriophage recovered from an avian strain of *Chlamydia psittaci*. *Ibid.*, p. 94.
8. SCHMEER, N. and KRAUSS, H. 1982. Purification of genus-specific chlamydial antigen and its separation into several components by ion-exchange chromatography. *J. clin. Microbiol.* **15:** 830–834.
9. EVERETT, K.D.E., ANDERSEN, A.A., PLAUNT, M. and HATCH, T.P. 1991. Cloning and sequence analysis of the major outer protein gene of *Chlamydia psittaci* 6BC. *Infect. Immun.* **59:** 2853–2855.
10. WINDSOR, D.K. JR and GRIMES, J.E. 1988. Relationship between infectivity and cytopathology for L-929 cells, membrane proteins and antigenicity of avian isolates of *Chlamydia psittaci*. *Avian Dis.* **35:** 421–431.

11. MAYER, K.F. 1967. The host spectrum of psittacosis–lymphogranuloma venereum (PL) agents. *Am. J. Opthal.* **63:** 1225–1246.
12. DAVIS, D.E., DELAPLANE, J.P. and WATKINS, J.R. 1957. The role of turkey eggs in the transmission of ornithosis. *Am. J. vet. Res.* **18:** 409–413.
13. GRIMES, J.E. and WYRICK, P.B. 1991. Chlamydiosis (Ornithosis). In: *Disease of Poultry,* pp. 311–325. CALNEK, B.E. (Ed.), Iowa State University Press, Ames.
14. BEVAN, B.J. and BRACEWELL, C.D. 1986. Chlamydiosis in birds in Great Britain. *J. Hyg. Camb.* **96:** 447–458.
15. CROSSE, B.A. 1990. Psittacosis; a clinical review. *J. Infect.* **21:** 251–259.
16. WARD, C. and WARD, A.M. 1974. Acquired valvular heart-disease in patients who keep pet birds. *Lancet* **1:** 734–736.
17. HODINKA, R.L. and WYRICK, P.B. 1986. Ultrastructural study of mode of entry of *C. psittaci* into L929 cells. *Infect. Immun.* **54:** 855–863.
18. EDDIE, B., MAYER, K.F., LAMBRECHT, F.L. and FURMAN, D.P. 1962. Isolation of ornithosis bedsoniae from mites collected in turkey quarters and from chicken lice. *J. infect. Dis.* **110:** 213–237.
19. PAGE, L.A. 1959. Experimental ornithosis in turkeys. *Avian Dis.* **3:** 67–79.
20. GALE, C., SANGER, V.L. POMEROY, B.S. 1960. The gross and microscopic pathology of an ornithosis virus of low virulence for turkeys. *Am. J. vet. Res.* **21:** 491–497.
21. AITKEN, I.D. 1981. Immunity to chlamydia. In: *Avian Immunology,* pp. 301–312. ROSE, M.E., PAYNE, L.N. and FREEMAN, B.M. (Eds), British Poultry Science Ltd, Edinburgh.
22. PAGE, L.A. and BANKOWSKI, R.A. 1960. Factors affecting the production and detection of ornithosis antibodies in infected turkeys. *Am. J. vet. Res.* **21:** 971–978.
23. BANKOWSKI, R.A. and PAGE, L.A. 1959. Studies of two epornitics of ornithosis caused by agents of low virulence. *Am. J. vet. Res.* **20:** 935–940.
24. PAGE, L.A., PATTERSON, J.M., ROEPKE, M.H. and GLASER, F.O. 1967. Studies on the biophysical characteristics of antibodies produced in birds and mammals in response to experimental chlamydial infection (psittacosis). *J. Immun.* **98:** 732–738.
25. BANKS, J., EDDIE, B., SUNG, M., SUGG, N., SCHACHTER, J. and MAYER, K.F. 1970. Plaque reduction technique for demonstrating neutralizing antibodies for chlamydia. *Infect. Immun.* **2:** 443–447.
26. PAGE, L.A. 1978. Stimulation of cell-mediated immunity of chlamydiosis in turkeys by inoculation of chlamydial bacterin. *Am. J. vet. Res.* **39:** 473–480.
27. GRIMES, J.E. 1985. Enigmatic psittacine chlamydiosis: Results of serotesting and isolation attempts, 1978 through 1983 and considerations for the future. *J. vet. Med. Ass.* **186:** 1075–1079.
28. EVANS, R.T., CHALMERS, W.S.K., WOOLCOCK, P.R., FARMER, H. and TAYLOR-ROBINSON, D. 1983. An enzyme-linked immunosorbent assay (ELISA) for the detection of chlamydial antibody in duck sera. *Avian Path.* **12:** 117–124.
29. ANDERSEN, A.A. and TAPPE, J.P. JR 1989. Chlamydiosis. In: *A Laboratory Manual for the Isolation and Identification of Avian Pathogens,* pp. 63–69. PURCHASE, H.G. (Ed.), Kendall/Hunt, Iowa.
30. GRIMES, J.E. 1989. Serodiagnosis of avian chlamydia infection. *J. Am. vet. Med. Ass.* **195:** 1561–1564.
31. PAUL, I.D. 1982. The growth of Chlamydia in McCoy cells treated with emetine. *Med. Lab. Sci.* **39:** 15–32.

32. Hewinson, R.G., Rankin, S.E.S., Bevan, B.J., Field, M. and Woodward, M.J. 1991. Detection of *Chlamydia psittaci* from avian samples using the PCR. *Vet. Rec.* **128:** 129–130.
33. Rasmussen, S. and Timms, P. 1991. Detection of *Chlamydia psittaci* using DNA probes and the polymerase chain reaction. *FEMS Microbiol. Lett.* **77:** 169–174.
34. Page, L.A. 1975. Stimulation of cell-mediated immunity to chlamydiosis in turkeys by inoculation of *chlamydial bacterin. Am. J. vet. Res.* **39:** 473–480.
35. Ashton, W.L.G. and Alexander, D.J. 1980. A two year survey on the control of the importation of captive birds into Great Britain. *Vet. Rec.* **106:** 80–83.

19

Ovine Chlamydial Abortion

I. D. AITKEN

Introduction

Abortion of ewes in late pregnancy as a consequence of placental necrosis is among the most dramatic and economically devastating manifestations of the pathogenicity of *Chlamydia psittaci*. Though chlamydial-induced abortion and production of weak offspring have been reported in sheep, goats and cattle it was in ewes that the ability of chlamydial agents to cause disease was first recognized. The transmissible nature of ovine enzootic abortion was established by Stamp and colleagues[1] in 1950 who demonstrated very large numbers of organisms resembling "rickettsiae and the psittacosis–lymphogranuloma group of infective agents" in the diseased fetal membranes of aborted lambs. Filtered (0.4 μm) suspensions of tissues from aborted fetuses inoculated into pregnant ewes reproduced the natural disease with all its characteristics. Associated field investigations[2] described the epidemiological features of enzootic abortion and experimental studies on immunity[3] led to the development of a vaccine to aid in control of the disease.[5,6]

With the notable exception of Australia and New Zealand chlamydial abortion has been encountered in most sheep-rearing areas of the world, particularly where flocks are closely herded. The organism responsible for ewe abortion presents a special zoonotic hazard for pregnant women who should avoid contact with sheep suspected of harboring chlamydial infection.[7]

A number of publications relevant to ovine chlamydial abortion have appeared in the last few years.[8–11]

Etiology

C. psittaci, the causative organism, is an obligate intracellular bacterium capable of infecting and parasitizing a wide range of avian and mammalian hosts, often without overt clinical effects. In its promiscuous infectivity and ease of transfer between host species, *C. psittaci* contrasts markedly with the restricted host range of the other members of the genus, *C. trachomatis* and *C. pneumoniae*, which are essentially human pathogens. Chlamydiae have an unusual but distinctive life cycle and are wholly dependent on an intracellular environment for their growth and multiplication. Adsorption to and penetration of susceptible cells by the compact infectious chlamydial elementary body is followed by its intravacuolar differentiation to a larger thin walled vegetative reticulate body that divides repeatedly by binary fission before reverting to the elementary body form. Rupture of the infected cell releases large numbers of infective particles to renew the cycle of infection. Details of the microbiology and life cycle of chlamydia are given in Chapter 2.

Though *C. psittaci* is described taxonomically as a single species it comprises a diversity of chlamydial types and there is growing biochemical, immunological and genetic evidence to justify its subdivision.[12,13] Isolates from cases of ruminant abortion constitute a discrete subgroup of *C. psittaci*. Though individual abortion isolates can vary in virulence there is no difference in polypeptide profiles to suggest antigenic differences between them.[14] Experimentally, avian and ruminant fecal isolates can induce ewe abortion but the extent to which this occurs under natural circumstances, if at all, is not known. However, at least one avian isolate has been shown to bear close resemblance to sheep abortion isolates[12] which could imply that some abortion strains have an avian origin.[13]

Epidemiology

Infection is normally introduced and maintained by sheep-to-sheep transmission although the possibility of occasional primary acquisition of chlamydial infection from other ruminants or birds must be borne in mind. In infected flocks the seasonal parturition period and congregation of ewes results in near synchronous expulsion of massive numbers of organisms by females with active placental infection and consequent heavy environmental contamination.

The main sources of infection are the expelled products of conception, postabortion uterine discharges, which may continue in diminishing volume for several days, and the soiled hindquarters of aborted ewes. Susceptible ewes and viable lambs in the immediate environment are at high risk of acquiring infection by inhalation of locally generated aerosols, by ingestion of contaminated food or bedding or by nuzzling aborted females. The viability of infective elementary bodies in the lambing environment is likely to vary according to prevailing circumstances, ranging from several days under temperate climatic conditions to several weeks at near-freezing temperatures.

The intestine is a common habitat for *C. psittaci* in a variety of hosts[10] and in sheep flocks which have experienced chlamydial abortion it is not uncommon to find evidence of intermittent fecal shedding. Intestinal isolates differ in several respects from those recovered from abortion material and their significance as a source of abortifacient infection is, at best, uncertain. Evidence has been sought but not found for significant postabortion excretion of chlamydiae in colostrum and milk[1,15,16] making it highly improbable that these secretions, unless externally contaminated, are vehicles for lamb infection. However, lambs fostered on to ewes which have aborted run the risk of acquiring *C. psittaci* infection from their contaminated fleece. However, it may be noted that direct inoculation of *C. psittaci* into the lactating mammary gland can induce an acute mastitis.[17]

C. psittaci has been isolated from the urogenital tract and semen of rams with orchitis and epidiyimitis in flocks experiencing chlamydial abortions[18,19] and seminal excretion of chlamydia occurs during the acute phase of experimentally established infection.[20,21] Both circumstantial and limited experimental evidence suggest that while venereal transmission of *C. psittaci* may occur it is an exceptional rather than a usual component of chlamydial epidemiology, particularly where males and females are segregated outwith the breeding season. Moreover, routine prebreeding examination of rams should result in the detection and removal of any with palpable abnormalities.

The introduction of *C. psittaci* to a fully susceptible breeding flock can provoke a major outbreak of abortions, stillbirths and delivery of weakly lambs with up to 30% of the ewes being affected. Thereafter, the disease tends to become enzootic with an annual incidence of 5–10%, principally among younger females and new flock entrants though this figure can be reduced by appropriate control measures. In most cases animals acquiring infection during the lambing season exhibit no immediate clinical signs. Inhaled or ingested *C. psittaci* may localize initially in the tonsils[22] before being disseminated to other sites where they remain quiescent until the host's subsequent pregnancy. There is a dearth of information about the tissue sites where chlamydia persist and their fate in those sites. In some cases the infection may be completely sequestered or eliminated as field studies indicate that only about one-third of ewe lambs from heavily infected flocks develop placental infection in their first breeding season (at 10 months of age) and that only some of those so infected will abort.[4] The specific factors that affect the outcome in individual animals are unknown nor has the influence of time between neonatal infection and first pregnancy been investigated. It is possible that the longer the interval, the greater will be the likelihood of systemic infection being eliminated and placentitis avoided.

In flocks with a naturally protracted lambing season of several weeks or if batch lambing of very large flocks is practised to facilitate management there is a risk of infection and abortion within the same pregnancy.[23] For ewes that are 90–100 days pregnant the interval between infection and abortion is about 35–40 days. Thus, abortions amongst the earliest lambing ewes can create an infectious hazard for cohort animals which are still several weeks away from normal parturition at 21 weeks.

C. psittaci can also cause, or contribute to, other disease syndromes in lambs such as conjunctivitis, arthritis and respiratory disease (see Chapter 20). However, there are seldom concurrent chlamydiae-related problems affecting lambs in flocks experiencing chlamydial abortion.

Pathology and Pathogenesis

Innovative studies in the pathology and pathogenesis of ovine chlamydial abortion have been reported by several workers[1,24–26] and the following overview is drawn from their observations and other interpretive accounts of the disease process.[8,10,27]

The cardinal gross pathological feature is a necrotic placentitis affecting the cotyledons and adjacent intercotyledonary areas, although in both natural and experimental infections the extent and severity of lesions is quite variable. Adjacent to affected cotyledons the periplacentome exhibits rough granular thickening and edematous change while the margins of the affected areas are hyperemic or hemorrhagic. Associated with the lesions is a turbid dirty pink exudate containing flakes of discolored necrotic material.

The primary placental lesion is initiated in the placentome, the intimate apposition of endometrical caruncle and chorionic cotyledon used for maternal–fetal transfer of oxygen and nutrients. From about 60 days of gestation the caruncular stroma is subjected to normal physiological invasion by chorionic villi while coincident hemorrhage from maternal vessels results in the formation of hematomata. These natural events provide the bridge that allows chlamydia from the maternal circulation to breach the placental barrier. Once that has happened the course of infection and pathogenesis in the conceptus proceeds independently of that in the dam which may cease to show evidence of systemic chlamydial infectivity.

However, there is a remarkable temporal restriction in the development of placental pathology. In a well controlled study Buxton and colleagues[26] demonstrated that ewes were susceptible to infection from early gestation and that the placenta could be invaded from about day 60 but, irrespective of the timing of early infection, placental pathology did not develop before 90 days. Though perhaps endocrine-dependent the underlying reasons for this restriction are not known but the observation is in accord with the consistent timing of ewe abortion induced by *C. psittaci*.

Following chlamydial invasion of the placentome intracytoplasmic chlamydial inclusions develop in the enlarged trophoblastic epithelial cells of the chorion, particularly at the hilar limbus. Continued expansion of the inclusions results in necrosis and shedding of infected cells and the adherence of necrotic debris and chlamydial material to adjacent unaffected epithelium. Progressive epithelial necrosis denudes the underlying villus which becomes edematous and infiltrated by neutrophils, macrophages and lymphoid cells. Necrotic changes also affect the tips of the caruncular septa and increasing amounts of cellular debris accumulate in the placentomal hematomas. The process duly extends to the periplacentome and intercotyledonary areas, resulting in infection and death of chorionic epithelial cells with inflammatory cell infiltration and fibrinous deposition within the underlying thickened mesenchyme. Blood vessels in the affected parts of the chorion show varying degrees of arteritis penetrating as far as the endothelium.

The fetal side of the chorion exhibits no chlamydial-induced changes but some pathology is evident in the endometrium directly apposed to affected areas of the chorion. The principal features are necrosis and sloughing of infected epithelial cells and an underlying mixed inflammatory cell response of variable intensity.

Aborted lambs are usually well grown and of fresh appearance though the fleece may show residues of placental debris or exudate. Some lambs may appear potbellied due to accumulation of blood-tinged fluid in the peritoneal cavity. Petechial hemorrhages can be detected in the subcutis and swelling of the liver and edema of lymph nodes may also be evident. Histologically, foci of inflammation or necrosis may be discerned in parenchymatous organs, lung, brain and lymph nodes. The lesion most commonly encountered is focal hepatic necrosis that may have an embolic origin. Lymph nodes may show cortical demarcation and development of follicles and germinal centres indicative of a fetal immune response.

The specific cause and effect relationships between pathological events and fetal expulsion remain to be ascertained. Contributing factors may be impairment of maternal–fetal exchange by disruption of placentomes, reduction in progesterone output consequent on destruction of chorionic epithelial cells,[28] the principal source of this key hormone in the latter half of ovine pregnancy, and direct effects of chlamydial infection on fetal viability.

Clinical Disease

Abortion in the last 2–3 weeks of pregnancy or the near term delivery of dead, moribund or weakly lambs are the main clinical features of ovine chlamydial abortion. Though some behavioral changes in the ewe and a vulval discharge may precede abortion these are unlikely to be detected under normal farming conditions. Unless carefully nursed, weak lambs are unlikely to survive. Intermittent uterine discharges may continue for several days but most ewes remain clinically normal. In a few cases secondary metritis may supervene and require treatment. The future breeding potential of ewes that have experienced chlamydial placentitis with or without abortion remains unimpaired.

Immunity

Like other intracellular pathogens chlamydia have a complex relationship with the host immune system, particularly because of their ability to infect and survive within phagocytic cells and to be disseminated by them. Various *in vitro* and *in vivo* models have been used to investigate aspects of immunity to chlamydia but variations within and between chlamydial species in respect of tissue tropism, pathogenicity and other characteristics influence the host's ability to recover from clinical disease, to eliminate infection and to resist reinfection. For more detailed information the reader is referred to Chapter 2 and to texts such as that by Barron.[29] This contribution will consider ovine immunity to chlamydia, a recently reviewed topic.[30]

For the individual animal, chlamydial abortion is a single episodic event from which most recover well. Similarly, most remain refractory to recurrence of the disease although exceptions have been recorded both experimentally and in field situations. These exceptions may reflect chlamydial virulence, weak or waning protective immunity or a combination of these factors. The extent to which recovered ewes are refractory to low grade, nonclinical, placental reinfection is not clear.

That chlamydial infection of ewes induces an antibody response is well established but neither complement-fixing nor neutralizing activities relate to protective immunity.[8] Postabortion sera detect up to eighteen surface antigens of *C. psittaci* including the 40 kDa major outer membrane protein (MOMP),[31] which is probably important in host immunity. The gene encoding MOMP has been cloned from an ovine abortifacient strain of *C. psittaci*[32] for further study. Other antigens of interest which react with ovine antibody are LPS, the genus-specific antigen exploited in the pan-chlamydial complement fixation test, three cysteine-rich proteins and two adhesins that may be responsible for binding chlamydial elementary bodies to host cells as a necessary prelude to infection.

Evidence from *in vitro* and laboratory animal studies points to an important role for cell-mediated immunity in chlamydial infections. That such events are induced in sheep is evident from the development of delayed type hypersensitivity in the postabortion period and most readily detected by intra-palpebral inoculation of antigen.[33,34] However, the phenomenon is not discernible following infection of nonpregnant animals perhaps because of the lower weight of systemic infection. Also relevant is the histological response of the draining lymph nodes following subcutaneous inoculation of susceptible nonpregnant sheep with *C. psittaci*.[35] Postinfection enlargement of the nodes was attributed mainly to expansion of medullary cords containing both B and T cells although, over the 18 day time course of the study, B cell activity was the more strongly stimulated.

Because the sheep is a manageable experimental species for which *C. psittaci* is a natural pathogen opportunities are available for detailed *in vivo* studies at the cellular and molecular level of the immunological events triggered by chlamydial infection. Experiments employing lymphatic cannulation techniques are likely to be particularly rewarding.[36]

Diagnosis

Clinical history, pathological findings and the demonstration of large numbers of small (300 nm) coccoid elementary bodies in stained smears of affected areas of placenta provide the basis for a firm diagnosis. Suitable staining procedures include modified Macchiavello, Giemsa, Brucella differential or modified Ziehl–Neelsen stains.[1] By the latter method organisms stain red against the blue background of cellular debris. Under darkground illumination the elementary bodies are pale green. In the absence of placental material smears made from vaginal swabs of aborted ewes or from the moist fleece of a recently aborted fetus are useful substitutes although chlamydial organisms may not be so abundant. The morphological and tinctorial similarities between *C. psittaci* and *Coxiella burnetii* (see Chapter 6) may require their immunological differentiation.

In tissue sections intracytoplasmic chlamydial inclusions can be demonstrated by Giemsa staining after fixation in Bouin or Carnoy fluids but more striking results are obtained by the direct immunoperoxidase technique.[37]

Isolation of the organism is most easily accomplished in cell cultures although the chick embryo yolk sac remains a reliable medium for primary isolation. A suitable transport medium and cell culture system have been described[38,39] and appropriate methodologies can be found in standard microbiological texts.

Retrospective confirmation of diagnosis can be obtained by serology for which the complement fixation (CF) test is still commonly used. Paired blood samples collected soon after abortion and 2–3 weeks later, will detect a postabortion rise in titer. However, it is advisable to take samples from more than one animal and to include serum from ewes which lambed normally so that the flock status can be more readily ascertained. Interpretation of low CF antibody titers, particularly in individual animals, is difficult because of the known cross reactions between *C. psittaci* and other Gram-negative bacteria and the uncertain significance of enteric chlamydial infection.

Alternative tests based on immunofluorescence or ELISA procedures are used also but tend to be restricted to specialist laboratories.

Treatment and Control

C. psittaci is susceptible to a number of antibiotics but, as an emergency treatment to counter an ongoing outbreak of chlamydial abortion, a long-acting tetracycline has been shown to be of value.[40–44]

Intramuscular doses (20 mg per kg) repeated at 10–14 day intervals until parturition are recommended. Treatment suppresses chlamydial growth and multiplication but does not eliminate infection. For that reason, recourse to antibiotic treatment should be restricted to emergency situations and not adopted as an annual routine. The net clinical effect in treated ewes is a reduction in the number of aborted or stillborn lambs compared to the outcome in the absence of treatment.

In Britain, early epidemiological investigations confirmed that ewes that had aborted once as a result of chlamydial infection rarely did so again.[2,4] The implicit acquisition of durable protective immunity prompted the development of an inactivated vaccine able to moderate the severity of both experimentally induced and naturally occurring disease.[3,5,45] That empirical vaccine, containing a specific field isolate (A22) at low passage number as seed material, has been in continuous use for almost 40 years albeit with some modification to the adjuvant[6] and the later addition of a more recent field isolate (S26/3).[46] In Germany, a multipassaged (170 times) A22 used for vaccine production, grows well in all chick embryo fluids and tissues, generating a higher yield per embryo. The vaccine has been successful both as a prophylactic measure and when used in the course of an outbreak.[47]

However, some workers[48] have obtained equivocal results after challenging the immunity of ewes given a commercial inactivated yolk sac vaccine, although the outcome varied with the route of challenge adopted.

Cell cultures are alternative substrates for growing chlamydia and inactivated vaccines prepared from organisms grown in this way have induced good protective immunity of pregnant ewes against experimental challenge.[49,50] For vaccine manufacture, cell cultures offer processing advantages over chick embryos and, once present limitations of chlamydial yield are overcome, cell culture will probably replace the chick embryo for this purpose.

Because the purified elementary bodies used by Anderson and colleagues[50] in their successful experimental vaccine elicited a strong antibody response to MOMP they proceeded to prepare a subcellular vaccine highly enriched for undenatured MOMP.[51] Within one month of mating, individual ewes were vaccinated subcutaneously with MOMP (20 μg protein/ewe). Challenge later in pregnancy caused 5 of 12 unvaccinated control ewes to abort and a further 2 to develop placental infection. All of the 11 vaccinated ewes lambed normally and in only one was chlamydial infection detected. These results give a strong indication that the constituents of MOMP can provide the basis for an effective chlamydial subunit vaccine. Further, as the MOMP gene for an established chlamydial vaccine strain (S26/3) has been cloned, sequenced[32] and expressed in bacterial vectors amenable to *in vitro* culture, a recombinant vaccine is now a distinct possibility.[52]

The use of *C. psittaci* strains adapted to chick embryos or cell cultures as "attenuated" live vaccines has been investigated but even after repeated passage these strains retain their pathogenicity for the ovine placenta and fetus.[8,53,54] On the other hand, two chemically-induced temperature-sensitive mutants of a virulent ovine abortifacient strain were attenuated for pregnant mice and ewes.[55,56] Infection of ewes prior to mating did not affect the ensuing pregnancy nor was any chlamydial excretion detected at lambing. Challenge of vaccinated and control ewes in the following year's pregnancy with the virulent parental strain of *C. psittaci* resulted in excretion by 9 of 10 controls but only 1 of 34 vaccinates. Similar results were obtained in goats.[57] One of the two induced mutants reverted to virulence for mice and was discarded. The other is undergoing assessment in naturally infected flocks but its genetic stability under field conditions remains to be demonstrated.

When chlamydial abortion is encountered attention must be paid to reducing the risk of within-flock transmission by removal and destruction of the products of conception, by cleaning and disinfecting the area where abortion occurred and by isolating ewes which have aborted for 2–3 weeks. If the number of aborting ewes is small they should be culled but if significant numbers are involved they may be retained for future breeding, preferably as a separately managed group. Options for longer term flock management in the wake of the outbreak have been described.[58]

Zoonotic Implications

C. psittaci of ovine origin has been responsible for a small number of sporadic cases of respiratory illness in laboratory and vaccine workers.[59,60] However, there is no reported evidence of an association between the lambing season and episodes of influenza-like illness in flock attendants. Novice assistants such as trainees and vacation students are most likely to be at risk, particularly if drawn from a nonrural background. However, a serological survey in an area of north west England, in which ovine chlamydial abortion is endemic, revealed no differences in antibody profiles amongst adults engaged in sheep production, in other types of farming or nonagricultural activities.[61]

Ovine abortifacient *C. psittaci* has an affinity for the human placenta and thus is a particular hazard for pregnant women. A link between lambing sheep and human abortion was suspected initially on circumstantial evidence[62] but has been fully authenticated by the isolation and genomic typing of *C. psittaci* from case material from farmers' wives who have been affected.[63,64] The specific nature of the risk and the life-threatening severity of the disease for the mother justify the recommendation that pregnant women should avoid working with sheep, especially at lambing time and seek prompt medical attention in the event of any influenza-like symptoms.[7]

References

1. Stamp, J.T., McEwen, A.D., Watt, J.A.A. and Nisbet, D.I. 1950. Enzootic abortion in ewes. I. Transmission of the disease. *Vet. Rec.* **62:** 251–254.

2. LITTLEJOHN, A.I. 1950. Enzootic abortion in ewes—an investigation into the naturally occurring disease. *Vet. Rec.* **62:** 571–577.
3. MCEWEN, A.D., STAMP, J.T. and LITTLEJOHN, A.I. 1951. Enzootic abortion in ewes. II. Immunization and infection experiments. *Vet. Rec.* **63:** 197–200.
4. MCEWEN, A.D., LITTLEJOHN, A.I. and FOGGIE, A. 1951. Enzootic abortion of ewes: some aspects of infection and resistance. *Vet. Rec.* **63:** 489–492.
5. LITTLEJOHN, A.I., FOGGIE, A. and MCEWEN, A.D. 1952. Enzootic abortion in ewes. Field trials of vaccine. *Vet. Rec.* **64:** 858–862.
6. FOGGIE, A. 1973. Preparation of vaccines against enzootic abortion of ewes. A review of the research work at the Moredun Institute. *Vet. Bull.* **43:** 587–590.
7. BUXTON, D. 1986. Potential danger to pregnant women of *Chlamydia psittaci* from sheep. *Vet. Rec.* **118:** 510–511.
8. STORZ, J. and KRAUSS, H. 1985. Chlamydia. In: *Handbuch der Bakteriellen Infectionen bei Tieren,* Vol. 5, pp. 447–531. BLOBEL, H. and SCHLIESSER, T. (Eds), Gustav Fischer Verlag, Stuttgart.
9. AITKEN, I.D. (Ed.) 1986. *Chlamydial Diseases of Ruminants,* CEC, Luxembourg.
10. STORZ, J. 1989. Overview of animal diseases induced by chlamydial infections. In: *Microbiology of Chlamydia,* pp. 167–192. BARRON, A.L. (Ed.), CRC Florida.
11. AITKEN, I.D. 1991. Enzootic (chlamydial) abortion. In: *Diseases of Sheep,* 2nd edn, pp. 43–49. MARTIN, W.B. and AITKEN, I.D. (Eds), Blackwells, Oxford.
12. FUKUSHI, H. and HIRAI, K. 1989. Genetic diversity of avian and mammalian *Chlamydia psittaci* strains and relation to host origin. *J. Bact.* **171:** 2850–2855.
13. HERRING, A.J. 1993. Typing *Chlamydia psittaci*—procedures and problems. *Br. Vet. J.,* in press.
14. MCCLENAGHAN, M., INGLIS, N.F. and HERRING, A.J. 1991. Comparison of isolates of *Chlamydia psittaci* of ovine, avian and feline origin by analysis of polypeptide profiles from purified elementary bodies. *Vet. Microbiol.* **26:** 269–278.
15. JONES, G.E. and ANDERSON, I.E. 1989. *Chlamydia psittaci* excretion in ovine milk tested. *Vet. Rec.* **124:** 618–619.
16. WILSMORE, A.J. 1989. Chlamydia in ovine milk. *Vet. Rec.* **124:** 618–619.
17. PAPADOPOULOS, O. and LEONTIDES, S. 1972. Mastitis produced experimentally in sheep with an ovine abortion chlamydia. *Zentbl. vet. Med. B.* **19:** 655–665.
18. RODOLAKIS, A. and BERNARD, K. 1977. Isolement de *Chlamydia ovis* des organs genitaux de beliers atteints d'epididymite. *Bull. Acad. vet. Fr.* **50:** 65–70.
19. PIENAAR, J.G. and SCHUTTE, A.P. 1975. The occurrence and pathology of chlamydiosis in domestic and laboratory animals: a review. *Onderstepoort J. vet Res.* **42:** 77–90.
20. STORZ, J., CARROLL, E.J., STEPHENSON, E.H., BALL, L. and EUGSTER, A.K. 1976. Urogenital infection and seminal excretion after inoculation of bulls and rams with chlamydiae. *Am. J. vet. Res.* **37:** 517–520.
21. APPLEYARD, W.T., AITKEN, I.D. and ANDERSON, I.E. 1985. Attempted venereal transmission of *Chlamydia psittaci* in sheep. *Vet. Rec.* **116:** 535–538.
22. JONES, G.E. and ANDERSON, I.E. 1988. *Chlamydia psittaci*: is tonsillar tissue the portal of entry in ovine enzootic abortion? *Res. vet. Sci.* **44:** 260–261.
23. BLEWETT, D.A., GISEMBA, F., MILLER, J.K., JOHNSON, F.W.A. and CLARKSON, M.J. 1982. Ovine enzootic abortion: the acquisition of infection and consequent abortion within a single lambing season. *Vet. Rec.* **111:** 499–501.
24. STUDDERT, M.J. 1968. *Bedsonia* abortion of sheep II. Pathology and pathogenesis with observations on the normal ovine placenta. *Res. vet. Sci.* **9:** 57–64.

25. Novilla, M.N. and Jensen, R. 1970. Placental pathology of experimentally induced enzootic abortion in ewes. *Am. J. vet. Res.* **31:** 1983–2000.
26. Buxton, D., Barlow, R.M., Finlayson, J., Anderson, I.E. and McKellar, A. 1990. Observations on the pathogenesis of *Chlamydia psittaci* infection of pregnant sheep. *J. comp. Path.* **102:** 221–237.
27. Storz, J. 1971. *Chlamydia and Chlamydia-Induced Diseases.* C.C. Thomas, Springfield, Illinois.
28. Leaver, H.A., Howie, A., Aitken, I.D., Appleyard, W.T., Anderson, I.E., Jones, G.E., Hay, L.A., Williams, J.T. and Buxton, D. 1989. Changes in progesterone, oestradiol 17B and intrauterine prostaglandin E2 during late gestation in sheep experimentally infected with an ovine abortion strain of *Chlamydia psittaci. J. gen. Microbiol.* **135:** 565–573.
29. Barron, A.L. (Ed.) 1988. *Microbiology of Chlamydia.* CRC Press, Boca Raton, Florida.
30. McCafferty, M.C. 1990. Immunity to *Chlamydia psittaci* with particular reference to sheep. *Vet. Microbiol.* **25:** 87–99.
31. Tan, T.W., Herring, A.J., McClenaghan, M., Huang, H.-S., Anderson, I.E., Inglis, N.F., Jones, G.E. and Buxton, D. 1988. Immunoblotting analysis of the humoral immune response in sheep infected with ovine abortion strain of *Chlamydia psittaci. Proc. Eur. Soc. Chlamydial Res.* p. 136. Soc. Editrice Esculapio, Bologna.
32. Herring, A.J., Tan, T.W., Baxter, S., Inglis, N.F. and Dunbar, S. 1989. Sequence analysis of the major outer membrane protein gene of an ovine abortion strain of *Chlamydia psittaci. FEMS Microbiol. Letts.* **65:** 153–158.
33. Wilsmore, A.J., Abduljahl, S.A., Parsons, V.H. and Dawson, M. 1984. Observations on a skin sensitivity test for ovine enzootic abortion. *Br. Vet. J.* **140:** 468–476.
34. Dawson, M., Zaghlone, A. and Wilsmore, A.J. 1986. Ovine enzootic abortion: experimental studies of immune responses. *Res. vet. Sci.* **40:** 59–64.
35. Huang, H.-S., Buxton, D. and Anderson, I.E. 1990. The ovine immune response to *Chlamydia psittaci*: histopathology of the lymph node. *J. comp. Path.* **102:** 89–97.
36. Huang, H.S., Buxton, D., Burrells, C., Anderson, I.E. and Miller, H.R.P. 1991. Immune responses of the ovine lymph node to *Chlamydia psittaci*: a cellular study of popliteal efferent lymph. *J. comp. Path.* **105:** 191–202.
37. Finlayson, J., Buxton, D., Anderson, I.E. and Donald, K.M. 1985. Direct immunoperoxidase method for demonstrating *Chlamydia psittaci* in tissue sections. *J. clin. Path.* **38:** 712–714.
38. Spencer, W.N. and Johnson, F.W.A. 1983. Simple transport medium for the isolation of *Chlamydia psittaci* from clinical material. *Vet. Rec.* **113:** 535–536.
39. Johnson, F.W.A., Clarkson, M.J. and Spencer, W.N. 1983. Direct isolation of the agent of enzootic abortion of ewes. (*Chlamydia psittaci*) in cell cultures. *Vet. Rec.* **113:** 413–414.
40. Rodolakis, A., Souriau, A., Reynaud, J.-P. and Brunault, G. 1980. Efficacy of a long acting tetracycline against chlamydial ovine abortion. *Ann. Rech. Vet.* **11:** 437–444.
41. Aitken, I.D., Robinson, G.W. and Anderson, I.E. 1982. Long-acting tetracycline in the treatment of enzootic abortion of ewes. *Vet. Rec.* **111:** 446.
42. Greig, A., Linklater, K.A. and Dyson, D.A. 1982. Long-acting tetracycline in the treatment of enzootic abortion of ewes. *Vet. Rec.* **111:** 445.
43. Brodie, T.A., Duncan, J.L. and Harvey, M.J.A. 1983. Role of enzootic

abortion and toxoplasmosis in an outbreak of abortion in a Scottish sheep flock. *Vet. Rec.* **113:** 437–440.

44. WILSMORE, A.J., DAWSON, M., ARTHUR, M.J. and DAVIES, D.C. 1986. The use of a delayed hypersensitivity test and long-acting tetracycline in a flock affected with ovine enzootic abortion. *Br. vet. J.* **142:** 557–561.
45. MCEWEN, A.D. and FOGGIE, A. 1956. Enzootic abortion in ewes. Prolonged immunity following the injection of adjuvant vaccine. *Vet. Rec.* **68:** 686–689.
46. AITKEN, I.D., ANDERSON, I.E. and ROBINSON, G.W. 1986. Ovine chlamydial abortion: limitations of inactivated vaccine. In: *Chlamydial Diseases of Ruminants,* pp. 67–70. AITKEN, I.D. (Ed.), CEC, Luxembourg.
47. FROST, J.W. and WACHENDORFER, G. 1986. Ten years' vaccination against chlamydial abortion of ewes. In: *Chlamydial Diseases of Ruminants,* pp. 67–70. AITKEN, I.D. (Ed.), CEC, Luxembourg.
48. RODOLAKIS, A. and SOURIAU, A. 1979. Clinical evaluation of a commercial vaccine against chlamydial abortion of ewes. *Ann. Rech. Vet.* **10:** 41–48.
49. WALDHELM. D.G., DELONG, W.J. and HALL, R.F. 1982. Efficacy of bacteria prepared from *Chlamydia psittaci* grown in cell culture for experimental immunization of ewes. *Vet. Microbiol.* **7:** 493–498.
50. ANDERSON, I.E., TAN, T.-W., JONES, G.E. and HERRING, A.J. 1990. Efficacy against ovine enzootic abortion of an experimental vaccine containing purified elementary bodies of *Chlamydia psittaci. Vet. Microbiol.* **24:** 21–27.
51. TAN, T.-W., HERRING, A.J., ANDERSON, I.E. and JONES, G.E. 1990. Protection of sheep against *Chlamydia psittaci* infection with a subcellular vaccine containing the major outer membrane protein. *Infect. Immun.* **58:** 3101–3108.
52. HERRING, A.J., TAN, T.-W. and BAXTER, S. 1990. Chlamydial abortion in sheep: molecular approaches to vaccination, pathogen detection and strain typing. *Proceedings of the 7th International Symposium on Human Chlamydial Infections,* pp. 378–382. Harrison Hot Springs, British Columbia.
53. BECERRA, V.M. and STORZ, J. 1974. Tissue culture adaptation and pathogenic properties of an ovine chlamydial abortion strain. *Zentralbl. Vet. Med* **21:** 288–299.
54. BECERRA, V.M., ATA, F.A. and STORZ, J. 1976. Studies on the response of ewes to live chlamydiae adapted to chicken embryos or tissue culture. *Can. J. comp. Med.* **40:** 46–51.
55. RODOLAKIS, A. 1983. *In vitro* and *in vivo* properties of chemically induced temperature-sensitive mutants of *Chlamydia psittaci* var *ovis*: screening in a murine model. *Infect. Immun.* **42:** 525–530.
56. RODOLAKIS, A. and SOURIAU, A. 1983. Response of ewes to temperature-sensitive mutants of *Chlamydia psittaci* (var. *ovis*) obtained by NTG mutagenesis. *Ann. Rech. Vet.* **14:** 155–161.
57. RODOLAKIS, A. 1976. Use of a live temperature-sensitive vaccine in experimental and natural infections. In: *Chlamydia Diseases of Ruminants,* pp. 71–77. AITKEN, I.D. (Ed.), CRC, Luxembourg.
58. AITKEN, I.D., CLARKSON, M.J. and LINKLATER, K.A. 1990. Disease update: chlamydial abortion of ewes. *Vet. Rec.* **126:** 136–138.
59. BARWELL, C.F. 1955. Laboratory infection of man with virus of enzootic abortion of ewes. *Lancet* **ii:** 1369–1371.
60. BAKER, C.C. and COOPER, N. 1983. A case of good management. *J. Infect.* **6:** 71–73.
61. HOBSON, D. and MORGAN-CAPNER, P. 1988. Chlamydial antibodies in farmers in north-west England. *Epid. Inf.* **101:** 397–404.

62. ROBERTS, W., GRIST, N.R. and GIROUD, P. 1967. Human abortion associated with infection of ovine abortion agent. *Br. Med. J.* **iv:** 37.
63. JOHNSON, F.W.A., MATHESON, B.A., WILLIAMS, H., LAING, A.G., JANDIAL, V., DAVIDSON-LAMB, R., HALLIDAY, G.J., HOBSON, D., WONG, S.Y., HADLEY, K.M., MOFFAT, M.A.J. and POSTLETHWAITE, R. 1985. Abortion due to infection with *Chlamydia psittaci* in a sheep farmer's wife. *Br. Med. J.* **290:** 592.
64. HERRING, A.J., ANDERSON, I.E., MCCLENAGHAN, M., INGLIS, N.F., WILLIAMS, H., MATHESON, B.A., WEST, C.P., RODGER, M. and BRETTLE, R.P. 1987. Restriction endonuclease analysis of DNA from two isolates of *Chlamydia psittaci* obtained from human abortions. *Br. Med. J.* **295:** 1239.

20

Diversity of Chlamydia-Induced Diseases

J. STORZ AND B. KALTENBOECK

History of Disease Diversity of Chlamydial Infections

The pathogenic role of chlamydiae of the species *Chlamydia* (C) *psittaci* in several diseases of domestic animals and man is well established.[1] Infections with agents now known to be chlamydiae were first identified as the cause of atypical pneumonia as well as several epidemics of severe pneumonia in human subjects late in the last and the early part of this century.[2] Psittacosis was the term given to these human infections because it was recognized that the infection was contracted from parrots.[3] These observations directed attention to chlamydial agents as a cause of respiratory disease in birds and domestic poultry.[4] The first naturally occurring pneumonic chlamydial infection in mammals was identified in cats[5] and in laboratory mice in 1942.[6,7] Today pneumonia is a recognized manifestation of respiratory chlamydial infection in domestic animals. McNutt[8] described in 1940 a sporadically occurring encephalomyelitis in cattle. He isolated the causative agent in guinea pigs, and it was later classified as a chlamydial agent. Stamp and coworkers proved in 1950 that placental lesions and abortions in sheep were associated with chlamydial infections.[9] The disease was called enzootic abortion of ewes. Conceptually, a novel pathogenic potential of chlamydial infections in animals was thus identified. Years later it was found that chlamydiae are transmitted in semen of bulls and rams affected with seminal vesiculitis and epididymitis and that these infections are involved in forms of reproductive failure other than abortions.[10–13] Furthermore, chlamydiae were detected by culture as well as by DNA amplification through polymerase chain reactions (PCR) in milk samples from cows with mastitis.[14,15] Mastitis was induced in cows following intracisternal inoculation of chlamydial isolates from ovine abortions,[16] sporadic bovine encephalomyelitis,[17] and intestinal infections.[18]

Detection of intestinal chlamydial infections of calves in 1951 represents another milestone.[19] This discovery initiated work on the importance of the intestinal habitat in perpetuating chlamydial infections in cattle, sheep, goats and swine, as well as in poultry and pet birds where this infection often is clinically inapparent and therefore of high epidemiological significance.[20] The arthropathogenic potential of specific chlamydial strains from sheep was recognized in the late fifties by Mendlowski and Segre.[21] Polyarthritis was seen particularly in sheep but also in calves.[22] While trachoma, a distinct disease in human subjects caused by chlamydial infections, had been recognized for centuries,[2] it was not until 1960 and later that chlamydial infections as a cause of conjunctivitis and other ocular diseases were differentiated in animals.[23] The first chlamydia-induced conjunctivitis was described in cats[23] and later in other domestic animal species including guinea pigs.[24] A severe form of keratoconjunctivitis associated with chlamydial infections was described in Australian koalas.[25] Records indicate that severe eye conditions associated with blindness and mortality of koalas leading to major die-offs were observed and recorded as long ago as 1887.[25] Additionally, koalas involved in the recent epidemics had genital infections leading to reproductive failure.[26] Epizootic die-offs among African clawed frogs in commercial operations were proven to be caused by chlamydial infections.[27] These ectothermic vertebrates had pyelogranulomatous inflammations leading to myocarditis, hepatitis, nephritis and lung lesions.[28]

Intestinal Infections and Enteritis

Epidemiology

Intestinal chlamydial infections may be found as persistent, clinically inapparent infection or as a cause of diarrhea in young animals; but they also function in initial events in the pathogenesis of other chlamydia-induced diseases.[1,20] They represent an epidemiological factor in perpetuating and spreading this infection in animal populations. Chlamydiae were first isolated from fecal and diarrhea fluid samples of calves in New York state in 1951. Calves as young as 2 days and adult cattle of various ages were found to excrete chlamydiae. Reports from Europe, Asia, Africa and Australia verified that intestinal chlamydial infections of cattle, sheep, and goats are worldwide.[20] Clinically normal goats and sheep harbored chlamydial agents in the intestines and excreted these organisms in readily detectable amounts. Chlamydiae were also isolated from feces of pigs in Austria and Germany.[29,30] Evidently, the intestinal chlamydial infection of mammals is comparable to the chlamydial infection of acutely, as well as inapparently infected, birds, which are known to excrete chlamydiae in feces or diarrhea fluids over long periods of time.[4] The infectious chain involving intestinal infections of animals is tightly linked to fecal shedding of infectious chlamydiae. Susceptible hosts may acquire the infection by ingesting contaminated fomites or by inhaling chlamydia-laden dust.

Properties of Chlamydiae from Intestinal Infections

Chlamydiae isolated from feces or intestinal samples of different animal species have antigenic properties of serovar 1, which also includes isolates from abortions of ewes and cows, and of serovars 2, 3, 4 and 9,[31] which are now classified as *C. pecorum*.[102] The strain S-45 of serovar 5 isolated from feces of pigs has properties of *C. trachomatis*.[32] Detection and differentiation by PCR involving the genes of the major outer membrane protein (MOMP) place intestinal chlamydial isolates into the psittacosis, polyarthritis and trachoma groups. The DNAs of MOMP genes of mammalian serovar 1 chlamydiae have a restriction fragment length polymorphism (RFLP) of avian strains[33] but differences in antigens and the molecular mass of MOMP exist between the B577 prototype of serovar 1 and some avian isolates.

Clinical Signs

The effect of oral inoculation of calves with chlamydiae depends on the age at the time of exposure.[34] Newborn calves in herds infected with serotype 1 chlamydiae may have episodes of watery to mucoid diarrhea, slight fever and nasal discharge. Calves with serovar 2 infections had yellow, watery feces and became dehydrated, anorectic and depressed. They also developed fever and leukocytosis. The majority of these calves died within 17 days of exposure.[34] Sheep and goats with intestinal chlamydial infections usually had normal feces, but this infection has not been studied sufficiently in the young of these species or in swine.[20]

Cytopathic Functions in Pathogenesis

The events of chlamydial infections leading to enteritis and diarrhea were studied in newborn calves.[34] Chlamydiae were isolated from mucosal scrapings of the abomasum, duodenum, jejunum, ileum, caecum and colon at various times after oral inoculation. Fluorescent antibodies revealed that the epithelial cells on the tips of the villi and in the intervillous zones as well as some cells in the crypts of Lieberkühn and the transition zones were infected.[35] Infection of intestinal cells occurred predominantly through the brush border. The host cell range included absorptive epithelial cells at the tips of the villi and the intervillous zones (Fig. 20.1), follicle-associated M cells, enterochro-

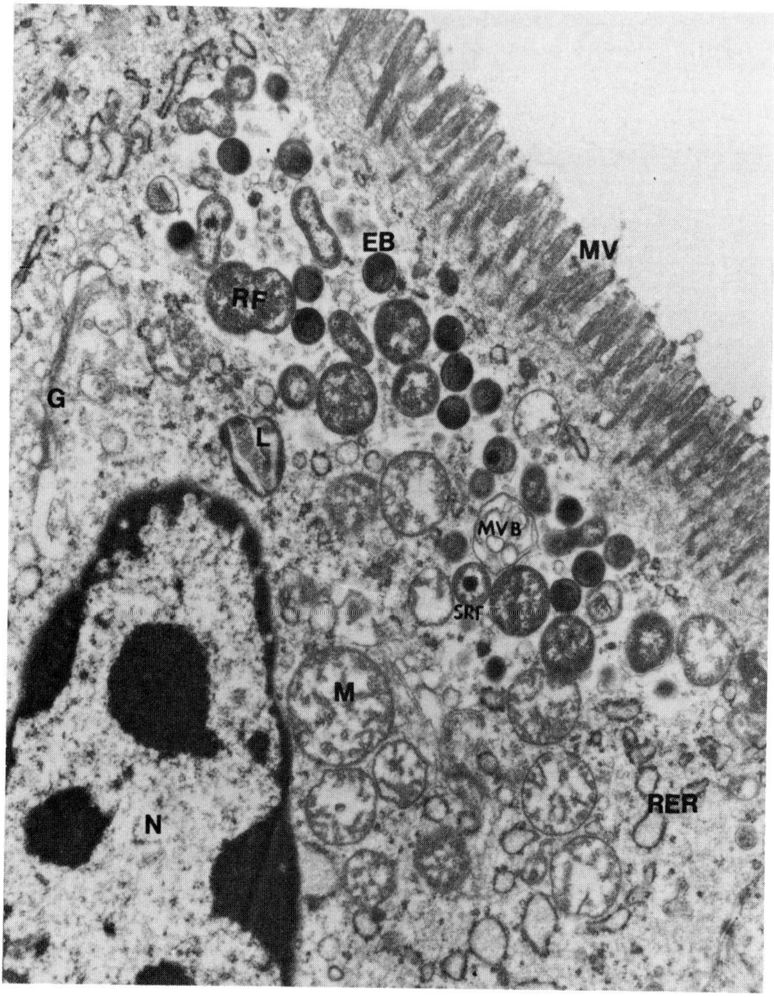

FIG. 20.1. Absorptive intestinal epithelial cell at a late stage of infection. Elementary bodies (EB) are more numerous than reticulate bodies (RB) and secondary reorganized or condensing forms (SRF). Mitochondria (M) are damaged, the rough endoplasmic reticulum (RER) and Golgi elements (G) are vesiculated, and the nucleus (N) is pycnotic. Lysosome-like structures (L) are present and microvilli (MV) are shortened. Uranyl acetate-lead citrate stain, ×5,600.[36]

maffin and goblet cells of the villi, and undifferentiated cells in the crypts, as well as macrophages and fibroblasts in the lamina propria and endothelial cells in the central lacteals.[36,37] Lysis of productively infected endothelial cells in the central lacteals released infectious chlamydiae into the circulating lymph and blood stream. Neutrophilic leukocytes rarely contained chlamydiae, but leukocytes pavement the vicinity of chlamydia-infected epithelial cells.[38,39]

When sequential stages of chlamydial development were correlated with ultrastructural lesions in infected intestinal cells, the earliest ultrastructural change was the space-occupying presence of the endosome containing the chlamydial dispersing form within deeper regions of the cytoplasm or in the Golgi region.[38] The rough endoplasmic reticulum remained near the inclusion, but the lysosomes appeared to migrate away and accumulated close to the cytoplasmic periphery. The number and prominence of free ribosomes and polysomes in the cytosol diminished in all types of cells infected. The mucus droplets became depleted in goblet cells. Chlamydial inclusions containing arrested reticulate bodies were located at the secreting face of the Golgi stacks and little mucus was formed. The specific granules of infected enterochromaffin cells, which supported productive chlamydial multiplication, decreased in number and electron density.[37–39]

The appearance of condensing forms and elementary bodies in infections of all cell types coincided with the beginning of severe degenerative changes characterized by cytoplasmic vesiculation, fragmentation of membranes and lysis of cellular organelles. The network of the smooth and rough endoplasmic reticulum dilated, became ill-defined and vacuolated. Golgi complexes became dilated and vesiculated. The nuclei were pyknotic or karyolytic after an initial loss of chromatin pattern and nucleoli, and separation of the membranes of the nuclear envelope. The chlamydial inclusion membranes ultimately ruptured, the plasmalemma lyzed, and chlamydiae were released.

Specialized organelles of infected cells such as microvilli and terminal webs of enterocytes were also affected (Fig. 20.2). The microvilli lost their uniform, regular spacing and became shorter, irregularly shaped, and vesiculated. Their rootlets were lost and the terminal web became ill-defined. Lateral junctional complexes were displaced and fragmented. The desmosomes persisted, and converging fibrils remained in their vicinity. Diarrhea resulted from the enterocytes' loss of absorptive and digestive functions, interference with cellular transport and energy generation, accelerated death of infected intestinal epithelial cells, edema and cellular infiltration of the lamina propria mucosae.[35,39]

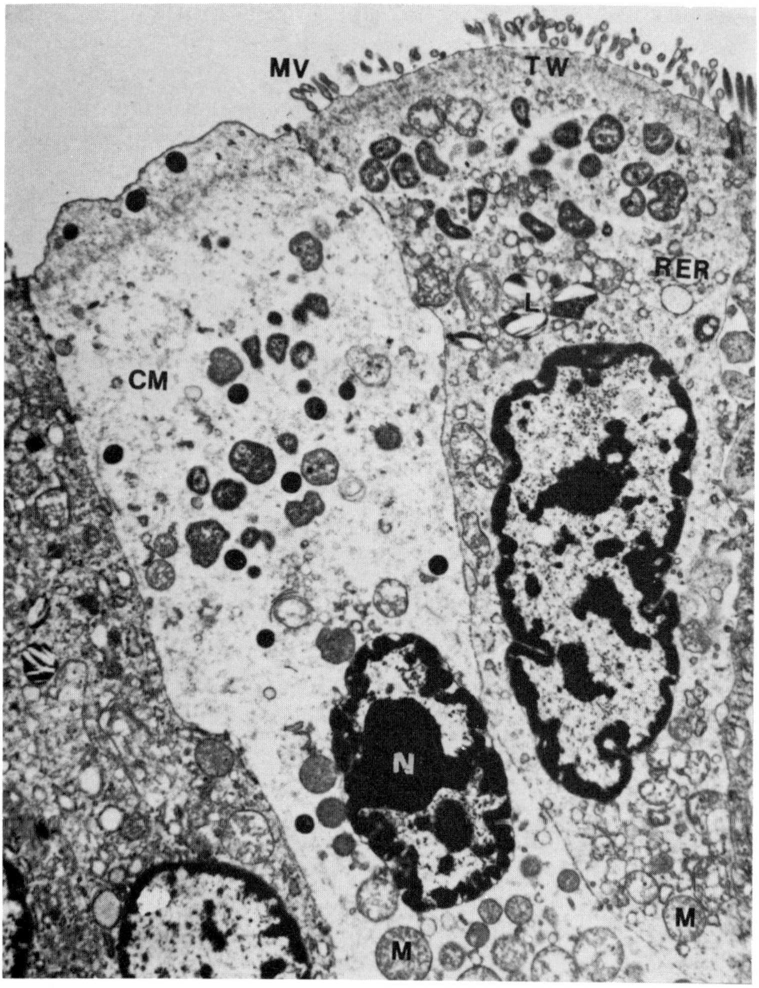

FIG. 20.2. Two absorptive intestinal epithelial cells in late stages of chlamydial infection. Nuclei (N) are pyknotic, the cytoplasmic matrix (CM) is dissolved, the terminal web (TW) is swollen lacking the rootlets of microvilli (MV). Uranyl acetate, lead citrate stain, × 11,520.[36]

Pathological Lesions

The serosal surfaces of the abomasum and small intestine of calves were dull and granular. Paint-brush hemorrhages were present in the duodenal and cecal serosa. The mucosa of the entire small intestine was congested and petechiated. The jejunal wall was thickened by edema. The terminal parts of the ileum were more severely affected than other gastrointestinal regions. The ileocecal valve was congested and often had numerous petechiae, while the cecal mucosa was hyperemic. Rugae of the colon were congested, and their free edges were slightly eroded. The mesenteric lymph nodes were enlarged, and the lymphatics of the mesentery were abnormally dilated.[40]

Histologically, the intestinal villi had a bulbous appearance caused by dilation of capillaries and central lacteals, edema and infiltration of mononuclear cells.[40] The inflammatory process spanned from the mucosal to the serosal surfaces in some instances. The epithelial cells desquamated extensively at many levels of the small intestine. Numerous crypts of Lieberkühn were distended by inflammatory leukocytes and sloughed, degenerated epithelial cells. The remaining epithelial cells lining such crypts were cuboidal rather than columnar. The Peyer's patches had lost their follicular architecture and contained necrotic centers, a feature also seen in the tonsils.

Diagnosis and Differentiation

The specific diagnosis must be established by demonstration of chlamydiae or chlamydial antigens or DNA in feces, diarrhea fluid or intestinal mucosal samples. The isolation of chlamydiae from fecal samples by the cell culture method is more sensitive and faster than the previously used propagation in yolk sacs of developing chicken embryos.[41] Demonstration of chlamydiae in intestinal sections after immunofluorescent staining provides a specific and rapid test.[35] Examination of diarrhea fluid by electron microscopic methods or ELISA for detecting chlamydiae has not been explored sufficiently, but these methods reveal most of the enteropathogenic viruses that must be considered for differential diagnosis. A sensitive tool to detect intestinal chlamydial infections will be PCR amplification of DNA of chlamydial MOMP genes with genus-specific oligonucleotide primers.[33]

The antibody response of newborn calves is weak following intestinal chlamydial infections. Newborn calves surviving the intestinal infection developed antibodies when they became 43–57 days old.[42] About 70% of clinically normal sheep that excreted chlamydiae in the feces did not have significant titers of antibodies, and the rest had low titers.[43]

Respiratory Infections and Pneumonia

Epidemiology

Chlamydia-induced pneumonia of different animal species was found to occur worldwide. A clinically inapparent respiratory chlamydial infection that can be activated to clinical pneumonia was first detected in mice.[6,7] The etiologic role of chlamydiae as a cause of pneumonia is established in cats, sheep, goats, cattle, swine, and domestic and wild rabbits.[1,5,44–46] Some horses affected with respiratory disease in Australia and in England had chlamydial infections.[47,48] The respiratory disease of calves from which chlamydiae were isolated has been recognized in the United States and Canada, in Germany and in England.[20] Similarly, enzootic pneumonia of swine was associated with chlamydial infections in Russia and Balkan countries.[46] Chlamydial pneumonia of cats, often associated with conjunctivitis and rhinitis, was described in the United States, Canada, England, Switzerland, and Australia.[1,20]

Complicating infections with *Pasteurella, Hemophilus,* or *Mycoplasma* spp, as well as viruses, were reported to lead to more serious clinical signs and lesions. The stress of shipping or crowding, abrupt changes in the weather, or adjustment to a new environment after weaning creates conditions favorable for chlamydial pneumonia.[20] Respiratory chlamydial infections of calves, sheep, and goats is linked closely to shedding of chlamydiae by carriers with clinically inapparent intestinal infections. Coughing by affected animals creates infectious aerosols, and chances for close contact with inhalation of chlamydiae-laden dust particles are important in transmission of the infection. Serial pulmonary passages probably enhance the virulence of the agent.

Airborne transmission and direct contact spread chlamydial infection from cat to cat. Droplet infection is facilitated by frequent coughing and sneezing of diseased cats, because the discharges from eyes and nose are highly infectious. Rapid airborne spread to cage mates established epizootics in animal hospitals and catteries. Queens infect their newborn kittens. Infected cats are a danger to human companions, who may contract ocular infections and conjunctivitis from chlamydia-infected cats.

Properties of Respiratory Chlamydiae

Few isolates from respiratory infections were characterized. The feline pneumonia strain falls into the separate serovar 7 which appears to be host specific.[31] The RFLP of the MOMP gene DNA confirmed this further.[32] An isolate from bovine pneumonia together with some porcine chlamydiae were typed as a serovar 6. The Nigg strain of mouse pneumonitis is the murine biotype of *C. trachomatis*.[49]

Clinical Signs

Calves with pneumonia and positive chlamydial cultures from respiratory tract samples have serous, mucous or mucopurulent nasal discharge. They usually are febrile and appear depressed, while a dry cough may be associated with dyspnea. Transient diarrhea is also observed. Often, pneumonic lesions are found incidentally at slaughter.

Lambs responded with a rise in temperature 24–48 h after intranasal or intratracheal inoculation with the chlamydial agent of ovine pneumonia. The fever remained high for about 2 days and then subsided to normal levels by the 6th day. During the febrile period, the lambs were depressed and anorectic and displayed signs of respiratory distress, with an occasionally dry cough. The uncomplicated experimental lung infection induced relatively mild symptoms. The disease was often observed after feeder lambs were gathered from different herds for fattening in feed lots or irrigated pastures.[45,51]

Goats with chlamydial pneumonia had symptoms similar to those of sheep. Clinical signs of pigs with respiratory chlamydial infections were typical of enzootic pneumonia.[46]

Cats affected with chlamydia-induced pneumonia sneeze, cough, have fever and are depressed and anorectic.[52] Mucopurulent discharge and excessive fluid flow from the eyes and nostrils as a result of conjunctivitis, rhinitis and pharyngitis. The cats recover in 2–4 weeks after infection, but they frequently remain asymptomatic carriers. The disease usually is not fatal, but very young or elderly cats may die of severe pneumonia. Sequelae to feline pneumonia are chronic conjunctivitis, sinusitis, bronchitis and tracheitis.[5]

Pathogenetic Events

The sequence of events in the genesis of chlamydial pneumonia was studied in sheep and in calves. Pulmonary infections of lambs with chlamydiae most likely are initiated in the bronchiolus and spread from there to the lung parenchyma.[50,51] Lung involvement was most severe on the 5th day after inoculation, then signs of regression became evident, and lungs were virtually normal after 30 days. Chlamydia-induced pneumonia of sheep was classified as an interstitial bronchopneumonia. The pulmonary lesions were also considered as hyperplastic pneumonia because of alveolar epthelialization.

Pathological Changes

Consolidations of the anterior lobes and in the hilus region of lungs are observed in naturally occurring cases of chlamydial-induced pneumonia of sheep and goats. Mature lesions consist of irregular but sharply defined areas of consolidation with a dull, grey–pink color. The lungs are heavy and fail to collapse. The consolidated areas are slightly elevated, lumpy and solid on palpation, and slightly opaque mucus appears in opened bronchioli. The mediastinal lymph nodes are usually enlarged. The lung lesions have streaky, irregular, dark-red bands during the evolving and resolving stages. These consist mostly of atelectatic regions that can not be distinguished from normal lung tissue by palpation alone.[50]

There was an early acute inflammatory response in terminal bronchioles and adjacent alveoli, followed by proliferation of alveolar cells and accumulation of macrophages within alveoli. Extensive alveolar epithelialization was present at the height of the pulmonary reaction 5 days after experimental injection. Reticulin stains revealed well-preserved alveolar architecture in densely consolidated regions which accounted, at least in part, for the ease with which resolution occurred.[50]

Diagnosis and Differentiation of Chlamydial Pneumonia

Clinical signs or the macroscopic pathologic changes are not specific enough to diagnose chlamydial pneumonia in animals and to differentiate them from viral or mycoplasma pneumonia. Impression smears from conjunctival and respiratory tract scrapings or from the margins of the pneumonic lesions provide a diagnosis if these preparations contain chlamydial elementary bodies or chlamydial inclusions in monocytes or conjunctival and respiratory epithelial cells. The use of fluorescent antibodies increases the diagnostic value of exfoliative cytologic findings.

Most reports on chlamydial pneumonia were based on an etiologic diagnosis with isolation and identification of the causative chlamydiae.[20,41] Chicken embryos were used as indicator hosts in the past, but cell culture methods are more sensitive and give earlier answers.[41] Samples from the reactive margins of the lung lesions contain viable chlamydial agent during the acute stage of the disease. Chlamydiae were isolated from nasal washings in bovine and equine pneumonia. Parallel testing of specimens for respiratory viruses on cultured animal cells and careful cultivating for bacterial and mycoplasmal species furnish the evidence needed for etiologic differentiation of the respiratory disease under study. Chlamydial pneumonia was diagnosed in calves from 4 out of 20 natural epizootics of pneumonia through a four-fold rise in the titer of genus-specific antibodies.[53]

Polyarthritis–Polyserositis

Epidemiology

Chlamydial polyarthritis of lambs is an acute febrile disease that occurs in epizootic proportions in the western and southern sheep-raising regions of the United States. The cause of the disease, which also is referred to as stiff lamb disease, was first identified by Mendlowski and Segre in 1960 as a chlamydial infection of the synovial tissues, with inflammation of most diarthrodial joints of the limbs, leading to stiffness and lameness.[21] A similar disease of calves was also recognized in the western United States.[54] Chlamydiae were isolated from the joints of calves affected with this disease.[22] Transmissible serositis of calves had previously been described in Australia.[55] Chlamydiae were isolated from synovial samples of swine suffering from polyarthritis in Austria.[29,56] The arthropathogenic potential was convincingly proven as yet another manifestation of chlamydial infections.

Chlamydial polyarthritis was observed in lambs out on ranges, as well as in lambs from farm flocks and feedlots; and morbidity ranged from 2 to 75%. Lambs that weighed 55–105 pounds appeared to be affected more often than smaller, younger lambs. The highest incidence of the disease among sheep on ranges was observed in July, August and September; while in feedlot lambs the disease is most prevalent in October, November and December.[21,54,57] The youngest calf that had naturally occurring chlamydial polyarthritis was 4 days old when the first signs of polyarthritis were detected. More commonly the calves are several weeks old. This condition is seen sporadically in individual calves in contrast to the disease in lambs. The agent is shed in feces, urine and also in conjunctival secretions.[22,58]

Properties of Arthropathogenic Chlamydiae

Isolates from joints of lambs, calves and swine as well as isolates from cattle with sporadic bovine encephalomyelitis belong to serovar 2 classified as *C. pecorum*.[31,102] The DNA of representative strains had less than 70% homology with DNA of other chlamydiae.[59–61] A multiple step PCR with primary genus specific and secondary group specific primers for the DNA of the MOMP gene also distinguished these strains as a distinct group of chlamydiae.[33] Infection with these strains is typically enhanced by cytoactive treatments of the cultured cells.[62] The effect on the cytoskeleton of infected cells distinguishes the serovar 2 strains as unique biovars.[62]

Several stable characteristics were thus identified that characterize the arthropathogenic chlamydiae as a separate chlamydial species.[102]

Clinical Signs

Rectal temperatures of affected lambs ranged from 39–42°C. The fever appeared to depend on the stage and acuteness of the disease. The lambs had varying degrees of stiffness, lameness and anorexia; and some had conjunctivitis (Fig. 20.3). Affected lambs were gaunt, depressed and reluctant to move or stand or bear weight on one or more limbs, and lingered behind the rest of the band; and many would lie down.[21,54,57]

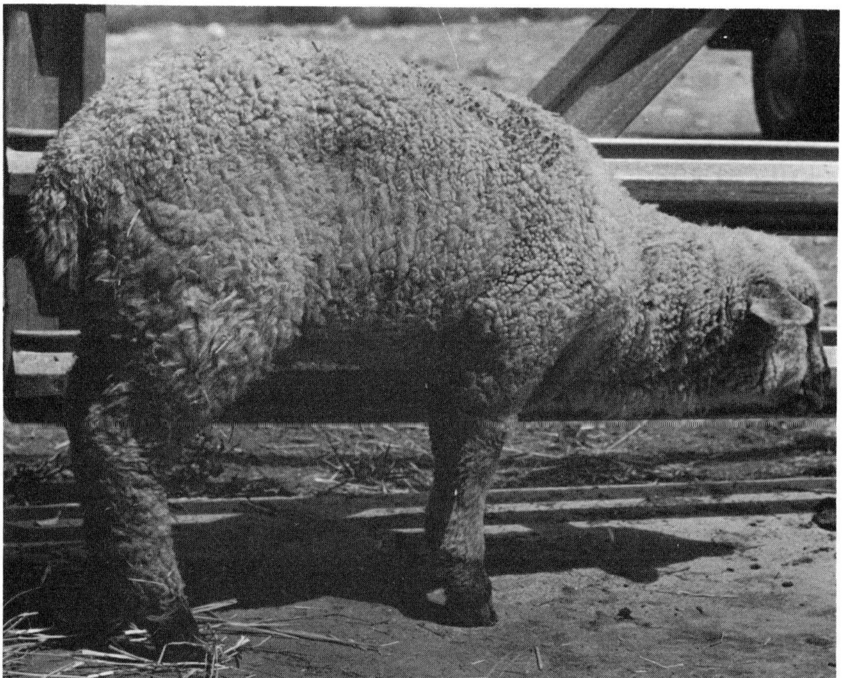

FIG. 20.3. Severe case of chlamydial polyarthritis in a lamb that is depressed, anorectic, gaunt, and reluctant to move.

Clinically affected calves are reluctant to move and they always have diarrhea. They usually are febrile, but they remain alert and nurse if carried to the dam and supported while they are suckling. Weight loss becomes evident within a few days. As the disease progresses the calves become depressed, favor their legs, and assume a hunched position while standing. When recumbent they extend their legs passively, and the joints and tendons of the limbs are painful when palpated. Umbilical lesions or signs of nervous disorders have not been associated with this syndrome. Younger calves usually die a week or two after appearance of clinical signs.[22,58]

Pathogenic Events

Chlamydiae were isolated from the sites of the major lesions, the affected joints of naturally occurring cases of chlamydial polyarthritis of lambs and calves. These agents were also isolated from different organs and body excretions that included synovial tissues and fluids; lungs, liver, spleen, kidneys, brain and lymph nodes; conjunctival scrapings; composite samples of mucosa and content from abomasum, duodenum, jejunum, ilium and caecum; and samples of blood, cerebrospinal fluid, urine and feces.[58,64]

A chlamydemic phase precedes infection of the synovial tissues in the pathogenesis of chlamydial polyarthritis.[58,64–66] Polyarthritis can readily be reproduced experimentally by inoculating lambs or calves via the oral, subcutaneous, intramuscular, intravenous, or intra-articular routes. Three days after intra-articular inoculation of lambs, the directly inoculated joint was severely inflamed and had high chlamydial infectivity. Lesions were not seen in other joints at this time, but chlamydiae were recovered from the blood and uninoculated joints. Three days after intramuscular or intravenous inoculation of lambs, chlamydial agents were isolated from several joints, although gross lesions were minimal at this time. Irrespective of the routes of inoculation, hip, knee, shoulder, and elbow joints of lambs examined on the 7th day of the experiment had moderate to severe inflammatory changes, and chlamydiae were isolated from the affected joints. Involvement of most joints of the experimental lambs remained evident 21 days after inoculation, and chlamydiae were cultured from the majority of the affected joints tested. Maximum chlamydial infectivity was present in the joints 7 and 14 days after inoculation of the lambs and decreased progressively thereafter to become negative after the 28th day.[64]

Calves inoculated orally or parenterally with serovar 2 isolates from joints developed polyarthritis and polyserositis, and chlamydiae were recovered from the affected joints, internal organs and intestinal tracts.[62] Oral infection is expected to occur under field conditions because the intestine was found to be infected in sheep and calves with naturally occurring chlamydial polyarthritis.[22,34,64] Infection and multiplication occurred in the mucosa of the small and large intestines, leading to primary diarrhea following oral inoculation of calves with chlamydial strains of polyarthritis. The intestinal barrier was breached by infection of endothelial cells of the central lacteals and release of infectious chlamydiae into the lymph flow.[38] Chlamydemia followed intestinal chlamydial multiplication and determined the further course of the disease.[65,66] Lesions were also evident in tonsils and Peyer's patches.

Pathological Changes

The most striking tissue changes were articular and periarticular in naturally occurring and experimentally induced chlamydial polyarthritis of lambs and calves.[64,67] Radiologically, there was no discernible malalignment of the limbs or joints. Periarticular, subcutaneous edema and fluid-filled, fluctuating synovial sacs contributed to joint enlargement of affected calves. The larger, freely movable, weight-bearing joints—such as hip, stiffle, tarsal, atlanto-occipital, shoulder, elbow and the carpal joints of calves—contained excessive, grayish-yellow, turbid synovial fluid. Grayish-yellow fibrin flakes and plaques of different sizes and shapes were found in joints with advanced lesions. The fibrin plaque in the recesses of the affected joints often adhered firmly to the synovial membranes, and the joint capsules were thickened. Erosions or evidence of marginal compensatory changes could not be found on the articular cartilage. The tendon sheaths of severely affected lambs and calves were distended and contained creamy, grayish-yellow exudate. Surrounding muscles were hyperemic and edematous having petechiae in their associated fascial planes. Calves also had enlarged spleens and swollen lymph nodes.[67,68]

Consistent and striking histopathological changes involved the synovial membranes, joint capsule, tendon sheaths, ligaments, periarticular connective tissue and muscles.[67] The inflammatory reaction in the synovium, tendon sheaths and subsynovial tissues progressed from initial serous to fibrinopurulent inflammation to, finally, accumulation of lymphoid cells and fibroplasia (Fig. 20.4). Dimorphic inflammatory responses with some leukocytes along the synovial surface and mononuclear cell infiltration in the subsynovial strains were prominent. Areas of the synovial membranes under the fibrinopurulent exudate were necrotic and heavily infiltrated with neutrophils and lymphocytes during the early stages of the infection. Involvement of subsynovial connective tissue and muscle was limited to accumulation of mononuclear cells in perivascular areas and increasing fibrosis. The joint capsule and tendon sheath of advanced cases had undergone marked fibrotic thickening, which was associated with an extensive inflammatory response that consisted primarily of infiltration by plasma cells, monocytes, lymphocytes, macro-

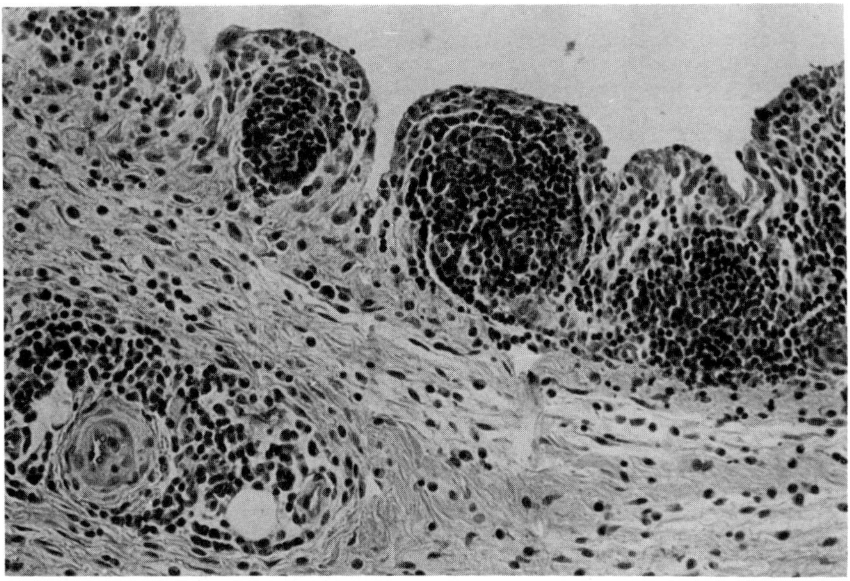

FIG. 20.4. Granulomatous lesions in synovial membrane of a lamb 21 days after intramuscular inoculation with an arthropathogenic chlamydial strain. Notice angiitis and perivascular infiltration. Hematoxylin and eosin stain, × 192.

phages and neutrophils. The synoviocytes became swollen and hyperplastic and assumed a pseudostratified appearance. The tendon sheaths had marked fibroblastic proliferation characterized by large, plump, round fibroblasts. Intra-articular masses of fibrin contained polymorphonuclear cells, monocytes and necrotic cellular debris. Chlamydial inclusions were found in fibroblasts, monocytes and endothelial and synovial cells in thin sections of affected joint tissues.[67]

Changes in muscles were periarticular and adjacent to tendinous insertions. These changes were best characterized as myositis because they consisted of infiltration with inflammatory cells and accumulation of edema fluid between individual muscle fibers and between muscle bundles.[67] Individual muscle fibers were intact and essentially normal, but hyperemia and hemorrhages were observed in muscles. The reactive processes in muscle tissues appeared to be dominated by fibroblastic proliferation suggestive of a musculo-tendofasciitis. Affected tendons and tendon sheaths contained edema fluid and were infiltrated by inflammatory cells.

Calves that were orally inoculated with chlamydial strains from polyarthritis harbored this infection in the kidneys and shed chlamydiae in high titers in the urine.[34,69] The kidneys of calves examined a week and later after inoculation had multiple, grayish-white nodules visible through the capsule. Focal renal tubular dilatation became severe and cystic, involving the distal convoluted tubules. The epithelial cells of such tubules were flattened. The lumen contained epithelial cell casts. Focal and interstitial inflammatory reactions of lymphocytes and plasma cells were dispersed throughout the cortex.[69]

The lesions were most pronounced 6 weeks postinoculation. Sagittal sections displayed these lesions as wedges of various depths in the cortex. The tissue changes advanced to a chronic focal nonsupporative nephritis. The cellular reactions involved the medulla but more often the cortex. Fibrous tissue became more prominent around tubules. Glomeruli surrounded by inflammatory reactions became atrophic, and their Bowman capsules had various degrees of fibrosis. The glomerular tufts had proliferative changes involving the epithelial, endothelial and mesangial cells, with little encroachment on the patency of the blood capillaries but leading to obliteration of the urinary space of glomeruli.[69]

Diagnosis and Differentiation

Isolation of chlamydiae from the site of the major lesion, the affected joints, provides a definitive diagnosis. Cytologic investigations on synovial fluids or tissues may reveal the presence of chlamydial inclusions in cells of affected joints. Bacteriologic cultures of affected joints were negative in samples from sheep, but *Escherichia coli* or streptococci were occasionally cultured from joints of calves that were chlamydia-infected.[22,58]

The clinical and pathological features distinguish chlamydial polyarthritis from other conditions that cause stiffness and lameness in lambs. Lambs with mineral deficiency, osteomalacia, or white muscle disease usually do not have fever, unless the fever is caused by secondary bacterial infection. Sheep with chronic, advanced cases of arthritis caused by *Erysipelas insidiosa* usually have eburnations, with compensatory marginal lipping and osteophyte formation. Laminitis caused by bluetongue virus infection can be differentiated clinically, pathologically and etiologically from chlamydial polyarthritis. Detailed microbiologic investigations are needed to differentiate arthritis and serositis caused by myoplasma.[41]

Humoral Antibody Response

The serological test most widely used in the past to detect chlamydial antibodies in animal infections was the CF test.[20,41] Active systemic chlamydial infections induce titers that have diagnostic significance if four-fold or higher antibody rises develop that are related to specific disease episodes. Since guinea pigs have naturally occurring chlamydial infections, guinea pig complement must be checked for freedom from chlamydial antibodies. Supplementation of guinea pig complement with fresh bovine serum free of chlamydial antibodies enhances the sensitivity of the CF test for bovine antibodies. The CF test has been virtually replaced by modern enzyme-linked immune assays.[41]

The antibody responses of cows experiencing chlamydial infections were recently analyzed with the enzyme linked immunosorbent assay (ELISA) and the indirect immunofluorescent antibody (IIFA) test.[42,70] The antibody responses were characteristic and diagnostically indicative. Partially purified elementary bodies were used to sensitize the test plates so that the predominant chlamydial antigens reactive in these tests were proteinaceous antigens of species-, type- and strain specificity. Heavy and light (H+L) chain specific conjugates were employed to detect all immunoglobulin isotypes. Interestingly, the chlamydia-specific antibody fraction of bovine serum contained high levels of noncomplement-binding IgG_2 when tested with the corresponding immunoglobulin subclass specific conjugates.[70–73] The ELISA can be set up with single serum dilutions of 1:100 if strictly quantitative evaluation and appropriate internal negative and positive controls are used.[71]

Treatment of Chlamydial Infections of Ruminants

The multiplication of chlamydiae in the cells of animals is inhibited or reduced by tetracyclines, chloramphenicol and erythromycin-like compounds, such as tylosin. To be effective the antibiotics must reach the intracellular sites where chlamydial multiplication occurs. When these antibiotics are used properly during the early stage of an infection, affected animals may respond favorably. The treatment usually does not eliminate chlamydial infections unless the antibiotics are given for an extended period.[19]

Dairy cattle of one closed breeding herd in which virtually all the animals had intestinal chlamydial infections, chlortetracycline (2 mg/kg body weight) was given to every animal orally for 7 days and then 1 mg/kg/day was given for the following 21 days. Though chlamydiae were not isolated from the feces of these cattle during the 2 weeks after treatment, a year later the cattle again shed chlamydiae in their feces even though the herd had remained closed. This was interpreted as a recurrence of the original infection.[74] There are no reports of specific studies of the effect of antibiotics on chlamydial enteritis during the neonatal period or on pneumonia in calves. The previously mentioned antibiotics should be given in addition to supportive therapy when chlamydial infections are suspected.

Favorable responses were obtained when lambs affected naturally with chlamydial polyarthritis were treated with long-lasting penicillins, oxytetracycline or tylosin. The lambs were intramuscularly given 200 mg of tylosin or 250 mg of oxytetracycline for 2 days or 300,000 units of penicillin G once, as soon as clinical signs of chlamydial polyarthritis became evident. Chlortetracycline or tylosin was effective in the treatment of calves with polyarthritis–serositis and calves with chlamydial meningo-encephalomyelitis. High doses of these antibiotics were given as early as possible in the course of the disease. They were injected parenterally for at least 4–5 days. The body temperature of treated animals dropped significantly within 24 h after initiation of the treatment.

The most effective antibiotics for treating chlamydial infections are tetracyclines, but even these antibiotics suppress only chlamydial growth and multiplication and do not eliminate the infection without intact defense mechanisms of the host. Tetracyclines block protein synthesis by interfering with the transfer of amino acids from the activated transfer RNA to the growing peptide chain on the ribosome. Different strains of chlamydiae may differ in susceptibility to tetracyclines.[75]

Sporadic Bovine Encephalomyelitis

Epidemiology

Some cattle may develop pronounced signs of nervous disease and encephalomelitis following infection with serovar 2 chlamydiae.[1,8,76] The causal agent was isolated in 1940 by intraperitoneal inoculation of guinea pigs and later identified to have chlamydial properties.[8,76] Tissue reactions in the brain and associated adverse neurological signs may be induced in the course of systemic chlamydial infections of other animal species, as well as man. Popek identified 27 cases of human chlamydiosis with nervous signs associated with meningitis, encephalitis and myelitis.[77] Opossums with naturally occurring chlamydial infections developed paralysis of the hind legs and convulsions.[78] Meningeal and encephalitic lesions were found histologically in chickens, pigeons and turkeys with chlamydial infections.[4,79]

The clinical encephalitic manifestations of chlamydial infections were investigated mainly in cattle. Sporadic bovine encephalomyelitis was proven to occur in cattle of many parts of the United States as well as in Japan, Czechoslovakia, Australia, Canada, Hungary and Germany.[1,20] Transmission by the oral–fecal route leads to this nervous disorder that affects cattle sporadically.[80] This disease is seen primarily in cattle younger than 2 years, although older animals may be affected. The morbidity is low, but the mortality of stricken cattle is 50–60%. Konrad and Bohac observed 100% mortality among SBE-affected cattle in Czechoslovakia.[81] The disease may remain enzootic in one herd, but, not infrequently, outbreaks follow introduction of susceptible cattle into established herds.

Clinical Signs

Depression and gradual loss of locomotor coordination are early clinical signs. The affected cattle become anorectic and develop a high fever approximately 2 weeks after exposure. Excessive salivation, dyspnea and mild diarrhea are signs in the early stages. Recovery may follow this stage, but in some instances the cattle develop neural involvement manifested by walking difficulties, a stiff gait and a tendency to stagger and circle, often falling over small obstacles. The limbs become progressively weaker, paralysis develops and the animals become recumbent and may exhibit opisthotonos. The course of the disease usually lasts from 10 to 14 days, but in some instances affected cattle may survive for a month.[8,80]

Pathogenesis and Pathological Changes

The dominant feature in the development of this disease is a generalized chlamydial infection. The chlamydial agent was isolated from blood, brain and cerebrospinal fluid and from liver, spleen, kidneys, lungs and peritoneal fluid.[76] Lesions in various organs are associated with vascular damage. The brain is the ultimate target organ, and the brain lesions usually are distributed through all parts of the brain, but they are regularly present in the medulla, pons and brain stem. The degree of brain involvement may well be the critical point that determines recovery or death. The arachnoid and ependymal tissues are favored sites of chlamydial multiplication. The factors that lead to the severe reaction in the brain are not well understood and could possibly involve immune-mediated injuries. Not all aspects of this disease have been reproduced experimentally; pathological changes of mild clinical cases have not been described, and fatal cases with no brain involvement are not on record. Although serositis was described, and fatal cases with no brain involvement are not on record. Although serositis was described often as a lesion in sporadic bovine encephalomyelitis, one should consider this nervous disease as a distinct clinical entity, separate from polyarthritis–serositis of calves, until certain clinical, pathological and pathogenetic differences are resolved.

Macroscopic lesions when visible in the central nervous system are primarily hyperemia and edema. After an acute course of the sickness, few gross lesions are found, but the serous cavities may contain an increased amount of yellowish fluid. Some chronic cases have serofibrinous exudate in serous cavities with peritonitis, pleuritis or pericarditis. Microscopically, all parts of the brain and spinal cord have vasculitis with perivascular cuffing and parenchymal foci of inflammation composed of lymphoid and mononuclear cells. Similar inflammatory reactions may be seen in the leptomeninges. Small foci of granulomatous inflammation are found in kidneys, lungs and livers. Acute and chronic bronchiolitis with focal areas of pneumonia are observed. Fibrin on visceral surfaces of abdominal organs undergoes organization.[80]

Diagnosis

Etiologic confirmation of the cause of this disease can be achieved by isolating chlamydiae from brain tissues or fluids. Pathological lesions and other encephalitic diseases of cattle, including listeriosis, rabies, pseudorabies, malignant catarrhal fever and encephalitis caused by the virus of infectious bovine rhinotracheitis, must be differentiated by clinical, etiological and histological examination.[77] Rising chlamydial antibody titers are supporting a clinical diagnosis of chlamydial meningoencephalomyelitis.[39]

Conjunctivitis and Ocular Diseases

Epidemiology

While trachoma and inclusion conjunctivitis of man have a long history as specific and distinct clinical entities caused by *C. trachomatis*,[2] the study of ocular chlamydial infections of animals is of rather recent history.[1] Ocular diseases are now known to be caused by *C. psittaci* and *C. pecorum* in several mammalian species. Conjunctivitis and ocular involvement have long been recognized as clinical signs of chlamydiosis in pigeons, ducks and geese.[5]

Yerasimides was the first to isolate and identify a chlamydial agent from conjunctival exudate of a cat suffering from acute catarrhal conjunctivitis.[23] An infectious agent with chlamydial properties was isolated from conjunctival samples of piglets affected with keratoconjunctivitis in Bulgaria.[82] Murray identified in 1964 inclusion conjunctivitis of guinea pigs as a prevalent chlamydial infection.[24]

The observation of chlamydial agents as the cause of contagious keratoconjunctivitis of sheep in England was based on cytologic examinations of conjunctival samples and on chemotherapeutic treatment of the infection.[83] Chlamydial agents were subsequently cultured in developing chicken embryos from conjunctival samples taken from sheep suffering from keratoconjunctivitis in the United States[84] and recently also from lambs in England.[85] Chlamydiae were also isolated from conjunctival scrapings of cattle afflicted with keratoconjunctivitis in Czechoslovakia and Germany.[20] Interestingly, Rowe and coworkers isolated chlamydiae in cultured cells from conjunctival samples of a calf from a free-living herd of African buffalos.[86] The studies of Cockram and Jackson are of unique interest because chlamydiae were isolated from eye samples of free-living koalas (*Phascolarctos cinereus*) severely affected with keratoconjunctivitis in Australia.[25]

Properties of Conjunctival Chlamydial Isolates

The isolates from cats belong to serovar 7 and those from guinea pigs are serovar 8. Serovar 2 isolates were recovered from conjunctivitis of lambs.[31,87] Serovar 7 and 8 infect L cells or other cultured cells readily while serovar 2 chlamydiae require infectivity enhancing conditions through treatment of cells with cytoactive compounds or centrifugation onto monolayers.[62,63]

Clinical Signs

Conjunctival chlamydial infections of different animal species probably lead to similar clinical signs. They have been studied in infections of cats, sheep and guinea pigs. The infection may become endemic in catteries, and cats may remain affected with conjunctivitis for as long as one year. Kittens born to affected or clinically recovered cats may have severe conjunctivitis at the time their eyelids normally open. Cats developed a severe conjunctivitis 3–5 days after conjunctival inoculation. On the 4th day, these cats invariably had fever, which lasted for 24 h. Chlamydial inclusion bodies were found in large numbers from the 3rd day after inoculation and persisted in decreasing numbers for 2 weeks. Many experimentally inoculated cats had clinical evidence of conjunctivitis for as long as 90 days.

Corneal involvement was not observed, but rhinitis and other signs of respiratory involvement were often seen.[52] Infections of the gastric mucosa was recently detected.[88,89] This site of infection appears to be an extension of the feline pneumonitis syndrome caused by chlamydiae. Mild gastritis was observed, but most cats with persistent gastric infection appeared clinically normal.

Early signs of chlamydial conjunctivitis of sheep consisted of chemosis and dilation of conjunctival vessels at the lid margins. Diffuse reddening was seen later in the lower fornices, where fine filaments of mucus were also present. The development of lymphoid follicles signaled intermediate stages of conjunctivitis involvement. Lymphoid follicles began as small, discrete, pale and elevated changes in the conjunctiva, enlarged to diameters of 3 mm and became confluent, forming delicate pink-to-red folds in the lower fornix and the 3rd eyelid. The bulbar surface of the 3rd eyelid had numerous follicles. Lymphoid follicles in the upper fornices developed into folds 2–4 mm high. Conjunctival hyperemia, edema and follicle development caused swelling of the periorbital tissues. Lacrimal drainage was compromised, epiphora was a common sign, and abundant seropurulent eye discharge was observed to seal the eye lids with a crust. Perilimbal edema of the cornea was associated with signs of severe inflammatory involvement of the bulbar conjunctiva and its extension into the cornea as keratitis (Fig. 20.5). Loops of blood vessels grew into the cornea at a rate of 1 mm per day. Neo-

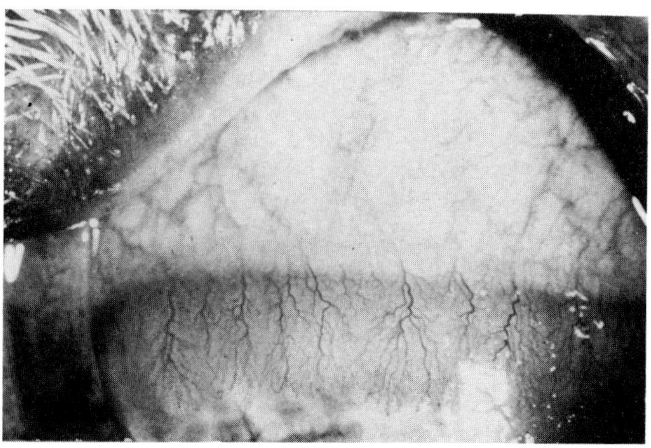

FIG. 20.5. Eye lesions of a lamb with chlamydial infection. Notice bulbar conjunctivitis, neovascularization and keratitis. Third eye lid is to the left.

vascularization of the cornea occurred in the upper limbus, often extended into the cornea for distances of 5 mm, and became completely perilimbal. Both eyes were found to be equally affected in 80% of the lambs. The disease was self-limiting in uncomplicated cases because full resolution of lesions was observed. Complications consisted of opacity of the entire cornea and corneal ulceration.[20,84,90]

Ten to eighty-five per cent of the lambs with conjunctivitis studied in the western United States had polyarthritis, and virtually all lambs with polyarthritis had conjunctivitis. Chlamydiae of serovar 2 were isolated from conjunctiva, blood and joint samples of affected lambs.[54,84] Goats experiencing chlamydial abortions also had keratoconjunctivitis.[91]

Chlamydial inclusion conjunctivitis affects many herds of guinea pigs and is predominantly found in 4–8 week old animals. A special effort is necessary to detect the inflammatory conjunctival reaction with its light, yellowish-white discharge. An intense conjunctivitis arises 3–6 days after experimental infection of guinea pig eyes which induces a watery to mucopurulent discharge, chemosis and follicular hypertrophy in the palpebral conjunctiva. Localized subepithelial cellular infiltrates are frequently seen in the peripheral cornea. Pannus or micropannus form in most inoculated guinea pigs as early as 5 days after exposure. The keratoconjunctivitis is self-limiting and clears up within 3–4 weeks.[24]

Pathogenesis and Pathological Changes

The development of chlamydial inclusion bodies in epithelial and monocytic cells was associated with mononuclear and heterophilic cellular responses in cats, lambs, piglets, and guinea pigs (Fig. 20.6). Inclusion bodies with chlamydial features were found in the conjunctival epithelial cells that also evidenced cytopathic changes and lysis.[24,53,90] The epithelium and subepithelial tissues of the conjunctiva were infiltrated with polymorphonuclear leukocytes in the early stages, while subepithelial collections of macrophages and mononuclear cells were found in the peripheral limbus, and mononuclear cells dominated the histological changes in the advanced stages. Persistent antigenic stimulation provoking chronic inflammations in chlamydial infections is considered to be one pathogenic mechanism. The guinea pig model of inclusion conjunctivitis was used in an elegant series of experiments to identify chlamydial fractions involved in the deleterious immune responses.[92] Triton X100 extracts of chlamydial elementary bodies elicited ocular hypersensitivity in immunized guinea pigs. This response was genus

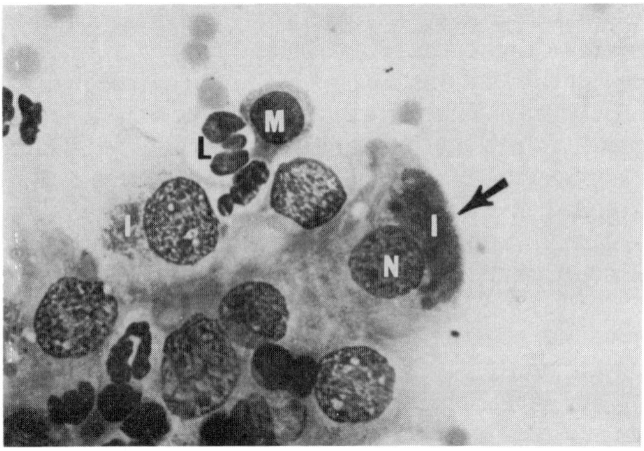

FIG. 20.6. Chlamydial inclusions (I) in conjunctival cells from lamb with conjunctivitis. Arrow points towards infected cells with nucleus (N). A monocyte (M) and numerous leukocytes (L) are present. Giemsa stain, ×600.

specific, but it was not elicited by purified LPS. A 57 kDa protein carried the function. This heat-stable antigen, associated with elementary and reticulate bodies of both chlamydial species, was identified as a member of stress–response proteins.[93]

Calves with systemic chlamydial infections leading to polyarthritis also developed conjunctivitis, and signs of blindness were observed in cattle with sporadic encephalomyelitis. Intraocular structures involved were the retina and the optic nerve. Optic papillitis consisted of mononuclear inflammatory reactions extending from the lamina cribosa to the head of the optic nerve. Histopathological alterations were present in the nerve fiber layer and the inner nuclear layer of the sensory retina. An inflammatory reaction extended towards the inner limiting membrane of the retina. Histiocytic cells, lymphocytes and a few polymorphonuclear leukocytes formed the inflammatory foci of granuloma-like appearance. Bilateral anterior uveitis was observed after intravenous inoculation of albino rabbits with a chlamydial strain isolated from muskrats. This uveitis disappeared about 10 days later, but iritis persisted longer, and mononuclear cells invaded the iris and the ciliary body.[94]

Diagnosis

Exfoliative cytologic examinations of conjunctival scrapings from subjects with conjunctivitis can give valuable diagnostic information.[40] The demonstration of cytoplasmic chlamydial inclusions in conjunctival epithelial cells or monocytes is an unequivocal indication of chlamydial infection (Fig. 20.6). Extracellular chlamydial elementary bodies can be distinguished in the background of such smears. Unfortunately, typical inclusions are present only in the early stages of the ocular chlamydial infection. Application of fluorescent antibody technique facilitates the detection of chlamydial conjunctivitis in animals. Monoclonal antibodies improved detection of this infection in conjunctival samples from cats.[95] Care should be taken to collect conjunctival samples for cytologic studies by scraping the conjunctival surface to collect fresh cells. Conjunctival cells in smears from affected eyes occur singly or in 2- to 3-cell groups, while cells in samples from normal eyes maintain their intercellular bridges to appear as sheets.[90]

The sampling techniques described in conjunction with attempts to express follicular contents are optimal for isolating chlamydiae from conjunctival lesions. The samples should be collected in a small volume of diluent. The developing chicken embryo, inoculated by the yolk sac route, is a good indicator host in isolating chlamydiae from ocular infections of several animal species.[83] Chlamydiae were isolated from conjunctival scrapings of 42% of the lambs affected with eye lesions.[87] Cell culture methods probably are even more sensitive, and they give definitive results within days instead of weeks. Bacterial contamination can be controlled by decontamination through differential centrifugation and use of specific antibiotics. Secondary infections with different kinds of bacteria or mycoplasma often are present in chronic stages of the disease. Viral infections of the conjunctiva must be differentiated by corresponding etiologic investigation.[40] Some information can be gained in this respect by cytologic examination of conjunctival smears if viral agents that induce specific inclusions are involved.

Vaccines to Prevent Feline Conjunctivitis and Pneumonia

Research on live and killed vaccines to prevent chlamydial infections of cats dates back to 1952.[96] These efforts gave insight into the challenges in preventing these infections in animals and are of interest because of the live chlamydial vaccine that was developed.[97] The chlamydiae were propagated in the yolk sacs of developing chicken embryos or recently in feline cell cultures. The live vaccine given intramuscularly afforded the best clinical protection of cats that were challenge-inoculated by the conjunctival and nasal routes.[98–101] Vaccination induced antibodies detected in the indirect immunofluorescent test and a cell-mediated immune response which were assessed in the lymphocyte blastogenesis test.[99]

Assessment of clinical signs appeared to be the most reliable method for evaluation of protection afforded by this vaccine.[98–101] Vaccinated cats did not develop fever after challenge-inoculation but test-infected controls had high fever after inoculation. Other clinical signs involving the upper respiratory tract and the eyes were significantly reduced in vaccinated cats. However, chlamydiae were shed in eye and respiratory secretion by some vaccinated cats following challenge inoculation. Shedding lasted from 5 to 9 days in vaccinates and 4 to 17 days in the controls. Killed chlamydial vaccines induced virtually no, or only inferior, protection to challenge inoculation and adjuvants did not change this measurably.[96,99]

References

1. Storz, J. 1971. *Chlamydia and Chlamydia Induced Diseases*. Charles C. Thomas, Publ. Co. Springfield, Ill. 358 pages.
2. Schachter, J. and Dawson, C.R. 1978. *Human Chlamydial Infections*. PSG Publishing Company, Inc. Littleton, MA.
3. Morange, A. 1895. De la psittacose, ou infection spediale determinée par des perruches. Thése Paris, Académie de Paris.
4. Meyer, K.F. 1967. The host spectrum of psittacosis–lymphogranuloma venereum (PL) agents. *Am. J. Ophthal.* **63:** 1225/199–1246/220.
5. Baker, J.A. 1942. A virus from a pneumonia of cats and its possible relation to the cause of atypical pneumonia in man. *Science* **96:** 475–476.
6. Gönnert, R. 1941. Die Bronchopneumonie, eine neue Viruskrankheit der Maus. *Zentbl. Bakt. I. Orig.* **147:** 161–174.
7. Nigg, C. 1942. Unidentified virus which produces pneumonia and systemic infection in mice. *Science* **95:** 49–50.
8. McNutt, S.H. 1940. A preliminary report on an infectious encephalomyelitis of cattle. *Vet. Med.* **35:** 228–231.
9. Stamp, J.T., McEwen, A.D., Watt, J.A.A. and Nisbet, D.J. 1950. Enzootic abortion in ewes. I. Transmission of the disease. *Vet. Rec.* **62:** 251–254.
10. Storz, J., Carroll, E.J., Ball, L. and Faulkner, L.C. 1968. Isolation of a psittacosis agent (*Chlamydia*) from semen and epididymis of bulls with seminal vesiculitis syndrome. *Am. J. vet. Res.* **29:** 549–555.
11. Rodolakis, A. and Bernard, K. 1977. Isolation of *Chlamydia ovis* from genital organs of rams with epididymitis. *Bull. Acad. vet. Fr.* **50:** 65–70.
12. Bowen, R.A., Spears, P., Storz, J. and Seidel, G.E. Jr 1978. Mechanisms of infertility in genital tract infections due to *Chlamydia psittaci* transmitted through contaminated semen. *J. infect. Dis.* **138:** 95–98.
13. Barron, A.L., White, H.J., Rank, R.G. and Soloff, B.L. 1979. Target tissues associated with genital infection of female guinea pigs by the chlamydial agent of guinea pig inclusion conjunctivitis. *J. infect. Dis.* **139:** 60–68.
14. Blanco-Loizelier, A. 1969. Aislamiento de un agente del grupo psittacosis linfogranuloma venereo (PLV) en mastitis bovinas. *Patronato Biol. Anim.* **13:** 179–186.

15. KALTENBOECK, B., KOUSOULAS, K.G. and STORZ. J. 1991. Detection and strain differentiation of *Chlamydia psittaci* mediated by a two-step polymerase chain reaction. *J. clin. Microbiol.* **29:** 1969–1975.
16. BOULANGER, P. and BANNISTER, G.L. 1959. Abortion produced experimentally in cattle with an agent of the psittacosis lymphogranuloma venereum group of virus. *Can. J. comp. med. vet. Sci.* **23:** 259–265.
17. ENRIGHT, J.B., SADLER, W.W. and ROBINSON, E.A. 1958. Sporadic bovine encephalomyelitis in California. *Proc. U.S. Livestock sanit. Ass.* **62:** 127–135.
18. RONSHOLT, L. and BASSE, A. 1981. Bovine mastitis induced by a common intestinal *Chlamydia psittaci* strain. *Acta vet. scand.* **22:** 9–22.
19. YORK, C.J. and BAKER, J.A. 1951. A new member of the psittacosis–lymphogranuloma group of viruses that causes infection in calves. *J. exp. med.* **93:** 587–604.
20. STORZ, J. and KRAUSS, H. 1985. Chlamydial infections and diseases of animals. In: *Handbook on Bacterial Infections in Animals,* Vol. V, p. 447–531. H. BLOBEL and T. SCHLEISSER (Eds), Fischer Verlag, Jena.
21. MENDLOWSKI, B. and SEGRE, D. 1960. Polyarthritis in sheep. I. Description of the disease and experimental transmission. *Am. J. vet. Res.* **21:** 68–73.
22. STORZ, J. SMART, R.A., MARRIOTT, M.E. and DAVIS, R.V. 1966. Polyarthritis in calves: Isolation of psittacosis agents from affected joints. *Am. J. vet. Res.* **27:** 633–641.
23. YERASIMIDES, T.G. 1960. Isolation of a new strain of feline pneumonitis virus from a domestic cat. J. infect. Dis. **106:** 290–296.
24. MURRAY, E.S. 1964. Guinea pig inclusion conjunctivitis virus. 1. Isolation and identification as a member of the psittacosis–lymphogranuloma–trachoma group. *J. infect. Dis.* **114:** 1–12.
25. COCKRAM, F.A. and JACKSON, A.R.B. 1981. Keratoconjunctivitis of the koala bear caused by chlamydial agents. *J. Wildlife Dis.* **17:** 497–504.
26. MCCOLL, K.A., MARTIN, R.W., GLEESON, L.J., HANDASYDE, K.A. and LEE, A.K. 1984. Chlamydia infection and infertility in the female koala *(Phascolarctos cinereus)*. *Vet. Rec.* **115:** 655–657.
27. NEWCOMER, C.E., ANVER, M.R., SIMMONS, J.L. WILCKE, B.W. JR and NACE, G.W. 1982. Spontaneous and experimental infections of *Xenopus laevis* with *Chlamydia psittaci*. *Lab. Anim. Sci.* **32:** 680–686.
28. WILCKE, B.W. JR, NEWCOMER, C.E., ANVER, M.R., SIMMONS, J.L. and NACE, G.W. 1983. Isolation of *Chlamydia psittaci* from naturally infected African clawed frogs *(Xenopus laevis)*. *Infect. Immun.* **41(2):** 789–794.
29. KÖLBL, O. 1969. Untersuchungen über das Vorkommen von Miyagawanellen beim Schwein. *Wiener Tierärztl. Monatsschr.* **56:** 332–335.
30. LEONHARD, I., WITTENBRINK, M.M. and BISPING, W. 1988. Nachweis von *Chlamydia psittaci* im Kot von Schweinen. *Berl. Münch. Tierärztl. Wschr.* **101:** 124–128.
31. PEREZ-MARTINEZ, J.A. and STORZ, J. 1985. Antigenic diversity of *Chlamydia psittaci* of mammalian origin determined by microimmunofluorescence. *Infect. Immun.* **50:** 905–910.
32. KALTENBOECK, B. and STORZ. J. 1992. Biological properties and genetic analysis of the ompA locus in chlamydiae isolated from swine. *Am. J. vet. Res.* **53:** 1482–1487.
33. KALTENBOECK, B., KOUSOULAS, K.G. and STORZ, J. 1992. Two-step polymerase chain reactions and restriction endonuclease analyses detect and differentiate ompA DNA of the genus *Chlamydia*. *J. clin. Microbiol.* **30:** 1098–1104.

34. Eugster, A.K. and Storz, J. 1971. Pathogenic events in intestinal chlamydial infections leading to polyarthritis in calves. *J. infect. Dis.* **123:** 41–50.
35. Eugster, A.K., Joyce, B.K. and Storz, J. 1970. Immunofluorescence studies on the pathogenesis of intestinal chlamydial infections in calves. *Infect. Immun.* **2:** 351–359.
36. Todd, W.J., Doughri, A.M. and Storz, J. 1976. Ultrastructural changes in host cellular organelles in the course of the chlamydial developmental cycle. *Zentlbl. Bakt. I. Orig.* **236:** 359–373.
37. Doughri, A.M., Altera, K.P. and Storz, J. 1973. Host cell range of chlamydial infection in the neonatal bovine gut. *J. comp. Path.* **83:** 107–114.
38. Doughri, A.M., Altera, K.P., Storz, J. and Eugster, A.K. 1973. Electron microscopic tracing of pathogenetic events in intestinal chlamydial infections of newborn calves. *Exp. molec. Path.* **18:** 10–17.
39. Doughri, A.M., Altera, K.P., Storz, J. and Eugster, A.K. 1973. Ultrastructural pathogenic changes in the chlamydia-infected ileal mucosa of newborn calves. *Vet. Path.* **10:** 114–123.
40. Doughri, A.M., Young, S. and Storz, J. 1974. Pathologic changes in intestinal chlamydial infections of newborn calves. *Am. J. vet. Res.* **35:** 939–944.
41. Storz, J. 1990. Rickettsia and chlamydia. In: *Diagnostic Procedures in Veterinary Bacteriology and Mycology*, pp. 309–331. Carter, G.R. and Cole, J.R. (Eds), Academic Press.
42. Perez-Martinez, J.A. and Storz, J. 1985. Chlamydial infections of cattle. *Modern Vet. Pract.* **66:** 517–522, 603–608.
43. Storz, J. and Thornley, W.R. 1966. Serologische und aetiologische Studien über die intestinale Psittakose-Lymphogranuloma-Infektion der Schafe. *Zentlbl. Vet.* **13:** 14–24.
44. Baker, J.A. 1944. Virus causing pneumonia in cats and producing elementary bodies. *J. exp. Med.* **79:** 159–172.
45. McKercher, D.G. 1952. A virus possibly related to the psittacosis–lymphogranuloma–pneumonitis group causing a pneumonia in sheep. *Science.* **115:** 543–544.
46. Tolybekow, A.S., Wischnajakowa, L.A. and Dobin. M.A. 1973. Die atiologische Bedeuteung eines Erregers aus der Bedsoniengruppe für die Enzootische Pneumonie der Schweine. *Monatsch. vet.* **28:** 339–344.
47. Moorthy, A.R.S. and Spradbrow, P.B. 1978. *Chlamydia psittaci* infection of horses with respiratory disease. *Equine vet. J.* **10:** 38–42.
48. Burrell, M.H., Chalmers, W.S.K. and Kewley, D.R. 1986. Isolation of *Chlamydia psittaci* from the respiratory tract and conjunctivae of thoroughbred horses. *Vet. Rec.* **119:** 302–303.
49. Moulder, J.W., Hatch, T.P., Juo, C.-C., Schachter, J. and Storz, J. 1984. Genus 1. Chlamydia Jones, Rake and Strearns 1945, pp. 729–739. In: Krieg, N.R. and Holt, J.G. (Eds), *Bergey's Manual of Systematic Bacteriology*. Vol. 1. The Williams and Wilkens Co., Baltimore.
50. Dungworth, D.L. and Cordy, D.R. 1962. The pathogenesis of ovine pneumonia. I. Isolation of a virus of the PL group. *J. comp. Path. Ther.* **72:** 49–76.
51. Dungworth, D.L. and Cordy, D.R. 1962. The pathogenesis of ovine pneumonia. II. Isolation of virus from faeces: Comparison of pneumonia caused by faecal, enzootic abortion and pneumonitis viruses. *J. comp. Path. Ther.* **72:** 71–79.
52. Cello, R.M. 1967. Ocular infections in animals wih PLT (Bedsonia) group agents. *Am. J. Ophthal.* **63:** 1270/224–1273/247.

53. HARBOURNE, J.F. 1966. Survey of bovine respiratory diseases with special references to the serological examination of paired serum samples. *Vet. Rec.* **78:** 749–752.
54. STORZ, J., SHUPE, J.L., JAMES, L.F. and SMART, R.A. 1963. Polyarthritis of sheep in the intermountain region caused by a psittacosis–lymphogranuloma agent. *Am. J. vet. Res.* **24:** 1201–1206.
55. LITTLEJOHNS, I.R., HARRIS, A.N.A. and HARDING, W.B. 1961. Sporadic bovine encephalomyelitis. *Aust. Vet. J.* **37:** 53–54.
56. KÖLBL, O., BURTSCHER, H. and HEBENSTREIT, J. 1970. Polyarthritis bei Schlachtschweinen. Microbiologische, histologische und fleisch-hygienische Untersuchungen und Aspekte. *Wien. Tierärztl. Monatsschr.* **57:** 355–361.
57. PIERSON, R.E. 1967. Polyarthritis in Colorado feedlot lambs. *J. Am. vet. Med. Ass.* **150:** 1487–1492.
58. STORZ, J., SHUPE, J.L, SMART, R.A. and THORNLEY, R.W. 1966. Polyarthritis of calves: Experimental induction by a psittacosis agent. *Am. J. vet. Res.* **27:** 987–995.
59. COX, R.L., KUO, C.-C., GRAYSTON, J.T. and CAMPBELL, L.A. 1988. Deoxyribonucleic acid relatedness of chlamydia sp. strain TWAR to *Chlamydia trachomatis* and *Chlamydia psittaci*. *Int. J. System. Bact.* **38(3):** 265–268.
60. TIMMS, P., EAVES, F.W., GIRJES, A.A. and LAVIN, M.F. 1988. Comparison of *Chlamydia psittaci* isolates by restriction endonuclease and DNA probe analyses. *Infect. Immun.* **56:** 287–290.
61. FUKUSHI, H. and HIRAI, K. 1989. Genetic diversity of avian and mammalian *Chlamydia psittaci* strains and relation to host origin. *J. Bact.* **171(5):** 2850–2855.
62. SPEARS, P. and STORZ, J. 1979. *Chlamydia psittaci*: Growth characteristics and enumeration of serotypes 1 and 2 in cultured cells. *J. infect. Dis.* **140:** 959–967.
63. SPEARS, P. and STORZ, J. 1979. Biotyping of *Chlamydia psittaci* based on inclusion morphology and response to DEAE-dextran and cycloheximide. *Infect. Immun.* **24:** 224–232.
64. STORZ, J., SHUPE, J.L., MARRIOT, M.E. and THORNLEY, W.R. 1965. Polyarthritis of lambs induced experimentally by a psittacosis agent. *J. infect. Dis.* **115:** 9–18.
65. STORZ, J., MARRIOTT, M.E. and THORNLEY, W.R. 1968. The dynamics of the blood infectious phase in psittacosis-induced abortions in animals. *J. infect. Dis.* **118:** 333–339.
66. ATA, F.A. and STORZ, J. 1974. Chlamydial blood clearance in convalescent sheep. *Cornell Vet.* **64:** 25–36.
67. SHUPE, J.L. and STORZ, J. 1964. Pathologic study of psittacosis lymphogranuloma polyarthritis of lambs. *Am. J. vet. Res.* **25:** 943–951.
68. CUTLIP, R.C. and RAMSEY, F.K. 1973. Ovine chlamydial polyarthritis: sequential development of articular lesions in lambs after intraarticular exposure. *Am. J. vet Res.* **34:** 71–75.
69. DOUGHRI, A.M., EUGSTER, A.K. and ALTERA, K.P. 1978. Pathological studies on chlamydial kidney infections in newborn calves. *Arab develop. Sci. Technol.* **1:** 10–18.
70. PEREZ-MARTINEZ, J., SCHMEER, N. and STORZ, J. 1986. Bovine chlamydial abortion: Serodiagnosis by modified complement fixation, indirect inclusion fluorescence, and enzyme-immunoassay. *Am. J. vet. Res.* **47:** 1501–1506.
71. SCHMEER, N., PEREZ-MARTINEZ, J.A., SCHNORR, K. and STORZ, J. 1987. Dominance of *Chlamydia psittaci*-specific IgG_2 isotypes in naturally and experimentally infected cattle. *Vet. Immun. Immunopath.* **15:** 311–322.

72. Schmeer, N., Schnorr, K.L., Perez-Martinez, J., Storz, J. and Krauss, H. 1987. Specific interaction of bovine IgG_1 and IgG_2 subclasses with different chlamydial antigens. *Zentlbl. Bakt. I. Orig.* **266:** 305–315.
73. Borovik, R.V., Kurbanov, I.A. and Terskikh, I.I. 1978. Specific activity of cattle immunoglobulins in experimental chlamydia infection. *Vop. Virusol.* **4:** 485–488.
74. Page, L.A., Matthews, P.J. and Smith, P.C. 1973. Natural intestinal infection with *Chlamydia psittaci* in a closed bovine herd: Serologic changes, incidence of shedding, antibiotic treatment of the herd, and biologic characteristics of the chlamydiae. *Am. J. vet. Res.* **34:** 611–614.
75. Jawetz, E. 1969. Chemotherapy of chlamydial infections. *Adv. Pharmac. Chemother.* **7:** 253–282.
76. Wenner, H.A., Harshfield, G.S., Chang, T.W. and Menges, R.W. 1953. Sporadic bovine encephalomyelitis. II. Studies on the etiology of the disease, isolation of nine strains of an infectious agent from naturally infected cattle. *Am. J. Hyg.* **57:** 15–29.
77. Popek, K. 1964. Komplikationen des Nervensystems bei der Ornithose des Menschen. *Arch. exp. Vet.* **18:** 201–209.
78. Rocca-Garcia, M. 1949. Viruses of the lymphogranuloma–psittacosis group isolated from opossums in Columbia, opossum virus A. *J. infect. Dis.* **85:** 275–289.
79. Pierce, K.R. and Moore, R.W. 1965. Meningoencephalitis in turkeys experimentally infected with ornithosis. *Avian Dis.* **9:** 266–271.
80. Harshfield, G.S. 1970. Sporadic bovine encephalomyelitis. *J. Am. vet. Med. Ass.* **156:** 466–477.
81. Konrad, J. and Bohac, J. 1959. Encephalomyelitis in cattle. *Vet. Casopis.* **8:** 228–238.
82. Pavlov, P., Milanov, M. and Tschilev, D. 1963. Recherches sur la rickettsiose keratoconjunctivale du porc en Bulgarie. *Ann. Inst. Pasteur.* **105:** 450–454.
83. Dickinson, L. and Cooper, B.S. 1959. Contagious conjunctivokeratitis of sheep. *J. Path. Bact.* **78:** 257–266.
84. Storz, J., Pierson, R.E., Marriott, M.E. and Chow, T.L. 1967. Isolation of psttacosis agents from follicular conjunctivitis of sheep. *Proc. Soc. exp. Biol. Med.* **125:** 857–860.
85. Wilsmore, A.J., Dagnall, G.J. and Woodland, R.M. 1990. Experimental conjunctival infection of lambs with a strain of *Chlamydia psittaci* isolated from the eyes of a sheep naturally affected with keratoconjunctivitis. *Vet. Rec.* **127:** 229–231.
86. Rowe, L.W.R., Hedger, R.S. and Smale, C. 1978. The isolation of a *Chlamydia psittaci*-like agent from a free-living African buffalo. *(Syncerus caffer)*. *Vet. Rec.* **103:** 13–14.
87. Stephenson, E.H., Storz, J. and Hopkins, J.B. 1974. Properties and frequency of isolation of chlamydiae from eyes of lambs with conjunctivitis and polyarthritis. *Am. J. vet. Res.* **35:** 177–180.
88. Hargis, A.M., Prieur, D.J. and Gaillard, E.T. 1983. Chlamydial infection of the gastric mucosa in twelve cats. *Vet. Path.* **20:** 170–178.
89. Gaillard, E.T., Hargis, A.M., Prieur, D.J., Evermann, J.F. and Dhillon, A.S. 1984. Pathogenesis of feline gastric chlamydial infection. *Am. J. vet. Res.* **45:** 2314–2323.
90. Hopkins, J.B., Stephenson, E.H., Storz, J. and Pierson, R.E. 1973. Clinical characteristics of eye lesions of lambs affected with chlamydial conjunctivitis and polyarthritis. *J. Am. vet. Med. Ass.* **163:** 510–513.

91. EUSTER, A.K., JONES, L.P. and GAYLE, L.G. 1977. Epizootics of chlamydial abortions and keratoconjunctivitis in goats. *Proc. Am. Ass. vet. Lab. Diag.* **20:** 59–78.
92. MORRISON, R.P., LYNG, K. and CALDWELL, H.D. 1989. Chlamydial disease pathogenesis. Ocular hypersensitivity elucidate by a genus-specific 57-kD protein. *J. exp. Med.* **169:** 663–675.
93. MORRISON, R.P., BELLAND, R.J., LYNG, K. and CALDWELL, H.D. 1989. Chlamydia disease pathogenesis. The 57-kD chlamydial hypersensitivity antigen is a stress response protein. *J. exp. Med.* **170:** 1271–1283.
94. DOUGHRI, A.M. and STORZ, J. 1978. Ocular histopathologic lesions in chlamydial infection of newborn calves. *Arab. develop. J. Sci. Technol.* **1:** 5–9.
95. WILLS, J.M., MILLARD, W.G. and HOWARD, P.E. 1986. Evaluation of a monoclonal antibody based ELISA for detection of feline *Chlamydia psittaci. Vet. Res.* **119:** 418–420.
96. MCKERCHER, D.G. 1952. Feline pneumonitis. I. Immunization studies in kittens. *Am. J. vet. Res.* **13:** 557–561.
97. BURCH, G.R., YORK, C.J., JOHNSTON, R.V. and MAYER, K. 1958. Feline pneumonitis vaccine. *Allied Vet.* **29:** 4–7.
98. MITZEL, J.R. and STRATING, A. 1977. Vaccination against feline pneumonitis. *Am. J. vet. Res.* **38:** 1361–1363.
99. SHEWEN, P.E., POVEY, R.C. and WILSON, M.R. 1980. A comparison of the efficacy of a live and 4 inactivated vaccine preparations for the protection of cats against experimental challenge with *Chlamydia psittaci. Can. J. comp. Med.* **44:** 244–258.
100. WILLS, J.M., GRUFFYDD-JONES, T.J., RICHMOND, S.D., GASKALL, R.M. and BOURNE, F.J. 1987. Effect of vaccination on infection due to feline *Chlamydia psittaci. Infect. Immun.*
101. KOLAR, J.R. and RUDE, T.A. 1977. Clinical evaluation of a commercial feline pneumonitis vaccine. *Feline Pract.* **7:** 47–50.
102. FUKUSHI, H. and HIRAI, K. 1992. Proposal of *Chlamydia pecorum* sp. nov. for *Chlamydia* strains derived from ruminants. *Int. J. Syst. Bact.* **42:** 306–308.

21

Public Health Significance of Animal Rickettsiae and Chlamydiae

Z. WOLDEHIWET AND G. R. SCOTT

Introduction

Most rickettsial and chlamydial infections of man have long been regarded as zoonoses. Human beings are considered to be incidental hosts which often get infected by accidently intruding into the cycle of infection between the arthropod vectors and their natural animal hosts.[1]

The etiological agents, their modes of transmission and the diseases they cause in animals have been covered in the relevant chapters. In this section, we will highlight the role of domestic and free-living animals as sources of rickettsial and chlamydial infections of humans. The most common rickettsial and chlamydial infections that could be acquired from animals and birds are shown in Table 21.1.

Q Fever

Although man is regarded as the only animal known to develop overt clinical signs following infections with *Coxiella burnetii*,[2] the disease is a zoonosis closely associated with animals and animal products.[3]

Sources of Infections

The first report of the disease was in abattoir workers.[3] It is now widely accepted that infected sheep, cattle and goats are the main sources of Q fever.[4] The organism has been isolated from other domestic animals such as cats, pigs, horses and dogs[5–9] but the frequency of transmission of the organism to humans from these

TABLE 21.1. *Rickettsial and Chlamydial Zoonoses and their Sources*

Rickettsia	Disease	Vector	Animal reservoir
C. burnetii	Q fever	ticks?	ruminants, cats
E. canis	ehrlichiosis	ticks	dogs
E. chaffeensis	ehrlichiosis	unknown	unknown
E. sennetsu	sennetsu disease	ticks?	
Chlamydia psittaci	psittacosis/ chlamydiosis		psittacine and other birds, other animals
R. akari	rickettsialpox	mites	house mice
R. australis	tick typhus	ticks	marsupials, rodents
R. conorii	boutonneuse or tick-bite fever	ticks	rodents, dogs, cattle
R. prowazekii	epidemic and sylvatic typhus	lice, fleas	flying squirrels
R. rickettsii	Rocky Mountain spotted fever	ticks	dogs, wild mice
R. sibirica	N. Asian tick typhus	ticks	rodents, birds?
R. tsutsugamushi	scrub typhus	(chiggers)	other mammals?
R. typhi (R. mooseri)	Murine typhus	fleas	rodents

animals is not well established. It may well be that camels and buffaloes are as important as the other domestic ruminants as sources of infection to man in countries where they are economically important.[2] Companion animals may also be an important reservoir of infection in some regions of the world. For example, in certain regions of Canada the cat is regarded as the main source of human infection.[5] Serological surveys in Germany[10] revealed that up to 26% of cats and 13% of dogs were seropositive, highlighting the importance of companion animals as a possible source of infection.

The organism has also been isolated from free-living animals, birds and a variety of fish[6] but the significance of these sources as reservoirs of infection has not been clearly established. Ticks are important for the maintenance of the organism in nature but not as vectors of human infection. However, the organism is shed in tick feces which may remain infectious for up to 586 days.[11] Marrie[12] hypothesized that there may be a cycle of infection involving ticks, rodents (moles), cats and people.

Large quantities of the organism are shed in body secretions of infected animals, particularly during the period of parturition. Because the organism is very resistant to physical and chemical agents, contaminated premises and the air continue to be dangerous sources of infections for periods which may exceed five months.[13] The main people at risk are those who come in contact with animals as part of their professional duty, including shepherds, animal attendants, veterinarians, farmers and wool shearers. Several outbreaks have been reported from research institutions using pregnant ewes.[14–16] The disease may also affect persons who are not in direct contact with animals or animal products but who may be exposed to wind-borne aerosols carrying the resistant rickettsiae during transport of infected animals, contaminated manure, hay or other products. For example, an explosive outbreak of Q fever affecting more than 400 residents of a valley in Switzerland was attributed to an indirect exposure to contaminated aerosols generated by infected sheep which regularly travelled through the valley.[17]

In the past human beings risked infection by drinking raw milk but rarely developed clinical signs.[18] Today ingestion of milk and other animal products is regarded as an uncommon source of human infection.[19]

Clinical Disease

The clinical signs are often described as "flu-like" but the illness may vary from self-limiting nonspecific fever to atypical pneumonia, endocarditis, hepatitis and neurological manifestations.[4] Often the disease appears as an acute febrile condition, usually described as "pyrexia of unknown origin".[4] Acute Q fever pneumonia is commonly accompanied by a very severe headache.[5] Q fever should be suspected when flu-like syndromes, atypical pneumonias or fevers of unknown origin occur, particularly in individuals working with parturient ruminants in farms and research centers or in persons living near such premises.[20] In individuals suffering from chronic cases of Q fever, the main symptom is an endocarditis for which an etiological agent cannot be readily identified but fever, malaise, weight loss, general fatigue and night sweats may also be present.[4] Splenomegaly and hepatomegaly are other common features of chronic Q fever.

Control and Treatment

Measures of prevention of Q fever include pasteurization or sterilization of milk, reduction of the build up of infectious coxiellae in areas where sheep and goats breed, to protect people handling these animals or those living near the area. In institutions where sheep are used for research purposes, regular testing and culling of seropositive animals should be considered. Vaccination of sheep, goats and cattle could also be used to reduce spread. In acutely infected individuals, treatment with chloramphenicol and chlortetracycline is effective.[21] Erythromycin is reported to be effective against acute *C. burnetii* pneumonia[22] and, in one trial, rifampin was reported to be effective against acute Q fever.[4] In individuals with chronic Q fever, a continuous treatment with more than one antibiotic is advocated. For example, it was reported that there were no relapses in eight patients with chronic Q fever after treatment for two years with tetracycline and cotrimoxazole.[4]

The Role of Animals on Human Rickettsiosis

Rickettsial diseases have been credited with influencing the history of man by decisively affecting the outcomes of many wars over the centuries.[23] Although the advent of antibiotics and better hygiene have significantly reduced epidemic outbreaks of typhus or spotted-type fevers, rickettsial infections still remain important in many parts of the world.

It was established early that the typhus and spotted-type fevers of man were transmitted by lice, fleas, ticks or mites and although initially some of them were thought to affect man alone, there was no doubt that animals play an important role in their epidemiology. Several of the agents naturally affect small mammals (rodents) and man while others may affect domestic animals. With very few exceptions, they do not cause clinical disease in domestic animals but free-living and domestic animals may serve as reservoirs of infection. *Rickettsia rickettsii*, the causative agent of Rocky Mountain spotted fever (RMSF) in man is now recognized as a cause of overt clinical disease in dogs[24] and it is also known that dogs infected with *R. conorii* may suffer severe clinical disease.[25] RMSF in the dog and the public health significance of infected dogs is discussed in Chapter 7.

Of the other spotted type fevers which affect man, several of them may have animals and/or birds as possible reservoirs of infection for the arthropod vectors which transmit disease (Table 21.1).

R. akari

This organism was first recognized as a cause of rickettsialpox in the United States in 1946.[26,27] During the same period the organism was isolated from household mice and hematophagous mites. It was later isolated from mites in the Soviet Union, Southern Africa and Korea.[27,28] In the U.S.A., the main animal reservoirs of infection are household mice while elsewhere other animals such as the bushveld in South Africa and the wild field vole in Korea are regarded as potential reservoirs.

R. australis

Queensland tick typhus appears to be a disease exclusively found in Australia.

The causative agent, *R. australis* was isolated from the blood of infected patients in Queensland, Australia in 1946.[29–31] The disease occurred in people who had a history of exposure to ticks but the exact nature of the vectors is not known.[31] Serological evidence indicates that rodents and several other free-living mammals such as opossums and bandicoots are possible reservoirs of infection.[31,32]

Control measure include the reduction of vectors and use of repellents in endemic areas. Persons entering tick-infested areas are advised to wear proper clothing, to reduce the possibility of tick bites.[31]

R. conorii

R. conorii causes "boutonneuse" fever in the Mediterranean and/or tick-bite fever in southern Africa. The same organism causes Indian tick typhus and East African tick typhus. The disease is characterized by a button-like rash with typical black spots or eschar and a very painful lymphadenitis. Transmission of the disease to man is through the bite of a tick infected with *R. conorii* or by accidental contamination of the conjunctiva with infected tick tissues or feces. In Africa south of the Sahara it is transmitted by several species of ixodid ticks. All stages of the ticks are involved and transovarian transmission occurs.[33] The significant natural reservoirs of infection in the bushveld of southern Africa are the arvicanthis rats (*Otomys irroratus*) and striped mouse (*Rhabdomys pumilio*),[28] the vectors being *Amblyomma hebraeum, Hyalomma aegyptium, Rhipicephalus appendiculatus, Rhipicephalus evertsi,* and perhaps, *Boophilus decoloratus.*[34] Heisch and his colleagues[35] in Kenya extended the list of vectors for East African tick typhus to include three further cattle ticks, *Amblyomma variegatum, Hyalomma albiparmatum* and *Rhipicephalus simus*. Philip and his team[36] working in Ethiopia also incriminated *A. variegatum* and *R. simus*. A few years later, Burgdorfer and his coworkers[37] isolated *R. conorii* from 17 *A. variegatum,* 14 *A. cohaerems* and 26 *A. gemma*. The natural reservoirs in the African urban niche are urban rats and dogs, the vector being the dog tick *Haemophysalis leachii.*[28] The other main vectors are ixodid ticks of the genera *Rhipicephalus, Amblyomma* and *Haemophysalis.*[38] In contrast, the vector of Mediterranean "boutonneuse" fever is *Rhipicephalus sanguineus.*[39] Indian tick typhus is transmitted by *Haemophysalis* spp. and other ixodid ticks.[25,38] Apart from dogs and cattle, other small free-living mammals such as rats, mice and shrews are believed to play an important role in the cycle of infection of vector ticks.[25,35]

Despite the apparent high prevalence of *R. conorii* in cattle ticks, the organism has not been isolated from cattle and a single experimental attempt to infect an ox failed.[40] French workers in equatorial Africa using Giroud's microagglutination technique[41] tested more than 1500 cattle sera and claimed to have detected specific antibodies in 36–47%.[42–44] Other smaller surveys of cattle in Ethiopia and Kenya failed to find antibodies although they were present in the sera of five out of six Ethiopian sheep[36] and three out of 30 Kenyan sheep.[35] The number of positive goat sera was small, being three out of ten and one out of eight in Ethiopia and Kenya respectively. A postulated role for small ruminants in the epidemiology of bushveld tick-borne fever is supported by experiments in which sheep infected with *R. conorii* developed fevers and Weil–Felix agglutinations.[45] The response was partially confirmed by Mason and Alexander[40] who succeeded in inducing fevers in some sheep injected with the Hare isolate of *R. conorii*. When challenged later with the Appleton isolate, the reacting sheep proved to be immune. Most people with tick-bite fever, Indian tick typhus or East African tick typhus acquire infection after travelling to tick-infested areas. Others may acquire the disease after deticking their dogs or other animals.[25] The disease is characterized by systemic signs such as fever and very painful headaches and lesions at the primary site of infection, the skin or conjunctiva. The lesions may begin as raised red papules on the skin, with a black centre, or as swellings of the eyelids, leading to the complete or partial closure of the eye.[25]

Control measures include reduction of tick vectors in general and use of repellents and proper clothings in endemic areas. Careful deticking procedures may reduce the number of affected people. In endemic areas, the methods of tick removal advocated by Needham[46] should be followed to reduce the possibility of tick hemolymph or other infected tick tissues spurting into the eyes. After removing ticks from affected dogs or other animals, hands should be washed thoroughly to avoid the inadvertent introduction of infected tick material into the conjunctivita. Severe disease could be prevented by starting treatment with tetracyclines as soon as the infective tick bite or signs of lymphadenitis are recognized.[25] The option of using vaccines as a measure of control has been boosted by the recent demonstration that a recombinant *R. conorii* vaccine protects guinea pigs from experimental "boutonneuse" fever.[47]

R. prowazekii

R. prowazekii causes epidemic typhus or louse-borne typhus. Over the years, this disease has been associated with heavy losses in human life in conditions of overcrowding, particularly during times of war. Unlike the other rickettsioses where man is regarded as an accidental host, *R. prowazekii* has man as its natural host and the host-specific body louse, *Pediculus humanus humanus*, as its natural vector.

An hypothesis that has not so far found favor was put forward by Dr Ruth J. Reiss-Gutfreund after she had detected antibodies in the sera of healthy Ethiopian cattle, goats, and sheep and had isolated *R. prowazekii* by injecting guinea-pigs with blood clot suspensions from domestic animals and suspensions of pools of ticks collected from domestic animals.[48] Therefore, she postulated that the transmission cycle of *R. prowazekii* in the annual epidemics of typhus in Ethiopia was man–louse–man and in the interepidemic periods was domestic animal–tick–domestic–animal.[49] Giroud and his colleagues[50] working in equatorial Africa had previously detected antibodies to *R. prowazekii* in the sera of cattle, dogs, donkeys and goats and suggested that domestic animals might be natural reservoirs of *R. prowazekii*. Reiss-Gutfreund[51] reported further isolations from a goat and from pools of *Amblyomma variegatum* ticks collected from zebu and a camel. International interest was aroused and an eminent team of investigators in collaboration with Reiss-Gutfreund collected 3,723 Ethiopian ticks belonging to five genera which they checked for rickettsias. Simultaneously sera from 45 domestic livestock were examined for antibodies. There was no evidence of the presence of *R. prowazekii* in the inoculated guinea pigs nor were there antibodies in the animal sera. *R. conorii* however, was isolated from a pool of *Rhipicephalus simus* ticks collected from cattle.[36] During the same period, serological surveys in Egypt revealed the presence of typhus antibodies in many sera from camels and donkeys and in a few sera from domestic buffaloes, goats, pigs and sheep.[52]

The case for incriminating domestic animals and their ticks was considered "unproven" and two further attempts were made to resolve the controversy. One found that the concentration of *R. prowazekii* in the blood of infected guinea pigs was too low to infect ticks[53] and the second merely confirmed that *R. conorii*, or a closely related agent, occurred in cattle ticks.[37]

Since then a natural reservoir of *R. prowazekii*, other than man and his lice, has been discovered in the eastern United States of America in southern flying squirrels (*Glaucomys volans L*).[54] These findings have introduced a new dimension to the epidemiology of *R. prowazekii* and it is now recognized that, in the United States, there may be two epidemiologically distinct diseases caused by the same organism, epidemic typhus and sylvatic typhus. Because the likely vectors of *R. prowazekii* associated with flying squirrels are not normal parasites of man, sylvatic typhus is likely to occur not as an epidemic but as a sporadic infection, occurring during periods of contact between flying squirrels and human habitations. Arthropods experimentally infected with *R. prowazekii* can transmit infection to flying squirrels.[55] Flying squirrels are believed to acquire *R. prowazekii* from the squirrel lice, *Neohaematopinus sciuropteri* and the squirrel flea, *Orthopeas howardii*[33] but the mechanism of transmission of *R. prowazekii* from flying squirrels to humans has not been elucidated.

R. sibirica

North Asian tick typhus was first recognized in the North Asian regions of the Soviet Union but is now known to occur in Japan and the Pacific Far East.[56] The organism has also been isolated in Czechoslovakia.[57] Various species of ixodid ticks naturally transmit the organism to a variety of rodents such as house mice, field mice, rats, voles and other vertebrates. Man is infected by accidental contact with infected ticks either through a tick bite or contamination of skin abrasions with infected tick tissues. Therefore, farmers, loggers, and other people who come in contact with tick-infected areas during their professional activities are likely to be affected. Urban dwellers may get infected during picnics and other occasional trips to tick-infested areas. Control measures are similar to those advocated for the other tick-borne rickettsioses.

R. tsutsugamushi

Scrub typhus is a disease of the Far East transmitted by the bite of red larval mites (tsutsugamushi) of the genus *Leptotrombidium*. Outbreaks of the disease occur within small localities because the mites have a tendency to aggregate in small clusters on dead dried grass stems or on stem, tips and edges of leaves in secondary forests and they do not actively seek their hosts.[58] Natural infections occur in rats, voles and birds. Birds could be heavily infected and it is possible that they may serve as vehicles of spread to vector mites from endemic areas.[58] The disease has been reported from Malaysia, India, Burma, Indonesia, Japan, Thailand, Afghanistan, Iran and

Australia.[58,59] Scrub typhus occurs in areas where the so called "zoonotic tetrad", which make up the four important ecological components are present.[59] According to Burgdorfer,[59] the zoonotic tetrad include *R. tsutsugamushi*, chiggers of the genus *Leptotrombidium*, rats of the genus *Rattus* and secondary or transitional forms of vegetation, which abound after cleared forests and formerly cultivated lands are allowed to turn into shrubs.

Rats, particularly of the genus *Rattus*, are the main hosts for the mites (chiggers) and in one study over 75% of all *R. tsutsugamushi* were isolated from rats and the rest from related voles.[60] However, chiggers can feed on a wide range of hosts and *R. tsutsugamushi* has been isolated from birds and a wide range of animals.[58,59]

Control measure include the reduction of vectors and reservoirs by the use of insecticides and antirodent measures.[58] Repellents and intentional infection followed by treatment with chloramphenicol have been used to protect individuals coming into endemic areas.[58]

R. typhus

Murine or endemic typhus is natural infection of urban rats.[61] The most important vector for human beings is the rat flea *Xenopsylla cheopis*, but it is transmitted between rats by the rat louse and by the tropical rat mite. People get accidently infected by contamination of skin abrasions with the feces of infected rat fleas when commensal rats abound in human dwellings and working premises such as ports.[62]

Because of the sporadic nature of the disease compared to epidemic typhus, it was suspected early in the history of the disease that natural reservoirs other than man were involved in the epidemiology of murine typhus.[63,64] The role of rats in the epidemiology of murine typhus was demonstrated when the causative agent was isolated from the flea, *Xenopsylla cheopis*, collected from rats and their nesting material and from the brains of *Rattus rattus*.[64,65] The disease occurs in many countries but is more common in warm climates and in ports and coastal areas where commensal rats are present. The role of other mammals as sources of human infection is not well established but it is possible for house mice, shrews, opposums, skunks and cats to acquire infection if they enter rat-infected premises.[66]

Antibody surveys of several hundred cattle in Chad,[42] Central African Republic[43] and Cameroon[44] using Giroud's microagglutination technique[41] gave point prevalence rates of *R. typhi* antibodies of 56, 50 and 44% respectively. In contrast, no antibodies were detected in small numbers of cattle sampled in Kenya[35] and Ethiopia.[36] Traub and his colleagues[61] attributed the discrepancies in the results to variations in the specificity and sensitivity of the different tests used, in particular, they considered the Giroud-type microagglutination test to be prone to give false positive reaction. Antibodies were also detected in the sera of 17 out of 200 Egyptian goats[52] and in 19 out of 135 Chadian goats.[42] Only one of 33 sheep sera, however, contained antibodies.[43] In Egypt, Imam and Alfy[52] included 200 camels and 50 donkeys in their survey and detected *R. typhi* antibodies in 23 and 13 respectively. The vectors acquire infection after feeding on infected hosts. *R. typhi* multiplies in the gut epithelium and is excreted with the feces after the rupture of infected cells. Infection of lice is fatal but fleas are not clinically affected, but they carry the rickettsiae for life.[66]

Control measures are directed at both the reservoir rats and the vector fleas. These include better environmental sanitation, control of rat populations and the use of insecticides to eradicate or reduce rat fleas in human habitations.

Human Ehrlichiosis

The recent recognition that *Ehrlichia canis* or a related organism may cause a disease in man has created a renewed interest in the ehrlichiae which have been known as important animal pathogens for over 50 years.

Until the recent demonstration of human ehrlichiosis in the U.S.A., the only recognized human disease due to an ehrlichial agent was sennetsu disease in Japan and Malaysia caused by *E. sennetsu*. The organism was first described as a human pathogen in Japan. It was isolated from the blood of patients suffering from fever, lymphoadenopathy and an increase in the number of circulating mononuclear cells.[67,68]

It is generally thought that the disease is transmitted by ticks but it is not known whether animal reservoirs serve as sources of infection to man.[69] However, the high incidence of sennetsu ehrlichiosis after consumption of some types of raw fish, has led some workers to suggest that fish may play some role in the epidemiology of the disease.[70] The organism is morphologically similar to other members of the genus *Ehrlichia* and its growth cycle in monocytes is similar to that of *E. canis*,[71] but *E. sennetsu* can infect mice and readily grows in other cell culture systems.[71,72] Recent phylogenetic studies indicate that *E. sennetsu* is more closely related to *E. risticii* than to the other members of the genus *Ehrlichia*.[73] Experimental infections of dogs with canine-monocyte adapted *E. sennetsu* showed that the organism may persist without apparent clinical signs, highlighting the possible existence of inapparent carriers.[71] More detailed information about the biology of the organism and the epidemiology of the disease is given in Chapter 9.

A case of human ehrlichiosis due to *Ehrlichia canis* was first reported in the U.S.A. in 1986 when a clinical case in which an organism similar to *Ehrlichia canis* was demonstrated and there was evidence of seroconversion to *Ehrlichia canis*.[74] No attempt was made to reproduce the disease by experimental infection of dogs. The morphology of the intracellular organism seen in cases subsequently reported was similar to that of *E. canis*. Limited serological,[75] clinical and laboratory[76] data also suggest that human infection with this or other ehrlichial agents may occur in parts of Africa where animal ehrlichiosis are enzootic.

Recently an agent causing human ehrlichiosis in the United States was isolated from a patient.[77] Because this agent is genetically different, but distantly related to *E. canis*, Anderson and his coworkers have proposed that it be recognized as a new species, *Ehrlichia chaffeensis*.[73]

It is not yet clear whether the reported cases of human ehrlichiosis attributed to *E. canis* were in fact caused by *E. chaffeensis*.

For a review of human ehrlichiosis in the U.S.A. see Chapter 9.

Psittacosis

Human psittacosis was recognized at the end of the last century but the association of the disease with psittacine birds was first established after the serious pandemic in 1929–1930 which affected many countries in Europe and America which imported exotic birds from South America.[78]

Sources of Human Infections

Although it was initially thought that psittacine species were the only source of human infections, it was later established that domestic chickens, ducks, turkeys and other domestic or free-living birds could be important reservoirs of infection. All avian species should, therefore, be regarded as possible sources of human psittacosis. The role of psittacine and other birds as sources of human psittacosis has been highlighted in Chapter 18.

The risk of acquiring infection is higher in persons likely to be in contact with infected birds as a result of their professional or recreational activities. These include persons working with cage birds, employees working in poultry processing plants, veterinarians attending cage birds and laboratory workers handling infected specimens. Because infected birds excrete *C. psittaci* in large numbers in their feces and the organism is very resistant to environmental factors, contaminated cages, breeding coops, and barns are important sources of infection. For purposes of surveillance of the disease, all avian species should be considered as possible sources of infection. Several avian species are believed to harbor the organism without showing clinical signs but when they are stressed, as a result of transport or due to dietary and environmental changes, they may shed chlamydia in large numbers. When chlamydial infections occur in conditions of overcrowding in breeding and other premises, explosive outbreaks of psittacosis can occur. It is very rare for patients suffering from severe and virulent forms of psittacosis to transmit infection to persons living with them or those looking after them but necessary precautions must be taken.

Disease and Treatment in Man

The disease may appear as a flu-like syndrome, or as severe atypical pneumonia. In some individuals, there may also be diarrhea and vomiting. Some individuals may develop latent infections which may last for prolonged periods.[79]

Tetracyclines are the antibiotics of choice in treating affected humans but the organism is also susceptible to erythromycin.

Prevention and Control

Several countries have import and export controls and quarantine regulations on psittacine birds. For example, although the disease is not notifiable, there are regulations in the United Kingdom which require for imported birds to be kept in quarantine for at least 35 days and for the detention and isolation of birds suspected of being infected. In the United States, several states have regulations which make it mandatory to report all cases of chlamydiosis[80] and the Surgeon General of the United States may declare an area "infected" with chlamydiosis if persons or psittacine birds are considered to have been infected with *C. psittaci*.[81]

Preventive measures against psittacosis include continuous surveillance of the disease in psittacine and other birds by regular serological surveys of psittacines, pigeons, turkeys and other likely reservoirs and adding specified amounts of antibiotics. The type and amount of antibiotics added into poultry feeds is usually governed by statutory regulations.

Postmortem examinations of birds suspected of psittacosis should be handled in safety cabinets.

Because of the danger to human health, it would be advisable not to attempt treating affected birds but rather to humanely euthanize them. However, appropriate quantities of antibiotics such as tetracyclines, erythromycin or tylosin could be added to the drinking water as a preventive measure. The use of antibiotics in the feeds of birds is an effective way of reducing the load of bacteria in the environment.

Other Chlamydial Infections

There have been some isolated incidents of chlamydial abortions, pneumonias and conjunctivitis in persons whose association with animals indicated that they acquired the infection from animal sources. Psittacosis of nonavian origin has also been described.[82]

Earlier epidemiological and serological data which suggested that strains of *C. psittaci* which cause enzootic abortion in ewes may cause human abortions[83,84] have recently been confirmed by the demonstration of bacterial antigens in human placenta,[85] by bacterial isolation[86] and by genomic typing.[87] The most common sources of human chlamydial abortions are infected ewes. The likely victims are pregnant women who come in direct contact with infected ewes during the lambing season.[86] Infected pregnant women often show flu-like symptoms, characterized by initial fever, headache, nausea and malaise, before the onset of spontaneous contractions three to eight days after the start of these symptoms.[85] Because of the special risk to pregnant women, it is advisable that they should not work with sheep during the lambing season.[85]

Very few cases of conjunctivitis and respiratory disease have been attributed to nonavian sources of *C. psittaci*. Personnel handling *C. psittaci* isolated from cases of enzootic abortion were reported to have developed respiratory disease similar to psittacosis or ornithosis.[88] Although people, other than pregnant women, handling infected ewes seldom develop respiratory or "flu-like" illness that could be attributed to aborting ewes, some public health reports indicate that other groups of persons, such as veterinarians, are more likely to develop chlamydial pneumonia.[89] It has been suggested that cattle with chlamydial pneumonia or enteritis are potentially an important source of human chlamydial pneumonia or bronchopneumonia.[78,90]

Feline pneumonitis agent is reported to cause conjunctivitis in human beings, and it has been suggested that there must be a high rate of exposure in individuals who have pets.[78] Several reports have implicated cats as sources of chlamydial conjunctivitis, bronchopneumonia or other conditions in man. An acute follicular conjunctivitis from which chlamydial agents were isolated was attributed to feline sources.[91,92] Other reports also implicated cats as sources of primary chlamydial infections resulting in severe endocarditis and glomerulonephritis.[93]

References

1. Burgdorfer, W. 1975. Introduction to the rickettsiosis. In: *Diseases Transmitted from Animals to Man,* 6th edn, pp. 382–386. Hubbert, W.T., McCulloch, W.F. and Schnurrenberger, P.R. (Eds), Charles C. Thomas, Springfield, Illinois.
2. Aitken, I.D. Clinical aspects and prevention of Q fever in animals. *Eur. J. Epidemiol.* **5:** 420–424.
3. Derrick, E.H. 1937. "Q" fever, new fever entity: clinical features, diagnosis and laboratory investigation. *Med. J. Aust.* **2:** 281–299.
4. Marrie, T.J. 1990. Q fever—A review. *Can. vet. J.* **31:** 555–563.
5. Marrie, T.J., Durant, H., Williams, J.C. and Yates. 1988. Exposure to parturient cats is a risk factor for acquisition of Q fever in maritime Canada. *J. infect. Dis.* **158:** 101–108.
6. Babudieri, B. 1959. Q fever: A zoonosis. *Adv. vet. Sci. comp. Med.* **5:** 81–181.
7. Stoker, M.G.P. and Thompson, J.F. 1953. An explosive outbreak of Q fever. *Lancet* **i:** 137–139.
8. George, J. and Marrie, T.J. 1987. Serological evidence of *Coxiella burnetii* infection in horses in Atlantic Canada. *Can. vet. J.* **28:** 425–426.
9. Willeberg, P., Ruppanner, R., Behymer, D.E., Haghighi, Kaneko, J.J. and Franti, C.E. 1980. Environmental exposure to *Coxiella burnetii*: A seroepidemiologic survey among domestic animals. *Am. J. Epidemiol.* **111:** 437–443.
10. Wereth, D., Schmeer, N., Muller, H.P., Karo, M. and Kraus, H. 1987. Nachweis von Antikorpen gegen Chlamydia psittaci und *Coxiella burnetii* bei Hunden und Ktzen: Vergleich zwischen Enzymimmuntest, Immunperoxidase-Tecknik, Komplement-bindungsreaction und Agargelprazipitationstest. *J. vet. Med. B* **34:** 165–176.
11. Ormsbee, R.A. 1972. In: *Viral and Rickettsial Infections of Man,* 4th edn, pp. 1144–1160. Horsfall, F.L.J.C. and Tamm, I. (Eds), J. B. Lippincott, Philadelphia.
12. Marrie, T.J. 1988. Q fever, clinical signs, symptoms and pathophysiology. In: *Biology of Rickettsial Diseases,* Vol. II, pp. 1–16. Walker D.H. (Ed.), CRC Press, Boca Raton, Florida.
13. Welsh, W.H., Lennette, E.H., Abinanti, F.R. and Winn, J.F. 1958. Airborne transmission of Q fever: The role of parturition in the generation of infective aerosols. *Ann. N.Y. Acad. Sci.* **70:** 528–540.
14. Curet, L.B. and Paust, J.C. 1972. Transmission of Q fever from experimental sheep to laboratory personnel. *Am. J. Obstet. Gynec.* **14:** 566–568.
15. Meiklejohn, G., Reimer, L.G., Graves, P.S. and Helmick, C. 1981. Cryptic epidemic of Q fever in a medical school. *J. infect. Dis.* **144:** 107–114.
16. Hall, C.J., Richmond, S.J., Caul, E.O., Pearce, N.H. and Silver, I.A. 1982. Laboratory outbreak of Q fever acquired from sheep. *Lancet* **i:** 1004–1006.
17. Dupuis, G., Petite, J., Peter, O. and Vouilloz, M. 1987. An important outbreak of human Q fever in Swiss Alpine Valley. *Int. J. Epidemiol.* **16:** 282–287.
18. Huebener, R.J., Jellison, W.L., Beck, M.D., Porter, R.R. and Shepard, C.C. 1948. Q fever studies in southern California. Recovery of Rickettsia burnetii from raw milk. *US publ. Hlth Rep.* **63:** 214–222.

19. BENSON, W.W., BROCK, D.W. and MATHER, J. 1963. Serological analysis of penitentiary group using raw milk from an infected herd. *Publ. Hlth Rep.* **78:** 707–710.
20. BEHYMER, D. and RIEMANN, H.P. 1989. Zoonosis update: *Coxiella burnetii* infection (Q fever). *J. Am. vet. Med. Ass.* **194:** 764–766.
21. TURK, W.P.G. Q fever. In: *Medical Microbiology and Infectious Diseases,* pp. 932–937. BRAUDE, A.I., DAVIS, C.E. and FIERES, J. (Eds), W. B. Saunders, Philadelphia.
22. YEAMAN, M.R. and BACO, O.G. 190. Antibiotic susceptibility of *Coxiella burnetii.* In: *Q Fever : The Disease,* pp. 213–223. MARRIE, T.J. (Ed.), CRC Press, Boca Raton, Florida.
23. WEISS, K. 1988. The role of rickettsioses in history. In: *Biology of Rickettsial Diseases,* Vol. I, pp. 1–14. WALKER, D.H. (Ed.), CRC Press, Boca Raton, Florida.
24. GREENE, C.E., BURGDORFER, W., CAVAGNOLO, R., PHILIP, R. and PEACOCK, M.G. 1985. Rocky Mountain spotted fever in dogs and its natural differentiation from canine ehrlichiosis. *J. Am. vet. Med. Ass.* **186:** 465–472.
25. GEAR, J.H.S. 1988. Other spotted fever group ricketsioses: Clinical signs, symptoms, and pathophysiology. In: *The Biology of Rickettsial Diseases,* Vol. I, pp. 101–113. WALKER, D.H. (Ed.), CRC Press, Boca Raton, Florida.
26. HUEBNER, R.J., JELLISON, W.L. and POMENARANTZ, CH. 1946. Rickettsialpox—a newly recognized rickettsial disease. IV. Isolation of a rickettsia apparently identical with the causative agent of rickettsialpox from *Allodermanyssus sanguineus,* a rodent mite. *Publ. Hlth Rep.* **61:** 2677–2682.
27. BURGDORFER, W. 1975. Rickettsialpox. In: *Diseases Transmitted from Animals to Man,* Sixth edn, pp. 405–409. HUBBERT, W.T., MCCULLOCH, W.F. and SCHNURRENBERGER, P.R. (Eds), Charles C. Thomas, Springfield, Illinois.
28. GEAR, J. 1954. The rickettsial diseases of Southern Africa. *S. Afr. J. clin. Sci.* **5:** 158–175.
29. ANDREW, R., BONNIN, J.M. and WILLIAMS, S. 1946. Tick typhus in North Queensland. *Med. J. Aust.* **2:** 253–258.
30. BRODY, J. 1946. A case of tick typhus in North Queensland. *Med. J. Aust.* **1:** 511–512.
31. BURGDORFER, W. 1975. Queensland tick typhus. In: *Diseases Transmitted fromAnimals to Man,* Sixth edn, pp. 415–417. HUBBERT, W.T., MCCULLOCH, W.F. and SCHNURRENBERGER, P.R. (Eds), Charles C. Thomas, Springfield, Illinois.
32. FENNER, F. 1946. The epidemiology of North Queensland tick-typhus: Natural mammalian hosts. *Med. J. Aust.* **2:** 666–668.
33. HAIG, D.A. 1955. Tick-borne rickettsioses in South Africa. *Adv. vet. Sci.* **11:** 307–325.
34. GEAR, J.H.S. 1941. The typhus group of fevers. *Leech* **12:** 7–15.
35. HEISCH, R.B., GRAINGER, W.E., HARVEY, A.E.C. and LISTER, G. 1962. Feral aspects of rickettsial infections in Kenya. *Trans. R. Soc. trop. Med. Hyg.* **56:** 272–282.
36. PHILIP, C.B., HOOGSTRAAL, H., REISS-GUTFREUND, R. and CLIFFORD, C.M. 1966. Evidence of rickettsial disease agents in ticks from Ethiopian cattle. *Bull. Wld. Hlth Ord.* **35:** 127–131.
37. BURGDORFER, W., ORMSBEE, R.A., SCHMIDT, M.L. and HOOGSTRAAL, H. 1973. A search for epidemic typhus agent in Ethiopian ticks. *Bull. Wld. Hlth Org.* **48:** 563–568.

38. MARCHETTE, N.J. 1966. Rickettsiosis (tick-typhus, Q fever, urban typhus) in Malaysia. *J. Med. Ent.* **2:** 339–371.
39. BRUMPT, E. 1932. Longevite du virus de la fievre boutenneuse (*Rickettsia conorii* n.sp.) chez le tique *Rhipicephalus sanguineus. Compte Rendus des Seances de la Soc. Biol.* **110:** 1119–1202.
40. MASON, J.H. and ALEXANDER, R.A. 1939. Studies of the rickettsias of the Typhus-Rocky-Mountain-Spotted-Fever group in South Africa III. The disease in the experimental animal. Cross immunity test. *Onderstepoort J. Vet. Sci. Anim. Indust.* **13:** 41–65.
41. GIROUD, P. 1951. Les rickettsioses en Afrique equatoriale. *Bull. Wld Hlth. Org.* **4:** 535–546.
42. GIDEL. R. 1965. Contribution a l'etude des rickettsioses au Tchad. *Rev. Elev. Med. vet. des Pays Trop.* **28:** 127–136.
43. MAURICE, Y. 1967. Contribution a l'etude des rickettsioses en Republique Centrafricaine. Enquete epidemiologique. *Rev. Elev. Med. vet. Pay. Trop.* **20:** 407–413.
44. MAURICE, Y., FERNEGUT, R. and GEROME, R. 1968. Contribution a l'etude des rickettsioses du Nord Cameroun enquete epidemiologique. Republique Centrafricaine. Enquete epidemiologique. *Rev. Elev. Med. vet. Pay. Trop.* **21:** 341–349.
45. PIJPER, A. and CROCKER, C.G. 1938. Rickettsioses of South Africa. *S. Afr. Med. J.* **12:** 613–630.
46. NEEDHAM, G.R. 1985. Evaluation of five popular methods for tick removal. *Pediatrics* **75:** 997–1002.
47. VISHWANATH, S., MCDONALD, G.A. and WATKINS, N.A. 1990. A recombinant *Rickettsia conorii* vaccine protects guinea pigs from experimental boutonneuse fever and Rocky Mountain spotted fever. *Infect. Immun.* **58:** 646–653.
48. REISS-GUTFREUND, R.J. 1955. Isolement de souches de *Rickettsia prowazekii* a partir du sang des animaux domestiques d'Ethiope et de leur tiques. *Bull. Soc. Path. Exot.* **48:** 602–606.
49. REISS-GUTFREUND, R.J. 1956. Un nouveau reservoir de virus pour *Rickettsia prowazekii* les animaux domestiques et leur tiques. *Bull. Soc. Path. Exo.* **49:** 946–1021.
50. GIROUD, P., LE GAC, P., BRIZARD, H. and LAURENT, C. 1952. Compartement de serums des divers animaux domestiques, de l'Oubabgui-Chari vis-a-vis de l'antigene epidemique. *Bull. Soc. Path. Exot.* **45:** 313–316.
51. REISS-GUTFREUND, R.J. 1961. Nouveaux isolements de reservoir *Rickettsia prowazekii* a partir d'animaux domestiques et de tiques. *Bull. Soc. Path. Exot.* **54:** 284–297.
52. IMAM, I.Z.E. and ALFY, L. 1966. Evidence of typhus infection in domestic animals in Egypt. *Bull. Wld Hlth. Org.* **35:** 123–126.
53. BURGDORFER, W., ORMSBEE, R.A. and HOOGSTRAAL, H. 1972. Ticks as vectors of *Rickettsia prowazekii*—a controversial issue. *Am. J. trop. Med. Hyg.* **21:** 989–998.
54. BOZEMAN, F.M., MASIELLO, S.A., WILLIAMS, M.S. and ELISBERG, B.L. 1975. Epidemic typhus rickettsiae isolated from flying squirrels. *Nature, Lond.* **255:** 545–547.
55. BOZEMAN, F.M., SONENSHINE, D.E., WILLIAMS, CHADWICK, D.P., LAUER, D.M. and ELISBERG, B.L. 1981. Experimental infection of ectoparasitic arthropods with *Rickettsia prowazekii* (GVF-16 strain) and transmission to flying squirrels. *Am. J. trop. Med. Hyg.* **30:** 253–263.
56. BURGDORFER, W. 1975. North Asian tick typhus (North Asian tick-borne rickettsiosis). In: *Diseases Transmitted from Animals to Man,* 6th edn, pp.

418–422. HUBBERT, W.T., MCCULLOCH, W.F. and SCHNURRENBERGER, P.R. (Eds), Charles C. Thomas, Springfield, Illinois.

57. BREZINA, R., REHACEK, J. and MAJERSKA, P.A.C. 1969. Two strains of rickettsiae of Rocky Mountain spotted fever group recovered from *Dermacentor marginatus* ticks in Czechoslovakia: results of preliminary serological identification. *Acta Virol.* **13:** 42–145.
58. BURGDORFER, W.1975. Scrub typhus. In: *Diseases Transmitted from Animal to Man,* 6th edn, pp. 423–429. HUBBERT, W.T., MCCULLOCH, W.F. and SCHNURRENBERGER, P.R. (Eds), Charles C. Thomas, Springfield, Illinois.
59. BURGDORFER, W. 1988. Ecological and epidemiological considerations of Rocky Mountain spotted fever and scrub typhus. In: *Biology of Rickettsial Diseases,* Vol. I, pp. 33–50. WALKER, D.H. (Ed.), CRC Press, Boca Raton, Florida.
60. TRAUB, R. and WISSEMAN, C.L., JR 1974. The ecology of chigger-borne rickettsiosis (scrub typhus). *J. med. Ent.* **11:** 237–303.
61. TRAUB, R., WISSEMAN, C.L., JR and AZAD, A.F. 1978. The ecology of murine typhus—a critical review. *Trop. Dis. Bull.* **75:** 237–317.
62. BURGDORFER, W. 1975. Murine (Flea-borne) typhus fever. In: *Diseases Transmitted from Animal to Man,* 6th edn, pp. 405–409. HUBBERT, W.T., MCCULLOCH, W.F. and SCHNURRENBERGER, P.R. (Eds), Charles C. Thomas, Springfield, Illinois.
63. MOOSER, H. 1928. Experiments relating to the pathology and etiology of Mexican typhus (Tabardillo). I. Clinical course and pathologic anatomy of Tabardillo in guinea pigs. *J. infect. Dis.* **43:** 241–260.
64. DYER, R.E., RUMREICH, A. and BADGER, L.F. 1931. Typhus fever. A virus of the typhus type derived from fleas collected from wild rodents. *Publ. Hlth Rep.* **46:** 334–338.
65. MOOSER, H., CASTANEDA, M.R. and ZINSSER, H. 1931. Rats as carriers Mexican typhus fever. *J. Am. med. Ass.* **97:** 231–232.
66. AZAD, A.F. 1988. Relationship of vector biology and epidemiology of louse- and flea-borne rickettsioses. In: *Biology of Rickettsial Diseases,* Vol. I, pp, 51–61. WALKER, D.H. (Ed.), CRC Press, Boca Raton, Florida.
67. MISAO, T. and KOBAYASHI, Y. 1954. Studies on infectious mononucleosis (glandular fever). I. Isolation of aetiologic agent from blood, bone marrow, and lymph node of patients with infectious mononucleosis by using mice. *Tokyo Iji Shinshi* **71:** 683–686.
68. FUKUDA, T., KITAO, T. and KEIDA, Y. 1954. Studies on the causative agent of Hyugaetsu disease. I. Isolation of agent and experimental infection. *Med. Biol.* **32:** 200–204.
69. MCDADE, J.E. 1989. Ehrlichiosis—A disease of animals and humans. *J. infect. Dis.* **161:** 609–617.
70. RIKIHISA, Y. 1991. The tribe *Ehrlichieae* and Ehrlichial diseases. *Clin. Microbiol. Rev.* **4:** 286–308.
71. HOLLAND, C.L., RISTIC, M. HUXSOLL, D.L., COLE, A.I. and KOKOMA, I. 1985. Adaptation of *Ehrlichia sennetsu* to canine blood monocytes: preliminary structural and serological studies with cell culture-derived *Ehrlichia sennetsu. Infect. Immun.* **48:** 366–371.
72. HOILIEN, G.A., RISTIC, M., HUXSOLL, D.L. and RAPMUND, G. 1982. *Rickettsia sennetsu* in human blood monocyte cultures: similarities to the growth cycle of *Ehrlichia canis. Infect. Immun.* **35:** 314–319.
73. ANDERSON, B.E., DAWSON, J.E., JONES, D.C. and WILSON, K.H. 1991. *Ehrlichia chaffeensis* a new species associated with human ehrlichiosis. *J. clin. Microbiol.* **29:** 2838–2842.

74. Maeda, K., Markowitz, N., Hawley, R.C., Ristic, M., Cox, D. and McDade, J.E. 1987. Human infection with *Ehrlichia canis*, a leuctytic rickettsia. *New Eng. J. Med.* **316:** 853–856.
75. Parzy, D., Davost, B., Bissuel, G. and Vidor, E. 1991. Human pathogenicity of *Ehrlichia canis. Lancet.* **337:** 1169.
76. Uhaa, I.J., MacLean, J.D., Greene, C.R. and Fishbein, D.B. 1992. A case of human ehrlichiosis acquired in Mali: Clinical and laboratory findings. *Am. J. trop. Med Hyg.* **46:** 161–164.
77. Dawson, J.E., Anderson, B.E., Anderson, D.B., Fishbein, J.L., Sanchez, C.S., Goldsmith, K.H., Wilson and Duntley, C.W. 1991. Isolation and characterization of an *Ehrlichia* spp. from a patient with human ehrlichiosis. *J. clin. Microbiol.* **34:** 379–412.
78. Schachter, J. 1989. Chlamydial infections—past, present future. *J. Am. vet. Med. Ass.* **195:** 1501–1506.
79. Meyer, K.F. and Eddie, B. 1951. Human carrier of the psittacosis virus. *J. infect. Dis.* **88:** 109.
80. Williams, L.P. 1989. Review of the epidemiology of chlamydiosis in the United States. *J. Am. vet. Med. Ass.* **195:** 1518–1521.
81. Garbe, J.L. 1989. Legal aspects of chlamydiosis in birds. *J. Am. vet. Med. Ass.* **195:** 1574–1576.
82. Anonymous 1984. Psittacosis of non-avian origin. *Lancet* **ii:** 442–443.
83. Roberts, W., Grist, N.R. and Giroud, P. 1967. Human abortion associated with infection by ovine abortion agent. *Br. Med. J.* **iv:** 37.
84. Beer, R.J.S., Bradford, W.P. and Hart, R.J.C. 1982. Pregnancy complicated by psittacosis acquired from sheep. *Br. Med. J.* **284:** 1156–1157.
85. Buxton, D. 1986. Potential danger to pregnant women of *Chlamydia psittaci. Vet. Rec.* **118:** 510–511.
86. Johnson, F.W.A., Matheson, B.A., Williams, H., Laing, A.G., Jandal, V., Davidson-Lamb, R., Halliday, G.J., Hobson, D., Wong, S.Y.M., Hadley, K.M., Moffat, M.A.J. and Postlethwaite, R. 1985. Abortion due to infection with *Chlamydia psittaci* in a sheep farmer's wife. *Br. Med. J.* **290:** 592–594.
87. Herring, A.J., Anderson, I.E., McClenaghan, M., Inglis, N.F., Matheson, B.A., West, C.P., Rodger, M. and Brettle, R.P. 1987. Restriction endonuclease analysis of DNA from two isolates of *Chlamydia psittaci* obtained from human abortions. *Br. Med. J.* **295:** 1239.
88. Barwell, C.F. 1955. Laboratory infection of man with virus of enzootic abortion of ewes. *Lancet.* **2:** 1369–1371.
89. Anonymous 1991. Animal-associated infections, England and Wales. *Commun. Dis. Rep.* **1:** 118.
90. Enright, J.B. and Sadler, W.W. 1954. Presence in human sera of complement fixing antibodies to virus of sporadic bovine encephalomyelitis. *Proc. Soc. exp. Biol. Med.* **85:** 466–468.
91. Ostler, H.B., Schachter, J. and Dawson, C.R. 1969. Acute follicular conjunctivitis of epizootic origin. Feline pneumonitis. *Arch. Ophthal., N.Y.* **82:** 587.
92. Schachter, J., Ostler, H.B. and Meyer, K.F. 1969. Human infection with the agent of feline pneumonitis. *Lancet* **1:** 1063–1065.
93. Regan, R.J., Dathan, J.R.E. and Treharne, J.D. 1979. Infective endocarditis with glomerulonephritis associated with cat chlamydia (*C. psittaci*) infection. *Br. Heart J.* **42:** 349–352.

Index

Page numbers in *italic* type indicate an illustration or table appearing on a different page to its text.